DEGENERATIVE DISORDERS OF THE BRAIN

Covering a wide range of diverse age-related disorders, *Degenerative Disorders of the Brain* addresses disabilities that occur or have their roots in the later stages of life. The book brings together an internationally recognised group of contributors to discuss frontostriatal, fronto-cerebellar and other major brain systems and structures which control and direct normal behaviour, and which can fail during the aging process, as well as addressing behavioural, clinical, pathophysiological and technical aspects.

Discussing the latest clinical and behavioural findings of disorders which are largely, though not necessarily entirely, age related, including Alzheimer's disease and other dementias, Parkinson's disease and related disorders, and Huntington's disease, the book covers information vital to the understanding, diagnosis, and management of degenerative disorders of the brain. It also considers the role of epigenetics, neural plasticity, and environmental enrichment in neurodegenerative disorders alongside the role of ground-breaking intervention methods, including transcranial magnetic stimulation and deep brain stimulation.

Degenerative Disorders of the Brain will be of great interest to, and use for, clinicians, researchers, students, lecturers, and affected individuals and their relatives.

Darren R. Hocking is Senior Research Fellow and ARC DECRA Fellow at La Trobe University, Australia.

John L. Bradshaw is Emeritus Professor of Neuropsychology at Monash University, Australia.

Joanne Fielding is Associate Professor in the Central Clinical School at Monash University, Australia.

DEGENERATIVE DISORDERS OF THE BRAIN

Edited by Darren R. Hocking,
John L. Bradshaw and
Joanne Fielding

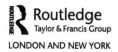
Routledge
Taylor & Francis Group

LONDON AND NEW YORK

First published 2019
by Routledge
2 Park Square, Milton Park, Abingdon, Oxon OX14 4RN

and by Routledge
52 Vanderbilt Avenue, New York, NY 10017

Routledge is an imprint of the Taylor & Francis Group, an informa business

British Library Cataloguing-in-Publication Data
A catalogue record for this book is available from the British Library

Library of Congress Cataloging-in-Publication Data
A catalog record has been requested for this book

ISBN: 978-0-8153-8224-9 (hbk)
ISBN: 978-0-8153-8226-3 (pbk)
ISBN: 978-1-351-20891-8 (ebk)

Typeset in Bembo
by Swales & Willis Ltd, Exeter, Devon, UK

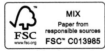

MIX
Paper from
responsible sources
FSC
www.fsc.org   FSC™ C013985

Printed in the United Kingdom
by Henry Ling Limited

CONTENTS

ACKNOWLEDGEMENTS

Darren dedicates his contribution to this book to his son, Matthew, and to his parents, Barry and Kathy, and to Claire, who have all in different ways provided inspiration, encouragement and unconditional support. He extends his utmost gratitude to his mentor and treasured friend, John Bradshaw, who provided so much guidance and support through the years.

John dedicates his contribution to this book to Judy, his beloved spouse of 52 years, now sadly in a nursing home after a catastrophic stroke; she helped him establish and run the Experimental Neuropsychology Unit at Monash University for nearly 20 years, and materially helped so many of his graduate students. He would also like to thank Ceri Mclardi for continuing support and encouragement over this and his two previous books published by Routledge.

Joanne dedicates her contribution to this book to David, her much beloved husband, who stands steadfastly by her side through the tumultuous journey that is academic life.

FOREWORD

In 2001, my book *Developmental Disorders of the Frontostriatal System: Neuropsychological, Neuropsychiatric and Evolutionary Perspectives* was published by Psychology Press/ Taylor and Francis. It continued to sell well, and in 2014 the publishers approached me for a second, updated edition. In view of the enormous amount of material which had been published since the turn of the century, I felt it advisable to propose an edited compilation instead, with chapters by recognised authorities for each syndrome and for material describing current cutting-edge techniques for studying relevant brain processes, and for manipulating them for therapeutic purposes. *Developmental Disorders of the Brain* duly appeared early 2017. With apparent early success, and in view of the fact that I and my lab had for many years also worked on degenerative as well as developmental pathologies, there being no up-to-date text to cover the former, *Degenerative Disorders of the Brain* was conceived as a companion volume. In this way we could address the latest theories, techniques and findings to cover pathologies evolving across the life span. Just as with the neurodevelopmental disorders, two great neural systems play a major, though not necessarily exclusive, role: the frontostriatal system (including the basal ganglia), and the fronto-parieto-cerebellar. At a purely motor level, and of course we cannot ignore the cognitive and emotional aspects of what it means to be human, we can roughly characterise the frontostriatal system as being perhaps more largely responsible for initiating and managing response sequences, and its companion, the fronto-parieto-cerebellar, as fine-tuning endpoint accuracy. Indeed, there are close analogues, especially in cognitive, thought and even emotional processes, of motor functions per se. This book is about the latest procedures and findings, neural and behavioural, diagnostic and management, of neurodegenerative disorders, with particular but not exclusive reference to these two great neural systems.

John L. Bradshaw, Monash University, 2018

CONTRIBUTORS

Smriti Agarwal, Brain and Mind Centre, University of Sydney, Australia

Jenny Bradshaw, School of Psychological Sciences, University of Melbourne, Australia

John L. Bradshaw, Monash Institute of Cognitive and Clinical Neurosciences, Monash University, Clayton, Australia

Jashelle Caga, Brain and Mind Centre, University of Sydney, Australia

Meaghan Clough, Department of Neuroscience, Central Clinical School, Monash University, Australia

Rachael C. Cvejic, Department of Developmental Disability Neuropsychiatry, School of Psychiatry, University of New South Wales, Australia

Mary Danoudis, Clinical Research Centre for Movement Disorders and Gait, Parkinson's Foundation Centre of Excellence, Monash Health, Kingston Centre, Australia

Thanuja Dharmadasa, Brain and Mind Centre, University of Sydney, Australia

Peter G. Enticott, School of Psychology, Deakin University, Australia

Joanne Fielding, Department of Neuroscience, Central Clinical School, Monash University, Australia

Alicia M. Goodwill, School of Psychology, Australian Catholic University, Australia

Anthony J. Hannan, Florey Institute of Neuroscience and Mental Health, Melbourne Brain Centre, University of Melbourne, Australia

Aileen K. Ho, School of Psychology and Clinical Language Sciences, University of Reading, UK

Darren R. Hocking, School of Psychology & Public Health, La Trobe University, Bundoora, Australia

William Huynh, Brain and Mind Centre, University of Sydney, Australia

Robert Iansek, Clinical Research Centre for Movement Disorders and Gait, Parkinson's Foundation Centre of Excellence, Monash Health, Kingston Centre, Australia

Sharna Jamadar, Monash Institute of Cognitive and Clinical Neurosciences, Monash University, Clayton, Australia

Matthew C. Kiernan, Central Clinical School, University of Sydney, Australia

Glynda Kinsella, School of Psychology & Public Health, La Trobe University, Bundoora, Australia

Isaline Mees, Florey Institute of Neuroscience and Mental Health, Melbourne Brain Centre, University of Melbourne, Australia

Kerryn Pike, School of Psychology & Public Health, La Trobe University, Bundoora, Australia

Thibault Renoir, Florey Institute of Neuroscience and Mental Health, Melbourne Brain Centre, University of Melbourne, Australia

Michael Saling, School of Psychological Sciences, University of Melbourne, Australia

Olivia Salthouse, School of Psychological Sciences, University of Melbourne, Australia

Wei-Peng Teo, Institute for Physical Activity and Nutrition, Deakin University, Australia

Harvey Tran, Florey Institute of Neuroscience and Mental Health, Melbourne Brain Centre, University of Melbourne, Australia

Julian N. Trollor, Department of Developmental Disability Neuropsychiatry, School of Psychiatry, University of New South Wales, Australia

1

BRAIN CIRCUITRY IN AGEING AND NEURODEGENERATIVE DISEASE

Sharna Jamadar

Introduction

As we age, our bodies undergo widespread and significant changes. Our hair greys and becomes thinner, our skin wrinkles, our eyesight and hearing become worse. Many people experience changes in their thinking as they get older, finding it more difficult to remember events and solve complex problems. It is not all doom and gloom for older people, however: older people have accumulated knowledge to help them solve many problems that may strike younger people as novel and complex (Salthouse, 2012); and many older people report a positive quality of life (Farquhar, 1995). Being retired, volunteer work, and social relationships with children, family and friends all have a positive impact on the older person's life (Netuveli, Wiggins, Hildon, Montgomery & Blane, 2006).

Since our bodies and cognitive abilities show clear evidence of age-related change, it is not surprising that our brain also shows signs of ageing. There are at least two reasons to study brain ageing. Firstly, cognitive decline is considered an inevitable consequence of the ageing process, and this decline is tightly locked to changes in the integrity of the brain. By understanding the influence of age on the brain, we will develop better mechanistic models of how some people seem to age more successfully than others, and whether we can develop interventions to counteract age-related cognitive decline. Secondly, brain ageing is a strong risk factor for many neurodegenerative and psychiatric illnesses, with age serving as the greatest risk factor for illnesses such as Alzheimer's disease (Guerreiro & Bras, 2015) and Parkinson's disease (Reeve, Simcox & Turnbull, 2014). It is important to understand brain ageing not only so we can understand the mechanism of age as a disease risk factor, but also so we can distinguish healthy from pathological ageing, thereby initiating therapeutic interventions earlier in the disease process.

In this chapter, we will review the effects of ageing on the human brain, with particular focus on cortico-basal ganglia and cortico-cerebellar networks.

Cortico-basal ganglia and cortico-cerebellar circuits: structure and function

Cortico-basal ganglia circuits

The basal ganglia comprise the striatum (caudate, putamen, nucleus accumbens), globus pallidus, substantia nigra, subthalamic nucleus and pons. The components of the basal ganglia are categorised according to their function within the cortico-basal ganglia circuits. The caudate, putamen and nucleus accumbens form the input nuclei of the basal ganglia; the globus pallidus pars interna and substantia nigra pars reticulata form the output nuclei; and the globus pallidus pas externa, subthalamic nucleus and substantia nigra pars compacta form the intrinsic or relay nuclei.

The output nuclei project to the thalamus and brain stem. The descending pallidal and nigral projections to the brainstem provide pathways for direct influence on motor circuits (e.g. oculomotor control via superior colliculus, locomotion via the pedunculopontine nucleus). The projections to the brainstem are also the likely location of cerebellar inputs to the basal ganglia via the pontine nuclei (Hoshi, Tremblay, Féger, Carras & Strick, 2005). Thalamic projections are directed to the ventral anterior, ventrolateral and intralaminar thalamic nuclei, which are then projected to the cortex (primarily frontal cortex). (Many excellent reviews of basal ganglia anatomy are available, including Lanciego, Luquin & Obeso, 2012; Wichmann & DeLong, 2013).

The basal ganglia form a number of segregated but parallel loops that originate in the cortex, innervate the thalamus via the basal ganglia, and then project back to the cortex. The cortico-basal ganglia motor loop is the best characterised, given that pathology within this network is associated with several major disorders of movement, including Parkinson's disease and Huntington's disease (see Chapters 3 and 4). A key feature of the cortico-basal ganglia networks is their closed-loop nature: the cortical regions that are the main inputs to the circuit are also the main target for outputs (Kelly & Strick, 2004). The circuits are labelled according to their functions, and include motor, oculomotor, executive and affective/motivation circuits (Figure 1.1A). Within each network, there are direct and indirect pathways of information flow (Figure 1.1B), with the direct pathway supporting activation and the indirect pathway supporting inhibition (DeLong & Wichmann, 2015). There is also evidence for a hyperdirect pathway within the motor circuit, which projects directly from the cortex to the subthalamic nucleus, conveying strong excitatory signals with faster velocity than the direct and indirect pathways (Nambu, 2008). This pathway seems to be important for cancelling motor plans (Nambu, Tokuno & Takada, 2002). Excitatory connections within the network (direct, indirect and hyperdirect) are glutamatergic, and inhibitory connections are GABAergic projections (ibid.). The opposing

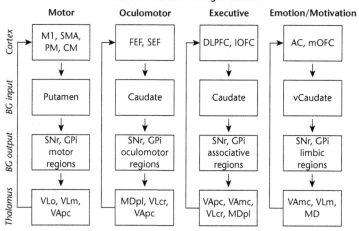

A. Four Cortico-Basal Ganglia Circuits

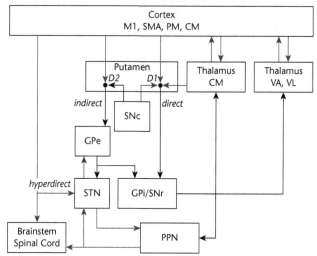

B. Direct, Indirect & Hyperdirect Pathways

FIGURE 1.1 Cortico-basal ganglia networks. (A) At least four cortico-basal ganglia networks have been described, and are labelled according to their presumed function (Wichmann & DeLong, 2013). (B) Direct, indirect and hyperdirect pathways of the motor cortico-basal ganglia network (DeLong & Wichmann, 2015; Nambu et al., 2002). Abbreviations: AC, anterior cingulate; CM, cingulate motor area; DLPFC, dorsolateral prefrontal cortex; FEF, frontal eye field; GPi, internal segment of the globus pallidus; lOFC, lateral orbitofrontal cortex; M1, primary motor cortex; MDpl, mediodorsal nucleus of thalamus, lateral part; mOFC, medial orbitofrontal cortex; PM, premotor cortex; SEF, supplementary eye field; SMA, supplementary motor area; SNr, substantia nigra pars reticulata; VAmc, ventral anterior nucleus of thalamus, magnocellular part; VApc, ventral anterior nucleus of thalamus, parvocellular part; VLcr, ventrolateral nucleus of thalamus, caudal part, rostral division; VLm, ventrolateral nucleus of thalamus, medial part; VLo, ventrolateral nucleus of thalamus, pars oralis.

Source: adapted from DeLong & Wichmann (2015); Wichmann & DeLong (2013)

behaviour of the direct and indirect pathway is established by differing response to dopamine: direct pathway neurons are facilitated by dopamine D1 receptors, whereas the indirect pathway is inhibited by dopamine, through activation of the D2 receptors (Wichmann & DeLong, 2013).

Cortico-cerebellar circuits

The cerebellum comprises a series of highly regular repeating units, each of which contains the same basic cellular organisation (see Haines & Mihailoff, 2018; Lisberger & Thach, 2013 for reviews). The cerebellum has a highly convoluted outer layer of grey matter, and internal core of white matter, containing four deep cerebellar nuclei: the fastigial, emboliform, globose and dentate nuclei. The cerebellar cortex is macroanatomically divided into the midline vermis, lateral hemispheres and flocculonodular lobes. Signals to and from the brain stem, spinal cord and cortex enter the cerebellum via the three cerebellar peduncles: the inferior, middle and superior cerebellar peduncles. Most of the output of the cerebellum project via the cerebellar deep nuclei to the cerebellar peduncles; projections from the flocculonodular lobe to the vestibular nuclei in the brainstem are the exception to this pattern. Unlike cortical and subcortical brain regions, which process somatosensory and motor input from contralateral regions of the body, the cerebellum processes input from ipsilateral sensory organs and limbs. Thus, when the cerebellum receives input from the body and sensory organs via the cortex, the signals must again cross the midline from the contralateral to the ipsilateral side, given the originally crossed representation in the sensorimotor cortex.

The cerebellum can also be divided into three systems or modules on the basis of their inputs and presumed function (Figure 1.2A). The *vestibulocerebellum* receives inputs from the ipsilateral vestibular system (via primary and secondary vestibulocerebellar fibres) and visual areas and projects directly through the flocculonodular lobe to the brainstem vestibular nuclei (via vestibulospinal and reticulospinal tracts). This system is important for balance and eye movements. The *spinocerebellum* covers the medial regions of the cerebellum, the vermis and the intermediate sections of the cerebellar hemispheres. The vermal spinocerebellar system receives visual, auditory, vestibular and somatosensory input from the body (via the posterior and anterior spinocerebellar tracts and the cuneocerebellar fibres) and projects via the fastigial nucleus to the brainstem and cortex. The vermal spinocerebellum is important for posture, locomotion and eye movements. The adjacent, more lateral intermediate hemispheric spinocerebellar system also receives somatosensory input from the limbs but also the motor cortex, and output neurons project to the brainstem via the emboliform and globose nuclei. This intermediate hemispheric spinocerebellar network is responsible for the control of distal muscles of the limbs and fingers. The *cerebrocerebellum* encompasses the lateral cerebellar hemispheres and receives almost all of its input from the contralateral cortex via the pontine nuclei (pontocerebellar fibres). Cerebrocerebellar output projects back to the cortex (motor, premotor, prefrontal) via the contralateral dentate nucleus. This module is responsible for the planning and control of fine motor movements, and in the timing of these movements. There is also significant evidence to suggest that cerebrocerebellar fine control and timing processes are also applied to cognitive functions, including working memory, executive function, and language (Buckner, 2013).

The repeating structure and similarity of the cellular organisation and physiology suggests that similar computational processes are carried out throughout the cerebellum. While it was once controversial to suggest that the cerebellum played a role in non-motor processes, it is now widely agreed that the structure plays a role in cognitive processes (Buckner, 2013; Koziol et al., 2014). The dysmetria of thought hypothesis (Schmahmann, 1991) draws upon evidence showing that the cerebellum modulates the rate, rhythm, force and accuracy of motor outputs, and proposes that the structure also regulates the speed, consistency, capacity and appropriateness of cognitive and limbic processes. This 'universal cerebellar transform' (Schmahmann, 2000) integrates multiple internal representations of the body and external environment with external stimuli and self-generated responses to optimise cognitive and motor actions according to the current context. Central to this theory is the concept of the 'internal model': neural representations that encode input–output relationships between motor commands and their consequences that are acquired through experience-dependent learning (Ramnani, 2006). The internal forward model (Figure 1.2B) encodes and updates representations of input–output mappings learned in real-world situations via error feedback. In this model, when a signal is sent to generate an action, an efference copy of this signal is also sent to the internal model. The internal model uses the efference copy to predict the ideal physical and sensory state after the action. The error between the current and predicted state after the movement is then fed forward to update the input–output mappings of the internal model. In this way, future repetitions of this action will be performed more accurately and appropriately. The concept of the dual processing streams (action and internal model) is consistent with the known architecture of the cerebellar modules (Miall & Wolpert, 1996), and is currently the leading hypothesis for how the cerebellum modulates and refines a broad range of cognitive and motor processes (Koziol et al., 2014).

Integration of cortico-basal ganglia and cortico-cerebellar circuits

The cortico-cerebellar and cortico-basal ganglia circuits have historically been considered to be anatomically and functionally distinct from one another (e.g. Doya, 2000). Any interaction between the two circuits was thought to occur only via the cortex. However, the cortico-cerebellar and cortico-basal ganglia circuits share a number of characteristics (Bostan & Strick, 2018): (a) the input nuclei of each circuit receives projections from widespread regions of the cortex; (b) the output nuclei of both circuits project to regions of the thalamus that innervate motor and non-motor regions of the cortex (Table 1.1); and (c) both

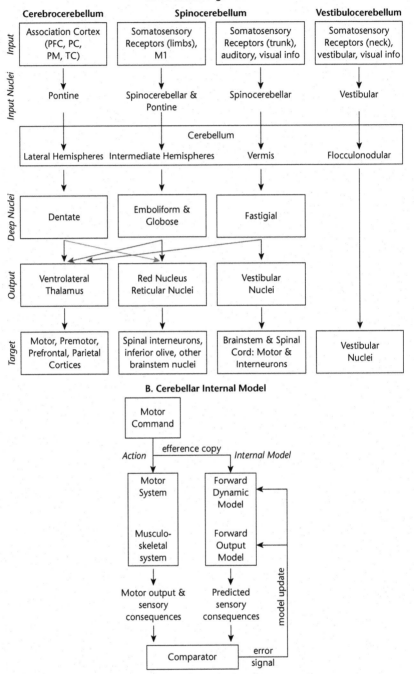

FIGURE 1.2 (A) Three functional modules of the cerebellum. (B) An internal forward model using the motor system as an example. Abbreviations: M1, primary motor cortex; PC, parietal cortex; PFC, prefrontal cortex; PM, premotor cortex; TC, temporal cortex.

Sources: (A) adapted from Lisberger & Thach (2013); (B) adapted from Ramnani (2006)

A. Integration of Basal Ganglia and Cerebellar Circuits

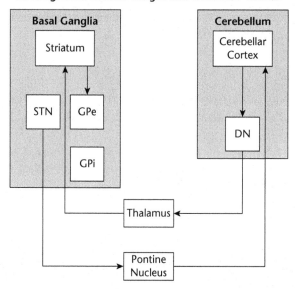

B. Houk's Model of Function of Basal Ganglia-Cerebellar Networks

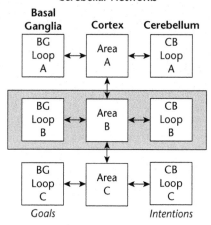

FIGURE 1.3 Integration of cortico-basal ganglia and cortico-cerebellar networks. (A) Connections between the cerebellum and basal ganglia. (B) One example model of the function of cortico-basal ganglia-cerebellar networks. In this model, reinforcement learning is achieved by basal ganglia loops, supervised learning is achieved by cerebellar loops, and Hebbian learning is achieved by interactions within the cortex. In this distributed processing modules model, a module comprises a basal ganglia loop, cortical area and cerebellar loop (shown by the grey rectangle). Abbreviations: BG, basal ganglia; CB, cerebellar; DN, dentate nucleus; GPe, external segment of the globus pallidus; GPi, internal segment of the globus pallidus; STN, subthalamic nucleus.

Sources: (A) adapted from Bostan & Strick (2018), based on data from Hoshi et al. (2005) and Bostan et al. (2010); (B) adapted from J. Houk, in Caligiore et al. (2017); see that consensus paper for alternate models)

cortico-cerebellar and cortico-basal ganglia circuits share a closed-loop structure, where regions of the cortex that are the major sources of input to the circuit are also the main targets of output.

It is now known that the basal ganglia and cerebellar networks form an interconnected network (Bostan & Strick, 2018; Figure 1.3A; Table 1.1). Neurons in the motor and non-motor regions of the cerebellar dentate nucleus project disynaptically (i.e. via an intermediary structure, in this case the pontine nucleus; Figure 1.3A) to the striatum and the globus pallidus pars externa. This suggests that the cerebellum modulates the motor and non-motor functions of the basal ganglia via the indirect pathway (Hoshi et al., 2005). In a similar manner, neurons in the motor and non-motor portions of the subthalamic nucleus project disynaptically (via the thalamus) to the cerebellum (Bostan, Dum & Strick, 2010), consistent with the conclusion that the subthalamic nucleus modulates motor and non-motor processes of the cerebellum.

While the anatomical results of Strick and colleagues provides strong evidence for cortico-basal ganglia and cortico-cerebellar network integration, the functional significance of this integration remains a matter of debate (Caligiore et al., 2017). One hypothesis (Caligiore et al., 2017; Houk et al., 2007; Figure 1.3B) draws upon the distributed processing modules framework to characterise a modular cortico-basal ganglia-cerebellar learning system. In this view, Hebbian learning is achieved via interactions between distinct cortical regions. Reinforcement learning is achieved via cortico-basal ganglia interactions and cortico-cerebellar interactions to achieve supervised learning. However, while the scientific consensus agrees that cortico-basal ganglia-cerebellar interactions are involved in learning and adaptation, the exact mechanism is a matter of ongoing theoretical development and experimental research (Caligiore et al., 2017).

TABLE 1.1 Cortical targets of basal ganglia and cerebellar outputs. Based on data from *Cebus* monkey. Numbers refer to cytoarchitectonic areas. Where required, human homologous regions are given in parentheses.

Target of both basal ganglia and cerebellar outputs	*Target of basal ganglia outputs but not cerebellar outputs*
9m, 9L (medial, lateral) (dorsal prefrontal)	46v (ventral) (ventrolateral prefrontal)
Pre-supplementary motor area	12 (ventrolateral prefrontal)
Supplementary motor area (arm)	Inferotemporal cortex
46d (dorsal) (dorsolateral prefrontal)	
Pre-dorsal premotor	
Frontal eye fields	
Dorsal premotor (arm)	
Ventral premotor (arm)	
M1 (face, arm, leg)	
Anterior intraparietal area (ventrolateral parietal)	
7b (dorsolateral parietal)	

Source: Bostan & Strick (2018)

The ageing brain: changes in structure, function, and metabolic integrity

Challenges in studying human brain ageing

While there are many thousands of studies examining human ageing, it is actually quite a challenging process to study. One of the primary challenges is its temporal duration: lifespan studies (birth to grave) require nine to ten decades; studies focusing only on older age (say 65+ years to death) may still require study durations of 20 to 30 years. Thus, to circumvent the issue of very long study durations, the vast majority of existing studies of the effects of age on the human brain are cross-sectional, rather than longitudinal. It is important to recognise however that cross-sectional designs, while more feasible for many researchers, fundamentally change the inferences that can be drawn on the basis of the results.

The challenges and advantages of cross-sectional and longitudinal designs in ageing research have been extensively discussed (see Rugg, 2017 for an excellent overview). Here, we will highlight two issues for each design to illustrate the methodological challenges of ageing research.

Firstly, cross-sectional designs can only allow inferences of age-related differences between younger and older samples, they cannot provide information about individual age-related changes (Salthouse, 2010). This is an important distinction, as younger and older samples are likely to differ substantially on a range of factors, including cohort differences in diet, access to education, life experiences (e.g. today's younger adults are likely to be more engaged in computer-based technologies than the young adults in the 1940s, 1950s and 1960s) and childhood socioeconomic and cultural environments; for example, compare the childhood environment of the 'baby boomers' (1940s, 1950s) to that of the 'millennial' generation (1990s, 2000s). It is very challenging to match young and older adults on all variables except age; and some studies have shown that apparent 'age-related' differences between younger and older groups are attributable to cohort differences (e.g. Rönnlund, Nyberg, Bäckman & Nilsson, 2005).

Secondly, cross-sectional and longitudinal designs may have different power to detect effects of ageing. Between-group differences between young and old subjects may have larger effect sizes than within-subject differences, particularly across short periods of time (1–2 years). On the other hand, longitudinal estimates are likely to be less noisy than cross-sectional estimates of age-related effects. Thirdly, older adults are likely to have physiological characteristics that are confounded with age. A clear example of this is the changes in neurovascular coupling and greater incidence of cardiovascular issues in older compared to younger samples. These physiological differences can pose a serious issue for fMRI studies that rely upon the blood oxygenation level-dependent (BOLD) response to measure brain activity. Importantly, this remains an issue even for longitudinal studies, however the magnitude of the effect is likely to be smaller in longitudinal than cross-sectional designs. Longitudinal brain imaging studies of ageing experience the same challenges as any other study of ageing using different methods (e.g. subject attrition, test–retest effects). However, brain imaging studies also have additional challenges in longitudinal designs, particularly changes to the imaging equipment (e.g. scanner upgrade, system deterioration and/or replacement), which will result in signal differences between time points unrelated to the characteristics of the subject.

There are no good solutions to any of these challenges of ageing research. Both cross-sectional and longitudinal designs can be very informative about the effect of age on the brain, and both designs have yielded important discoveries. Researchers should be aware of the challenges and caveats of ageing studies, regardless of their design, and evaluate the effects such issues may have on the inferences that can be drawn from any given study.

Structural changes in the aged brain

The volume of the brain progressively becomes smaller from mid-to-late life; estimates of around 5% per decade after 40 years (Svennerholm, Boström & Jungbjer, 1997), with the rate of decline increasing after 70 years (Scahill et al., 2003). In a systematic review of age-related effects on brain morphometry, Fjell and Walhovd (2010) concluded that while variability between cross-sectional studies is high, evidence suggests that the hippocampus, amygdala, striatum, pallidum, thalamus and accumbens show linear reductions with age. The cerebellum shows a non-linear effect of ageing, with accelerated reduction in very old age. Age accounts for a large proportion of the variance in the volume of brain structures (Table 1.2), with a large (46%) proportion of the variance in putamen volume explained by age. Age accounts for a smaller, but still substantial, proportion of the variance in cerebellar grey (25%) and caudate (38%) volume.

Grey matter consists largely of neuronal cell bodies, neuropil and glia. Grey matter volume and thickness is reduced with age (Courchesne et al., 2000; Good et al., 2001). Age-related grey matter reductions are largest in the hippocampus, frontal cortex, cerebellum and striatum (Jernigan et al., 2001). Findings from cross-sectional designs suggest a linear decrease in grey matter volume with age, however longitudinal studies suggest a non-linear effect of age, with grey matter volumes showing relative stability in middle age (30–50 years) and accelerated decline after the age of 60 (Cabeza, Nyberg & Park, 2017). In a review of 56 studies of ageing, including data from 2211 subjects aged 2–95 years (at baseline), Hedman, van Haren, Schnack, Kahn, and Hulshoff Pol (2012) found evidence for small decreases (0.2–0.5%) in grey matter volume per year between 35 and 60 years, with more marked (>0.5%) annual loss after 60 years. While it was once thought that age-related grey matter shrinkage reflected neuronal loss or death, it is now recognised that it is due to shrinkage in cell body size, loss of dendrites, and reduction in dendritic spine complexity (Dickstein et al., 2007).

White matter comprises largely of myelinated axons, which form tracts to connect grey matter regions. White matter is important for the integration of activity between distributed regions of the brain. White matter volume typically increases early in life up until 40–50 years; after this time there is an accelerated

TABLE 1.2 Proportion of variance in brain volume explained by age in 1143 healthy adults aged 18–94 years.

Structure	Proportion (%) of variance in volume explained by age
Lateral ventricles	46
Putamen	46
Total brain volume	43
Third ventricle	42
Inferior lateral ventricles	38
Thalamus	37
Nucleus accumbens	36
Hippocampus	33
Cerebral white matter	32
Amygdala	29
Pallidum	28
Cerebellar grey matter	25
Caudate	18
Cerebellar white matter	14
Brain stem	5
Fourth ventricle	3

Sources: Fjell & Walhovd (2010); Fjell et al. (2009)

loss of volume, possibly more rapid than is seen in grey matter (Jernigan et al., 2001; Salat et al., 2009). White matter volume loss is greatest in regions typically associated with age, including the orbitofrontal cortex and superior frontal gyrus; but is also significant in regions not usually associated with age including the fusiform, inferior temporal and middle frontal gyrus (Salat et al., 2009).

In addition to changes in white matter volume, the integrity (or health) of the white matter also changes with age. White matter integrity, as measured using diffusion tensor imaging (DTI), shows a non-linear relationship with age: measures of white matter health (axonal density, axonal health and myelin thickness; measured by fractional anisotropy, axial diffusion, mean diffusion) show an accelerated decrease in middle age (Walhovd, Johansen-Berg & Karadottir, 2014). Age-related change in white matter integrity follows an anterior-posterior axis, with greater effects of age found in the anterior regions of the brain (genu of corpus callosum and pericallosal white matter) than posterior regions (Bennett & Madden, 2014). White matter hyperintensities (also known as white matter lesions or leukoaraioses) are regions of damaged white matter that occur most often in the periventricular regions, although they may also occur in the deep white matter. Estimates of prevalence in the general population range from 39 to 96% (reviewed in Prins & Scheltens, 2015). The pathological significance of white matter hyperintensities is still unclear, however they are most likely related to vascular effects, particularly small local ischaemic events (Young, Halliday & Kril, 2008). White matter hyperintensities increase in prevalence with age (Vernooij et al., 2007), and are linked to declining cognitive performance with age (Maillard et al., 2012). The progression of white matter hyperintensities over time is associated with increased dementia risk (see Prins & Scheltens, 2015 for a recent review of white matter hyperintensities and cognitive decline).

Functional changes in the aged brain

There are widespread differences in functional brain activity in response to a task between older and younger adults. Task-based fMRI studies have revealed that older adults show a pattern of brain activity that is significantly different from younger adults, with both relative increases and decreases in brain activity across the brain. Compared to younger adults, older adults show: (a) a posterior-to-anterior shift in fMRI activity, particularly in medial parietal and prefrontal areas ('posterior-to-anterior shift in ageing', or 'PASA' effect; Davis, Dennis, Daselaar, Fleck & Cabeza, 2007); (b) a reduction in hemispheric lateralisation, particularly in prefrontal areas ('hemispheric asymmetry reduction in old age' or 'HAROLD' effect; Cabeza, 2002); and (c) over-recruitment of task-relevant regions and additional recruitment of non-task-relevant regions during performance. The regional hyperactivity effect in older adults has been attributed to both a 'compensation' effect (Reuter-Lorenz & Cappell, 2008) and a 'dedifferentiation' effect (Rajah & D'esposito, 2005). The compensation hypothesis states that older adults recruit more brain resources to compensate for functional deficits elsewhere in the brain, to perform the same tasks as younger people. The dedifferentiation hypothesis states that recruitment of additional brain regions and loss of hemispheric lateralisation is related to the loss of functional specificity in the brain. Both models have found support in the literature, and it is likely that hyperactivity in older vs. younger adults is due to a combination of compensatory and dedifferentiation effects. There are several influential reviews of the large body of task-related activity in brain ageing, particularly Grady (2012).

In the last decade or so, there has been a shift of brain imaging research away from examining the role of discrete brain regions in task-related processing, towards using connectivity measures to study the networks of the brain. The current focus on network connectomics has been motivated by the recognition that the majority of functions are supported by coordinated activity between spatially distinct regions, as well as from substantial advances in computational power and the application of complex systems approaches to neuroscience (Fornito, Zalesky & Breakspear, 2015). The majority of connectomics studies have used resting-state fMRI to study the brain at rest, with the assumption that resting-state connectivity reflects the intrinsic connectivity of the brain, upon which all task and goal-related activity builds. In other words, resting-state connectivity is thought to index the 'baseline' connectivity of the brain.

Resting-state connectivity studies can be categorised as those that examine specific, known, resting-state networks of the brain, including the default mode network, dorsal attention network and the salience network (among others, see Laird et al., 2009 for a meta-analysis of primary resting-state networks). These studies often rely on independent components analysis (ICA) or seed-based approaches to define the networks. ICA is a multivariate computational approach that separates a signal into its underlying subcomponents. In seed-based approaches, a region-of-interest is chosen as the 'seed' region, and the timeseries of the seed region is correlated with the timeseries of all other voxels in the brain. Alternatively, network approaches apply graph theory to examine network organisation across the brain. Graph theory approaches model the brain as a complex network that is comprised as nodes (brain regions) and edges (connections between brain regions). Functional connectivity analyses using graph theory generally parcellate the brain into a set of regions (nodes) at a much finer decomposition than used in ICA approaches (see Wang et al., 2010 for a review).

The default mode network is the most studied resting-state network, and is believed to underlie introspection, self-referential thought, and projection of the self through retrospective and prospective memory (e.g. Andrews-Hanna, Smallwood & Spreng, 2014; Buckner, Andrews-Hanna & Schacter, 2008). The intrinsic connectivity of the default mode network correlates with better cognitive outcomes (e.g. Damoiseaux et al., 2007; Jamadar, Egan, Calhoun, Johnson & Fielding, 2016; Mak et al., 2017). Importantly, this network is usually anti-correlated with task-relevant networks like the dorsal attention and salience networks (Fox, Laird & Lancaster, 2005), and the strength of this anti-correlation is associated with better performance (e.g. Kelly et al., 2009). In other words, the default mode network activity must be down-regulated for accurate task performance. Ageing is associated with reduced intrinsic connectivity within the default mode network (e.g. Allen et al., 2011; Andrews-Hanna et al., 2007; Tomasi & Volkow, 2012). Reduced default mode connectivity becomes evident in middle age and the rate of decline becomes faster in older age (Mak et al., 2017). Age is also associated with reduced capacity to down-regulate the default mode network during task processing (e.g. Grady, Springer, Hongwanishkul, McIntosh & Winocur, 2006; Lustig et al., 2003; Sambataro et al., 2010), and this is associated with poorer task performance (Sambataro et al., 2010). In other networks, reduced intrinsic connectivity in older vs. younger adults has been reported in the dorsal attention network (e.g. Tomasi & Volkow, 2012; Zhang et al., 2014), salience network (e.g. Betzel et al., 2014; Onoda, Ishihara & Yamaguchi, 2012; Zhang et al., 2014) and frontoparietal network (Campbell, Grady, Ng & Hasher, 2012; Geerligs, Renken, Saliasi, Maurits & Lorist, 2014). On the other hand, greater activity has been reported in sensorimotor and subcortical networks in older vs. younger adults (Allen et al., 2011; Meier et al., 2012).

Network theory proposes two features of brain function: functional segregation and functional integration (Sporns, 2013). Functional segregation is a modular connectivity profile, where there are strong connections between nodes within a network and weaker connections between nodes from different modules. Functional integration refers to connections between modules, which allows communication between modules and integration of information across modules.

A fine balance between functional segregation and integration must be maintained for optimal brain (and cognitive) function. The intrinsic connectivity profile of the default mode network and its interactions with other resting-state networks is a good example of the fine balance between functional segregation and integration. The most consistent finding of network connectivity in ageing is of lower within-network connectivity and higher between-network connectivity in older vs. younger adults (e.g. Grady, Sarraf, Saverino & Campbell, 2016; Spreng, Stevens, Viviano & Schacter, 2016; see Damoiseaux, 2017 for a review); in other words, older adults show less network segregation than younger adults (Chan, Park, Savalia, Petersen & Wig, 2014). Consistent with these findings, other studies have shown that older adults show less network modularity and lower local efficiency (efficiency of information transfer to nearby nodes within a network) compared to younger adults (Cao et al., 2014; Geerligs, Rubinov & Henson, 2015). No differences were reported in network global efficiency (the efficiency of information transfer among all nodes of a network) in older vs. younger adults. So-called 'rich club' connectivity (where highly interconnected nodes [or 'hubs'] within a network are more densely connected with other highly connected nodes) also decreases with age, with a reduction evident after 40 years (Cao et al., 2014). Together, the results from network measures of connectivity in ageing suggest that older adults have lower within- and higher between-network connectivity profiles compared to younger adults. This may explain the compensatory effect, where older adults show less task-related functional activity in task-relevant regions, and greater activity in non-task-relevant regions compared to younger adults.

Metabolic and molecular changes in the aged brain

The field of cognitive neuroscience has focused primarily on structural and functional consequences of ageing; however, the ageing process has widespread effects on the brain beyond these macroscopic changes. Indeed, structural and functional brain changes can be considered a consequence of organismal-level changes, which affect every level, including the molecular, cellular and systems-level (i.e. whole-brain or whole-organ). Each of these levels is in turn modulated by genetic, epigenetic, lifestyle and environmental factors. A full review of the multifactorial contributors to brain ageing is beyond the scope of this review, but interested readers should consult recent reviews by Khan, Singer, and Vaughan (2017), Yin, Sancheti, Patil, and Cadenas (2016), and Cole, Marioni, Harris, and Deary (2018). In this section, we will focus on evidence of the metabolic and molecular changes in the ageing brain in humans from in vivo positron emission tomography (PET) imaging. PET is an imaging technique that uses radionuclides to examine a broad range of metabolic targets in vivo, including glucose metabolism, neurotransmitter receptor uptake and transportation, protein deposition and inflammatory markers.

The human brain is a metabolically hungry organ, requiring a continual and reliable supply of glucose to maintain its functions. Although small compared to the rest of the body, the brain accounts for 20% of the total energy consumption in the human body (Kety, 1957; Sokoloff, 1960), of which 70–80% is used by neurons during synaptic activity (Harris, Jolivet & Attwell, 2012). It is increasingly recognised that maintaining a reliable neural energy supply is paramount to maintaining brain health. Imaging studies using 18-[F]-fludeoxyglucose PET (FDG-PET) have shown that older adults have widespread decreases in glucose metabolism, particularly in frontal, anterior cingulate and parietal regions (e.g. Chételat et al., 2013; Kalpouzos et al., 2009). Technological advances are beginning to allow FDG-PET to be used to study network connectivity in a manner similar to fMRI (Chen et al., 2018). Recent results suggest that older adults show high metabolic connectivity both within and between networks (Arnemann, Stöber, Narayan, Rabinovici & Jagust, 2018), consistent with results from functional connectivity studies (Damoiseaux, 2017). Cerebral glucose hypometabolism is an indicator of more widespread deterioration of the molecular integrity of the brain, including mitochondrial hypometabolism, altered insulin signalling, changes in glucose receptors, and inflammation (Bishop, Lu & Yankner, 2010; Yin et al., 2016).

Extra-cellular accumulation of amyloid-beta (Aβ) plaques is the hallmark pathology of Alzheimer's disease. Aβ accumulates throughout the lifespan, even in healthy ageing, but is more rapid in Alzheimer's disease, where it is believed that Aβ clearance mechanisms are impaired. According to the amyloid hypothesis (Hardy & Selcoe, 2002), Aβ aggregation disrupts cellular communication and activates an inflammatory response, which eventually results in neuron death. Amyloid imaging using PET (for review of available Aβ tracers see Chen et al., 2018) has shown that around 20–30% of older adults with no symptoms of Alzheimer's disease have substantial amyloid burden (Aizenstein et al., 2008; Jack et al., 2014; Jansen et al., 2015). Amyloid burden increases with age, with around 10–20% of cognitively normal order adults aged 60–70 years classified as Aβ+, increasing to 20–30% for those 70–80 years, and 30–40% aged 80–90 years (Baker et al., 2017). However, not all Aβ+ cognitively normal adults will progress to Alzheimer's disease: either because amyloid is not sufficient to progress to Alzheimer's disease, or because individuals have protective factors against Aβ toxicity, or because a large number of Aβ+ individuals pass away before developing Alzheimer's disease. It is not yet known which of these factors mediates the relationship between Aβ load and Alzheimer's disease onset (e.g. Sperling et al., 2011).

In a recent meta-analysis of amyloid imaging studies of 5005 cognitively normal older adults across 30 cross-sectional and longitudinal studies, Baker et al. (2017) concluded that Aβ+ is associated with subtle but non-specific cognitive decline. Aβ+ was most significantly associated with decline of episodic memory, semantic memory, visuospatial function and global cognition. Compared to Aβ– older adults, cognitively normal Aβ+ older adults show: reduced cortical thickness, particularly in the parietal lobe, precuneus and posterior cingulate (Becker et al., 2011; Doré et al., 2013); smaller hippocampal volumes (which appears related with Aβ burden in the precuneus; Apostolova et al., 2010); and aberrant default mode and central executive network connectivity (Lim et al., 2014; Sheline et al., 2010).

Aβ also seems to mediate the neural compensation effect, with higher levels of Aβ associated with greater activity in task-relevant networks (Elman et al., 2014).

In addition to amyloid, misfolding and aggregation of the tau protein into neurofibrillary tangles is a second hallmark feature of Alzheimer's disease. According to the tau hypothesis, tau aggregates within the soma of neurons until it covers the whole cell and eventually kills the cell (Maccioni et al., 2010). Like amyloid, aggregated tau proteins also accumulate in the brains of cognitively normal older adults (Bennett et al., 2006), particularly in the medial temporal lobe, even in the absence of amyloid (Braak, Thal, Ghebremedhin & Del Tredici, 2011). The spread of tau tangles beyond the medial temporal lobe is associated with the co-occurrence of amyloid plaques (Price & Morris, 1999). PET tracers to study tau in vivo have been recently developed (in the last 5 years; Chen et al., 2018), and results from large-scale studies and clinical trials are forthcoming (Villemagne, Fodero-Tavoletti, Masters & Rowe, 2015). However, recent studies have confirmed that cognitively normal Aβ– subjects show tau deposition only in medial temporal lobes, with tau accumulation outside of the medial temporal lobe (particularly in precuneus) appearing in cognitively normal Aβ+ individuals (Schöll et al., 2016). Increasing age predicted tau accumulation in the medial temporal lobe and ventral frontal cortex, and tau accumulation in the medial temporal lobe was associated with poorer episodic memory. Tau deposits in the inferior and medial temporal lobes and orbitofrontal areas are also associated with widespread grey matter reductions (Sepulcre et al., 2016).

The neurotransmitter system also undergoes changes during the ageing process. Ageing is associated with decreasing levels of serotonin receptors and serotonin transporter (Iyo & Yamasaki, 1993; Wong et al., 1984; Yamamoto et al., 2002), which may be a primary contributor to late-life depression (Alexopoulos & Kelly, 2017). Loss of serotonin receptor density appears greatest in the striatum and frontal cortex, and serotonin transporter is decreased in the midbrain and thalamus. Gamma-aminobutyric acid (GABA) concentrations decline with age (Gao et al., 2013; Porges et al., 2017), and age-related GABA reductions in the frontal cortex is associated with poorer cognitive outcome (Porges et al., 2017). Lastly, ageing is associated with widespread reductions of neural dopamine, with a 5–10% loss of dopamine concentration and cell density for cognitively healthy older adults per decade after age 50 (Bäckman, Lindenberger, Li & Nyberg, 2010; Reeves, Bench & Howard, 2002). A recent meta-analysis of 45 human imaging studies of dopamine in ageing concluded that age has a negative effect on striatal dopamine transporter, and striatal and frontal cortical D1 and D2 dopamine receptors (Karrer, Josef, Mata, Morris & Samanez-Larkin, 2017).

Differences in chronological versus brain age

It is widely acknowledged that there is a mismatch between a person's chronological age and the level of cognitive impairment and neural deterioration. Figure 1.4 (see also Plate 1 in the colour section) shows the T1 structural MRI of three cognitively healthy men aged 71–80 years. It is apparent from this figure that two of the men (the 71-year-old and 80-year-old) show clear signs of cortical brain ageing (ventricular enlargement and cortical thinning), whereas the third man (the 76-year-old) shows less indication of cortical ageing, but some signs of cerebellar thinning. As the previous review has highlighted, these men are also likely to differ in localised grey and white matter integrity, intrinsic functional connectivity and functional responses to tasks, glucose metabolism, protein deposition and neurotransmitter system integrity. Thus, the 'brain age' of the individual is not clearly linked to their chronological age, due to inter-individual differences in genotypes, cognitive and social environment, and lifestyle choices (Jia, Zhang & Chen, 2017). Research is ongoing to

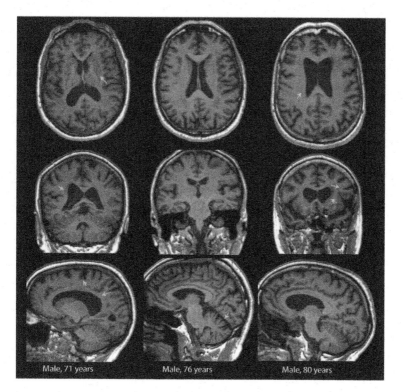

Male, 71 years   Male, 76 years   Male, 80 years

FIGURE 1.4 Mismatch between chronological age and brain age. Structural T1 MR images of three cognitively healthy older men. Brain ageing is immediately apparent as cortical thinning and ventricular enlargement, as highlighted by the arrows. The youngest (left) and oldest (right) men show substantial ventricular enlargement and cortical thinning. The 76-year-old man shows relative sparing of the cortex, but may show some evidence of cerebellar thinning. Thus, signs of brain ageing are variable between individuals, and are not tightly linked to the individual's chronological age.

formally define 'biological age' as a predictive mechanism for non-normal cognitive decline (DeCarlo, Tuokko, Williams, Dixon & MacDonald, 2014). It is hoped that these multivariate and mechanistic definitions of biological age will lead to more accurate prediction of age-related cognitive decline, and risk for age-related neurodegenerative illnesses.

Cortico-basal ganglia and fronto-cerebellar networks in ageing and neurodegeneration

Much of our knowledge of the structure and function of the cortico-basal ganglia and cortico-cerebellar networks comes from studies of neurodegenerative illnesses that are selective to those networks. For example, disturbances of the cortico-basal ganglia motor circuit are associated with hypokinetic (e.g. Parkinson's disease, progressive supranuclear palsy) and hyperkinetic (e.g. Huntington's disease, dystonia, hemiballism) disorders. Disturbances of the cerebellum are associated with ataxia (e.g. Friedreich's ataxia, spinocerebellar ataxia), hypotonia, astasia-abasia (inability to stand or walk), and cerebellar cognitive affective syndrome. While it is most common to study cortico-basal ganglia and cortico-cerebellar disturbances in neurodegenerative illnesses, evidence suggests that these networks also deteriorate with age (Seidler et al., 2010). Older adults show a range of motor difficulties, including coordination difficulty, increased variation of movement, motor slowing, and difficulties with balance and gait (ibid.). The motor symptoms with the highest prevalence in older adults includes bradykinesia (37%), gait disturbance (51%), and rigidity (43%; Bennett et al., 1996). Older adults also show reduced learning on sensorimotor adaptation and motor sequence tasks (Anguera, Reuter-Lorenz, Willingham & Seidler, 2011; Bo, Peltier, Noll & Seidler, 2011) as well as deficits with timing (Craik & Hay, 1999). While some of these disturbances are related to decline of the sensory receptors, muscles and peripheral nerves, deterioration of the cortico-basal ganglia and cortico-cerebellar circuits plays a role.

Chapters 2–9 comprehensively explore the degeneration of these circuits in neurodegenerative disease. In the present chapter, we will review the evidence that cortico-basal ganglia and cortico-cerebellar circuitry deteriorates with age, and highlight similarities between neurodegenerative illnesses and ageing that support the contention that these networks decline in ageing.

Age-related deterioration of cortico-basal ganglia circuits

There is a great deal of evidence to support the contention that cortico-basal ganglia circuits deteriorate with age. Ageing is associated with grey matter reductions in prefrontal cortex (e.g. Jernigan et al., 2001), premotor and primary motor cortex (Good et al., 2001; Salat et al., 2004; but see Raz et al., 1997) and basal ganglia (Langenecker, Briceno, Hamid & Nielson, 2007; Raz et al., 2005). The basal ganglia show reduced task-related activity in older compared to younger adults (Langenecker et al., 2007), and reduced task-related functional connectivity with the cortex (Marchand et al., 2011; Taniwaki et al., 2007). Older adults show reduced task-related activity in the basal ganglia (Langenecker et al., 2007) but increased prefrontal activity during motor tasks (Heuninckx, Wenderoth, Debaere, Peeters & Swinnen, 2005; Heuninckx, Wenderoth & Swinnen, 2008) compared to younger adults. These results have been taken as evidence that the prefrontal cortex may compensate for basal ganglia deterioration in ageing (Seidler et al., 2010). Cortical regions within the basal ganglia motor network also show HAROLD and PASA effects during motor tasks: with older adults showing increased inter-hemispheric connectivity (Langan et al., 2010; Michely et al., 2018; Solesio-Jofre et al., 2014) and prefrontal-premotor activity compared to younger adults (Michely et al., 2018). Lastly, age-related dopamine disturbance affects distributed nodes within the cortico-basal ganglia network, including the caudate nucleus, putamen and substantia nigra (Haycock et al., 2003; Kish, Shannak, Rajput, Deck & Hornykiewicz, 1992; Severson, Marcusson, Winblad & Finch, 1982).

Basal ganglia intrinsic connectivity reduces with age (Griffanti et al., 2018). Notably, one recent study suggests that structural and functional connectivity within the cortico-basal ganglia network may be an important predictor of brain age. In a sample of $n = 155$ healthy individuals aged 10–80 years, Bonifazi et al. (2018) examined whole-brain structural (white matter integrity; DTI) and functional (resting-state) connectivity across 2514 brain regions. They found that reduced structural and functional connectivity within a fronto-thalamic-basal ganglia network accurately predicted chronological age. They concluded that structural and functional connectivity within this network can be used as a metric of 'brain connectome age', suggesting that this network is critically important for brain ageing.

Additional evidence for deterioration of cortico-basal ganglia circuitry comes from the study of the relationship between Parkinson's disease and ageing. The primary pathology in Parkinson's disease is loss of dopaminergic cells within the substantia nigra, and results in shaking, rigidity, slowness of movement, sleep problems, emotional problems and dementia. Ageing is the largest risk factor for Parkinson's disease (see Reeve et al., 2014 for a review of common pathologies shared between ageing and Parkinson's disease). Of older adults without Parkinson's disease, around one third show mild to severe neuronal loss within the substantia nigra (Buchman et al., 2012; Rudow et al., 2008), with estimates of cell loss between 5% and 10% per decade (Fearnley & Lees, 1991; Ma, Röytt, Collan & Rinne, 1999). Iron accumulation in the substantia nigra is thought to be an important contributor to loss of neurons in the substantia in Parkinson's disease, and this also occurs in ageing (Daugherty & Raz, 2013). Thus, shared pathology between Parkinson's disease and ageing is compatible with the argument that cortico-basal ganglia circuitry deteriorates with age.

Age-related deterioration of cortico-cerebellar circuits

Like cortico-basal ganglia circuits, there is strong evidence for deterioration of cortico-cerebellar networks in ageing (see Bernard & Seidler, 2014 for a comprehensive review). The cerebellum becomes smaller with age, decreasing around 1.2% per year (Tang, Whitman, Lopez & Baloh, 2001), with more rapid reductions in advanced age (Walhovd et al., 2011). The anterior lobe of the cerebellum appears most affected by ageing, with degeneration also apparent in the superior cerebellum and posterior motor area (Hulst et al., 2015). The posterior cerebellum appears to be relatively spared in ageing (ibid.). Reduced cerebellar volumes are associated with a range of age-related behavioural impairments, including eyeblink conditioning (Woodruff-Pak et al., 2001), slower walking speed (Rosano, Aizenstein, Studenski & Newman, 2007), poor balance (ibid.), and cognitive function (reading, processing speed and executive function; Miller et al., 2013). Cerebellar white matter integrity reduces with age (Bennett, Madden, Vaidya, Howard & Howard Jr, 2010; Giorgio et al., 2010), as does cerebellar white matter volume (Fjell et al., 2013). The cerebellar peduncles, the white matter tracts of the cerebellum which connects the structure to the rest of the brain, are also reduced in integrity in ageing (Cavallari et al., 2013; Kafri et al., 2013). Finally, like the cortex and basal ganglia, the cerebellum shows reduced hemispheric asymmetry in ageing, as predicted by HAROLD (Ward & Frackowiak, 2003).

Strikingly, emerging evidence suggests it is the interaction between cerebellum and prefrontal cortex that is the most important in ageing. Grey matter reductions in the frontal cortex and thalamus covary with reduced grey matter in the cerebellum (Alexander et al., 2006; Su et al., 2012). Cerebellar motor deficits are associated with reductions in both the grey and white matter of the prefrontal cortex and cerebellum (Rosano et al., 2007; Eckert, Keren, Roberts, Calhoun & Harris, 2010), such that the cerebellum tracks the patterns and relationships of the prefrontal cortex in ageing (Bernard & Seidler, 2014). Cortico-cerebellar functional connectivity reduces with age (Wu et al., 2007; Bernard et al., 2013), with poorer connectivity strength predicting poorer motor (dexterity, timing, balance) and cognitive (working memory) outcomes (Bernard et al., 2013). Importantly, this study also found reduced connectivity within cortico-basal ganglia-cerebellar loops in ageing, with reduced cerebellar connectivity with the striatum and default mode network associated with poorer motor and cognitive performance in older adults (ibid.).

Ageing is also associated with ataxia. Cerebellar ataxia accounts for 8% of gait disorders in ageing (Sudarsky & Ronthal, 1983), most commonly due to cerebrovascular disease (Safe, Cooper & Windsor, 1992). On the other hand, at least one form of ataxia may be related to premature ageing. Ataxia-Telangiectasia is a neurodegenerative autosomal recessive condition characterised by movement and coordination problems (ataxia, oculomotor apraxia, slurred or slowed speech) but also signs of premature ageing. Adolescents and young adults with Ataxia-Telangiectasia show an array of conditions not usually seen until older age, including premature greying and thinning of hair and skin, osteoporosis, increased incidence of cancer, particularly in the solid organs (stomach, oesophagus, liver, skin, breast, lung), fatty liver, and diabetes (reviewed in Shiloh & Lederman, 2017). The link between this form of genetic neurodegenerative cerebellar ataxia and ageing is compatible with the contention that cortico-cerebellar circuits deteriorate with age.

In conclusion, while most research into cortico-basal ganglia and cortico-cerebellar connectivity is focused on dysconnectivity in neurodegenerative diseases, substantial evidence suggests both networks deteriorate in healthy ageing.

Concluding remarks

Unlike the disorders reviewed in the remainder of this volume, ageing is not pathological – although it serves as a strong risk factor for many neurodegenerative disorders. In some conditions (e.g. Alzheimer's disease, Parkinson's disease), it can be difficult to discriminate between these conditions and healthy ageing, with early stages of these diseases showing very subtle impairments compared to healthy ageing. This is an active area of research, as is the topic of how to predict a person's 'brain age' – the trajectory towards successful ageing, cognitive decline or dementia. Cortico-basal ganglia, cortico-cerebellar circuits and the interaction between them support important motor and non-motor cognitive processes. These circuits deteriorate with age, resulting in subtle but similar impairments to those found in neurodegenerative illnesses.

Abbreviations

Aβ	amyloid-beta
Aβ+	amyloid-beta positive
Aβ–	amyloid-beta negative
DTI	diffusion tensor imaging
FDG	fludeoxyglucose
fMRI	functional magnetic resonance imaging
HAROLD	hemispheric asymmetry reduction in old age
ICA	independent component analysis
PASA	posterior to anterior shift in ageing
PET	positron emission tomography

Further reading

Bernard, J. A. & Seidler, R. D. (2014). Moving forward: age effects on the cerebellum underlie cognitive and motor declines. *Neuroscience & Biobehavioral Reviews*, *42*, 193–207.

Bostan, A. C. & Strick, P. L. (2018). The basal ganglia and the cerebellum: nodes in an integrated network. *Nature Reviews Neuroscience*, doi:10.1038/s41583-018-0002-7

Haines, D. & Mihailoff, G. (2018). The pons and cerebellum. In D. Haines & G. Mihailoff (eds), *Fundamental Neuroscience for Basic and Clinical Applications*, vol. 5 (pp. 172–182). Oxford: Elsevier.

Wichmann, T. & DeLong, M. R. (2013). The basal ganglia. In E. Kandel, J. Schwartz, T. Jessell, S. Siegelbaum & A. Hudspeth (eds), *Principles of Neural Science* (pp. 982–998). New York: McGraw Hill.

References

Aizenstein, H. J., Nebes, R. D., Saxton, J. A., Price, J. C., Mathis, C. A., Tsopelas, N. D., ... Houck, P. R. (2008). Frequent amyloid deposition without significant cognitive impairment among the elderly. *Archives of Neurology, 65*(11), 1509–1517.

Alexander, G. E., Chen, K., Merkley, T. L., Reiman, E. M., Caselli, R. J., Aschenbrenner, M., ... Teipel, S. J. (2006). Regional network of magnetic resonance imaging gray matter volume in healthy aging. *Neuroreport, 17*(10), 951–956.

Alexopoulos, G. S. & Kelly, R. E. (2017) Late-life depression: translating neurobiological hypotheses into novel treatments. In R. Cabeza, L. Nyberg & D. C. Park (eds), *Cognitive Neuroscience of Ageing*. New York: Oxford University Press.

Allen, E. A., Erhardt, E. B., Damaraju, E., Gruner, W., Segall, J. M., Silva, R. F., ... Kalyanam, R. (2011). A baseline for the multivariate comparison of resting-state networks. *Frontiers in Systems Neuroscience, 5*, 2.

Andrews-Hanna, J. R., Snyder, A. Z., Vincent, J. L., Lustig, C., Head, D., Raichle, M. E. & Buckner, R. L. (2007). Disruption of large-scale brain systems in advanced aging. *Neuron, 56*(5), 924–935.

Andrews-Hanna, J. R., Smallwood, J. & Spreng, R. N. (2014). The default network and self-generated thought: component processes, dynamic control, and clinical relevance. *Annals of the New York Academy of Sciences, 1316*(1), 29–52.

Anguera, J. A., Reuter-Lorenz, P. A., Willingham, D. T. & Seidler, R. D. (2011). Failure to engage spatial working memory contributes to age-related declines in visuomotor learning. *Journal of Cognitive Neuroscience, 23*(1), 11–25.

Apostolova, L. G., Hwang, K. S., Andrawis, J. P., Green, A. E., Babakchanian, S., Morra, J. H., ... Shaw, L. M. (2010). 3D PIB and CSF biomarker associations with hippocampal atrophy in ADNI subjects. *Neurobiology of Aging, 31*(8), 1284–1303.

Arnemann, K. L., Stöber, F., Narayan, S., Rabinovici, G. D. & Jagust, W. J. (2018). Metabolic brain networks in aging and preclinical Alzheimer's disease. *NeuroImage: Clinical, 17*, 987–999.

Bäckman, L., Lindenberger, U., Li, S.-C. & Nyberg, L. (2010). Linking cognitive aging to alterations in dopamine neurotransmitter functioning: recent data and future avenues. *Neuroscience & Biobehavioral Reviews, 34*(5), 670–677.

Baker, J. E., Lim, Y. Y., Pietrzak, R. H., Hassenstab, J., Snyder, P. J., Masters, C. L. & Maruff, P. (2017). Cognitive impairment and decline in cognitively normal older adults with high amyloid-β: a meta-analysis. *Alzheimer's & Dementia: Diagnosis, Assessment & Disease Monitoring, 6*, 108–121.

Becker, J. A., Hedden, T., Carmasin, J., Maye, J., Rentz, D. M., Putcha, D., ... Salloway, S. (2011). Amyloid-β associated cortical thinning in clinically normal elderly. *Annals of Neurology, 69*(6), 1032–1042.

Bennett, D., Schneider, J., Arvanitakis, Z., Kelly, J., Aggarwal, N., Shah, R. & Wilson, R. (2006). Neuropathology of older persons without cognitive impairment from two community-based studies. *Neurology, 66*(12), 1837–1844.

Bennett, D. A., Beckett, L. A., Murray, A. M., Shannon, K. M., Goetz, C. G., Pilgrim, D. M. & Evans, D. A. (1996). Prevalence of parkinsonian signs and associated mortality in a community population of older people. *New England Journal of Medicine, 334*(2), 71–76.

Bennett, I. J. & Madden, D. J. (2014). Disconnected aging: cerebral white matter integrity and age-related differences in cognition. *Neuroscience, 276*, 187–205.

Bennett, I. J., Madden, D. J., Vaidya, C. J., Howard, D. V. & Howard Jr, J. H. (2010). Age-related differences in multiple measures of white matter integrity: a diffusion tensor imaging study of healthy aging. *Human Brain Mapping, 31*(3), 378–390.

Bernard, J. A., Peltier, S. J., Wiggins, J. L., Jaeggi, S. M., Buschkuehl, M., Fling, B. W., . . . Seidler, R. D. (2013). Disrupted cortico-cerebellar connectivity in older adults. *NeuroImage*, *83*, 103–119.

Bernard, J. A. & Seidler, R. D. (2014). Moving forward: age effects on the cerebellum underlie cognitive and motor declines. *Neuroscience & Biobehavioral Reviews*, *42*, 193–207.

Betzel, R. F., Byrge, L., He, Y., Goñi, J., Zuo, X.-N. & Sporns, O. (2014). Changes in structural and functional connectivity among resting-state networks across the human lifespan. *NeuroImage*, *102*, 345–357.

Bishop, N. A., Lu, T. & Yankner, B. A. (2010). Neural mechanisms of ageing and cognitive decline. *Nature*, *464*(7288), 529.

Bo, J., Peltier, S., Noll, D. & Seidler, R. (2011). Age differences in symbolic representations of motor sequence learning. *Neuroscience Letters*, *504*(1), 68–72.

Bonifazi, P., Erramuzpe, A., Diez, I., Gabilondo, I., Boisgontier, M. P., Pauwels, L., . . . Cortes, J. M. (2018). Structure-function multi-scale connectomics reveals a major role of the fronto-striato-thalamic circuit in brain aging. *Human Brain Mapping*, *39*(12), 4663–4677.

Bostan, A. C., Dum, R. P. & Strick, P. L. (2010). The basal ganglia communicate with the cerebellum. *Proceedings of the National Academy of Sciences*, *107*(18), 8452–8456.

Bostan, A. C. & Strick, P. L. (2018). The basal ganglia and the cerebellum: nodes in an integrated network. *Nature Reviews Neuroscience*, 1.

Braak, H., Thal, D. R., Ghebremedhin, E. & Del Tredici, K. (2011). Stages of the pathologic process in Alzheimer disease: age categories from 1 to 100 years. *Journal of Neuropathology & Experimental Neurology*, *70*(11), 960–969.

Buchman, A. S., Shulman, J. M., Nag, S., Leurgans, S. E., Arnold, S. E., Morris, M. C., . . . Bennett, D. A. (2012). Nigral pathology and parkinsonian signs in elders without Parkinson disease. *Annals of Neurology*, *71*(2), 258–266.

Buckner, R. L. (2013). The cerebellum and cognitive function: 25 years of insight from anatomy and neuroimaging. *Neuron*, *80*(3), 807–815.

Buckner, R. L., Andrews-Hanna, J. R. & Schacter, D. L. (2008). The brain's default network. *Annals of the New York Academy of Sciences*, *1124*(1), 1–38.

Cabeza, R. (2002). Hemispheric asymmetry reduction in older adults: the HAROLD model. *Psychology and Aging*, *17*(1), 85.

Cabeza, R., Nyberg, L. & Park, D. C. (2017). *Cognitive Neuroscience of Aging Linking Cognitive and Cerebral Aging*. Oxford: Oxford University Press.

Caligiore, D., Pezzulo, G., Baldassarre, G., Bostan, A. C., Strick, P. L., Doya, K., . . . Jörntell, H. (2017). Consensus paper: towards a systems-level view of cerebellar function: the interplay between cerebellum, basal ganglia, and cortex. *The Cerebellum*, *16*(1), 203–229.

Campbell, K. L., Grady, C. L., Ng, C. & Hasher, L. (2012). Age differences in the frontoparietal cognitive control network: implications for distractibility. *Neuropsychologia*, *50*(9), 2212–2223.

Cao, M., Wang, J.-H., Dai, Z.-J., Cao, X.-Y., Jiang, L.-L., Fan, F.-M., . . . Dong, Q. (2014). Topological organization of the human brain functional connectome across the lifespan. *Developmental Cognitive Neuroscience*, *7*, 76–93.

Cavallari, M., Moscufo, N., Skudlarski, P., Meier, D., Panzer, V. P., Pearlson, G. D., . . . Guttmann, C. R. (2013). Mobility impairment is associated with reduced microstructural integrity of the inferior and superior cerebellar peduncles in elderly with no clinical signs of cerebellar dysfunction. *NeuroImage: Clinical*, *2*, 332–340.

Chan, M. Y., Park, D. C., Savalia, N. K., Petersen, S. E. & Wig, G. S. (2014). Decreased segregation of brain systems across the healthy adult lifespan. *Proceedings of the National Academy of Sciences*, *111*(46), E4997–E5006.

Chen, Z., Jamadar, S. D., Li, S., Sforazzini, F., Baran, J., Ferris, N., . . . Egan, G. F. (2018). From simultaneous to synergistic MR-PET brain imaging: a review of hybrid MR-PET imaging methodologies. *Human Brain Mapping*, *39*(12), 5126–5144.

Chételat, G., La Joie, R., Villain, N., Perrotin, A., de La Sayette, V., Eustache, F. & Vandenberghe, R. (2013). Amyloid imaging in cognitively normal individuals, at-risk populations and preclinical Alzheimer's disease. *NeuroImage: Clinical*, *2*, 356–365.

Cole, J. H., Marioni, R. E., Harris, S. E. & Deary, I. J. (2018). Brain age and other bodily 'ages': implications for neuropsychiatry. *Molecular Psychiatry*, 1. doi: 10.1038/s41380-018-0098-1.

Courchesne, E., Chisum, H. J., Townsend, J., Cowles, A., Covington, J., Egaas, B., . . . Press, G. A. (2000). Normal brain development and aging: quantitative analysis at in vivo MR imaging in healthy volunteers. *Radiology*, *216*(3), 672–682.

Craik, F. I. & Hay, J. F. (1999). Aging and judgments of duration: effects of task complexity and method of estimation. *Perception & Psychophysics*, *61*(3), 549–560.

Damoiseaux, J. S. (2017). Effects of aging on functional and structural brain connectivity. *NeuroImage*, *160*, 32–40.

Damoiseaux, J. S., Beckmann, C., Arigita, E. S., Barkhof, F., Scheltens, P., Stam, C., . . . Rombouts, S. (2007). Reduced resting-state brain activity in the 'default network' in normal aging. *Cerebral Cortex*, *18*(8), 1856–1864.

Daugherty, A. & Raz, N. (2013). Age-related differences in iron content of subcortical nuclei observed in vivo: a meta-analysis. *NeuroImage*, *70*, 113–121.

Davis, S. W., Dennis, N. A., Daselaar, S. M., Fleck, M. S. & Cabeza, R. (2007). Que PASA? The posterior–anterior shift in aging. *Cerebral Cortex*, *18*(5), 1201–1209.

DeCarlo, C. A., Tuokko, H. A., Williams, D., Dixon, R. A. & MacDonald, S. W. (2014). BioAge: toward a multi-determined, mechanistic account of cognitive aging. *Ageing Research Reviews*, *18*, 95–105.

DeLong, M. R. & Wichmann, T. (2015). Basal ganglia circuits as targets for neuromodulation in Parkinson disease. *JAMA Neurology*, *72*(11), 1354–1360.

Dickstein, D. L., Kabaso, D., Rocher, A. B., Luebke, J. I., Wearne, S. L. & Hof, P. R. (2007). Changes in the structural complexity of the aged brain. *Aging Cell*, *6*(3), 275–284.

Doré, V., Villemagne, V. L., Bourgeat, P., Fripp, J., Acosta, O., Chételat, G., . . . Masters, C. L. (2013). Cross-sectional and longitudinal analysis of the relationship between Aβ deposition, cortical thickness, and memory in cognitively unimpaired individuals and in Alzheimer disease. *JAMA Neurology*, *70*(7), 903–911.

Doya, K. (2000). Complementary roles of basal ganglia and cerebellum in learning and motor control. *Current Opinion in Neurobiology*, *10*(6), 732–739.

Eckert, M. A., Keren, N. I., Roberts, D. R., Calhoun, V. D. & Harris, K. C. (2010). Age-related changes in processing speed: unique contributions of cerebellar and prefrontal cortex. *Frontiers in Human Neuroscience*, *4*, 10.

Elman, J. A., Oh, H., Madison, C. M., Baker, S. L., Vogel, J. W., Marks, S. M., . . . Jagust, W. J. (2014). Neural compensation in older people with brain amyloid-β deposition. *Nature Neuroscience*, *17*(10), 1316.

Farquhar, M. (1995). Elderly people's definitions of quality of life. *Social Science & Medicine*, *41*(10), 1439–1446.

Fearnley, J. M. & Lees, A. J. (1991). Ageing and Parkinson's disease: substantia nigra regional selectivity. *Brain*, *114*(5), 2283–2301.

Fjell, A. M. & Walhovd, K. B. (2010). Structural brain changes in aging: courses, causes and cognitive consequences. *Reviews in the Neurosciences*, *21*(3), 187–222.

Fjell, A. M., Walhovd, K. B., Fennema-Notestine, C., McEvoy, L. K., Hagler, D. J., Holland, D., . . . Dale, A. M. (2009). One-year brain atrophy evident in healthy aging. *Journal of Neuroscience, 29*(48), 15223–15231.

Fjell, A. M., Westlye, L. T., Grydeland, H., Amlien, I., Espeseth, T., Reinvang, I., . . . Walhovd, K. B. (2013). Critical ages in the life course of the adult brain: nonlinear subcortical aging. *Neurobiology of Aging, 34*(10), 2239–2247.

Fornito, A., Zalesky, A. & Breakspear, M. (2015). The connectomics of brain disorders. *Nature Reviews Neuroscience, 16*(3), 159.

Fox, P. T., Laird, A. R. & Lancaster, J. L. (2005). Coordinate-based voxel-wise meta-analysis: dividends of spatial normalization. Report of a virtual workshop. *Human Brain Mapping, 25*(1), 1–5.

Gao, F., Edden, R. A., Li, M., Puts, N. A., Wang, G., Liu, C., . . . Zhao, C. (2013). Edited magnetic resonance spectroscopy detects an age-related decline in brain GABA levels. *NeuroImage, 78,* 75–82.

Geerligs, L., Renken, R. J., Saliasi, E., Maurits, N. M. & Lorist, M. M. (2014). A brain-wide study of age-related changes in functional connectivity. *Cerebral Cortex, 25*(7), 1987–1999.

Geerligs, L., Rubinov, M. & Henson, R. N. (2015). State and trait components of functional connectivity: individual differences vary with mental state. *Journal of Neuroscience, 35*(41), 13949–13961.

Giorgio, A., Santelli, L., Tomassini, V., Bosnell, R., Smith, S., De Stefano, N. & Johansen-Berg, H. (2010). Age-related changes in grey and white matter structure throughout adulthood. *NeuroImage, 51*(3), 943–951.

Good, C., Johnsrude, I., Ashburner, J., Henson, R., Friston, K. & Frackowiak, R. (2001). A voxel-based morphometric study of ageing in 465 normal adult human brains. *NeuroImage, 14*(1 Pt 1), 21–36.

Grady, C. (2012). The cognitive neuroscience of ageing. *Nature Reviews Neuroscience, 13*(7), 491.

Grady, C., Sarraf, S., Saverino, C. & Campbell, K. (2016). Age differences in the functional interactions among the default, frontoparietal control, and dorsal attention networks. *Neurobiology of Aging, 41,* 159–172.

Grady, C. L., Springer, M. V., Hongwanishkul, D., McIntosh, A. R. & Winocur, G. (2006). Age-related changes in brain activity across the adult lifespan. *Journal of Cognitive Neuroscience, 18*(2), 227–241.

Griffanti, L., Stratmann, P., Rolinski, M., Filippini, N., Zsoldos, E., Mahmood, A., . . . Kivimäki, M. (2018). Exploring variability in basal ganglia connectivity with functional MRI in healthy aging. *Brain Imaging and Behavior, 12*(6), 1822–1827

Guerreiro, R. & Bras, J. (2015). The age factor in Alzheimer's disease. *Genome Medicine, 7*(1), 106.

Haines, D. & Mihailoff, G. (2018). *Fundamental Neuroscience for Basic and Clinical Applications,* vol. 5. Oxford: Elsevier.

Hardy, J. & Selcoe, D. J. (2002). The amyloid hypothesis of Alzheimer's disease: progress and problems on the road to therapeutics. *Science, 297,* 353–356.

Harris, J. J., Jolivet, R. & Attwell, D. (2012). Synaptic energy use and supply. *Neuron, 75*(5), 762–777.

Haycock, J. W., Becker, L., Ang, L., Furukawa, Y., Hornykiewicz, O. & Kish, S. J. (2003). Marked disparity between age-related changes in dopamine and other presynaptic dopaminergic markers in human striatum. *Journal of Neurochemistry, 87*(3), 574–585.

Hedman, A. M., van Haren, N. E., Schnack, H. G., Kahn, R. S. & Hulshoff Pol, H. E. (2012). Human brain changes across the life span: a review of 56 longitudinal magnetic resonance imaging studies. *Human Brain Mapping, 33*(8), 1987–2002.

Heuninckx, S., Wenderoth, N., Debaere, F., Peeters, R. & Swinnen, S. P. (2005). Neural basis of aging: the penetration of cognition into action control. *Journal of Neuroscience*, *25*(29), 6787–6796.

Heuninckx, S., Wenderoth, N. & Swinnen, S. P. (2008). Systems neuroplasticity in the aging brain: recruiting additional neural resources for successful motor performance in elderly persons. *Journal of Neuroscience*, *28*(1), 91–99.

Hoshi, E., Tremblay, L., Féger, J., Carras, P. L. & Strick, P. L. (2005). The cerebellum communicates with the basal ganglia. *Nature Neuroscience*, *8*(11), 1491.

Houk, J., Bastianen, C., Fansler, D., Fishbach, A., Fraser, D., Reber, P., . . . Simo, L. (2007). Action selection and refinement in subcortical loops through basal ganglia and cerebellum. *Philosophical Transactions of the Royal Society of London B: Biological Sciences*, *362*(1485), 1573–1583.

Hulst, T., van der Geest, J. N., Thürling, M., Goericke, S., Frens, M. A., Timmann, D. & Donchin, O. (2015). Ageing shows a pattern of cerebellar degeneration analogous, but not equal, to that in patients suffering from cerebellar degenerative disease. *NeuroImage*, *116*, 196–206.

Iyo, M. & Yamasaki, T. (1993). The detection of age-related decrease of dopamine D1, D2 and serotonin 5-HT2 receptors in living human brain. *Progress in Neuro-psychopharmacology & Biological Psychiatry*, *17*(3), 415–421.

Jack, C. R., Wiste, H. J., Weigand, S. D., Rocca, W. A., Knopman, D. S., Mielke, M. M., . . . Preboske, G. M. (2014). Age-specific population frequencies of cerebral β-amyloidosis and neurodegeneration among people with normal cognitive function aged 50–89 years: a cross-sectional study. *The Lancet Neurology*, *13*(10), 997–1005.

Jamadar, S. D., Egan, G. F., Calhoun, V. D., Johnson, B. & Fielding, J. (2016). Intrinsic connectivity provides the baseline framework for variability in motor performance: a multivariate fusion analysis of low-and high-frequency resting-state oscillations and anti-saccade performance. *Brain Connectivity*, *6*(6), 505–517.

Jansen, W. J., Ossenkoppele, R., Knol, D. L., Tijms, B. M., Scheltens, P., Verhey, F. R., . . . Alcolea, D. (2015). Prevalence of cerebral amyloid pathology in persons without dementia: a meta-analysis. *Journal of the American Medical Association*, *313*(19), 1924–1938.

Jernigan, T. L., Archibald, S. L., Fennema-Notestine, C., Gamst, A. C., Stout, J. C., Bonner, J. & Hesselink, J. R. (2001). Effects of age on tissues and regions of the cerebrum and cerebellum. *Neurobiology of Aging*, *22*(4), 581–594.

Jia, L., Zhang, W. & Chen, X. (2017). Common methods of biological age estimation. *Clinical Interventions in Aging*, *12*, 759.

Kafri, M., Sasson, E., Assaf, Y., Balash, Y., Aiznstein, O., Hausdorff, J. M. & Giladi, N. (2013). High-level gait disorder: associations with specific white matter changes observed on advanced diffusion imaging. *Journal of Neuroimaging*, *23*(1), 39–46.

Kalpouzos, G., Chételat, G., Baron, J.-C., Landeau, B., Mevel, K., Godeau, C., . . . Eustache, F. (2009). Voxel-based mapping of brain gray matter volume and glucose metabolism profiles in normal aging. *Neurobiology of Aging*, *30*(1), 112–124.

Karrer, T. M., Josef, A. K., Mata, R., Morris, E. D. & Samanez-Larkin, G. R. (2017). Reduced dopamine receptors and transporters but not synthesis capacity in normal aging adults: a meta-analysis. *Neurobiology of Aging*, *57*, 36–46.

Kelly, C., de Zubicaray, G., Di Martino, A., Copland, D. A., Reiss, P. T., Klein, D. F., . . . McMahon, K. (2009). L-dopa modulates functional connectivity in striatal cognitive and motor networks: a double-blind placebo-controlled study. *Journal of Neuroscience*, *29*(22), 7364–7378.

Kelly, R. M. & Strick, P. L. (2004). Macro-architecture of basal ganglia loops with the cerebral cortex: use of rabies virus to reveal multisynaptic circuits. *Progress in Brain Research*, *143*, 447–459.

Kety, S. S. (1957). The general metabolism of the brain in vivo. In *Metabolism of the Nervous System* (pp. 221–237). Oxford: Elsevier.

Khan, S. S., Singer, B. D. & Vaughan, D. E. (2017). Molecular and physiological manifestations and measurement of aging in humans. *Aging Cell*, *16*(4), 624–633.

Kish, S. J., Shannak, K., Rajput, A., Deck, J. H. & Hornykiewicz, O. (1992). Aging produces a specific pattern of striatal dopamine loss: implications for the etiology of idiopathic Parkinson's disease. *Journal of Neurochemistry*, *58*(2), 642–648.

Koziol, L. F., Budding, D., Andreasen, N., D'Arrigo, S., Bulgheroni, S., Imamizu, H., . . . Parker, K. (2014). Consensus paper: the cerebellum's role in movement and cognition. *The Cerebellum*, *13*(1), 151–177.

Laird, A. R., Eickhoff, S. B., Li, K., Robin, D. A., Glahn, D. C. & Fox, P. T. (2009). Investigating the functional heterogeneity of the default mode network using coordinate-based meta-analytic modeling. *Journal of Neuroscience*, *29*(46), 14496–14505.

Lanciego, J. L., Luquin, N. & Obeso, J. A. (2012). Functional neuroanatomy of the basal ganglia. *Cold Spring Harbor Perspectives in Medicine*, a009621.

Langan, J., Peltier, S., Bo, J., Fling, B. W., Welsh, R. C. & Seidler, R. D. (2010). Functional implications of age differences in motor system connectivity. *Frontiers in Systems Neuroscience*, *4*, 17.

Langenecker, S. A., Briceno, E. M., Hamid, N. M. & Nielson, K. A. (2007). An evaluation of distinct volumetric and functional MRI contributions toward understanding age and task performance: a study in the basal ganglia. *Brain Research*, *1135*, 58–68.

Lim, H. K., Nebes, R., Snitz, B., Cohen, A., Mathis, C., Price, J., . . . Aizenstein, H. J. (2014). Regional amyloid burden and intrinsic connectivity networks in cognitively normal elderly subjects. *Brain*, *137*(12), 3327–3338.

Lisberger, S. & Thach, T. (2013). The cerebellum. In E. Kandel, J. Schwartz, T. Jessell, S. Siegelbaum & A. Hudspeth (eds), *Principles of Neural Science* (pp. 960–981). New York: McGraw Hill.

Lustig, C., Snyder, A. Z., Bhakta, M., O'Brien, K. C., McAvoy, M., Raichle, M. E., . . . Buckner, R. L. (2003). Functional deactivations: change with age and dementia of the Alzheimer type. *Proceedings of the National Academy of Sciences*, *100*(24), 14504–14509.

Ma, S., Röytt, M., Collan, Y. & Rinne, J. (1999). Unbiased morphometrical measurements show loss of pigmented nigral neurones with ageing. *Neuropathology and Applied Neurobiology*, *25*(5), 394–399.

Maccioni, R. B., Farias, G., Morales, I., Navarrete, L. (2010). The revitalised tau hypothesis on Alzheimer's disease. *Archives of Medical Research*, *41*, 226–231.

Maillard, P., Carmichael, O., Fletcher, E., Reed, B., Mungas, D. & DeCarli, C. (2012). Coevolution of white matter hyperintensities and cognition in the elderly. *Neurology*, *79*(5), 442–448.

Mak, L. E., Minuzzi, L., MacQueen, G., Hall, G., Kennedy, S. H. & Milev, R. (2017). The default mode network in healthy individuals: a systematic review and meta-analysis. *Brain Connectivity*, *7*(1), 25–33.

Marchand, W. R., Lee, J. N., Suchy, Y., Garn, C., Johnson, S., Wood, N. & Chelune, G. (2011). Age-related changes of the functional architecture of the cortico-basal ganglia circuitry during motor task execution. *NeuroImage*, *55*(1), 194–203.

Meier, T. B., Desphande, A. S., Vergun, S., Nair, V. A., Song, J., Biswal, B. B., . . . Prabhakaran, V. (2012). Support vector machine classification and characterization of age-related reorganization of functional brain networks. *NeuroImage*, *60*(1), 601–613.

Miall, R. C. & Wolpert, D. M. (1996). Forward models for physiological motor control. *Neural Networks, 9*(8), 1265–1279.

Michely, J., Volz, L. J., Hoffstaedter, F., Tittgemeyer, M., Eickhoff, S. B., Fink, G. R. & Grefkes, C. (2018). Network connectivity of motor control in the ageing brain. *NeuroImage: Clinical, 18*, 443–455.

Miller, T. D., Ferguson, K. J., Reid, L. M., Wardlaw, J. M., Starr, J. M., Seckl, J. R., . . . MacLullich, A. M. (2013). Cerebellar vermis size and cognitive ability in community-dwelling elderly men. *The Cerebellum, 12*(1), 68–73.

Nambu, A. (2008). Seven problems on the basal ganglia. *Current Opinion in Neurobiology, 18*(6), 595–604.

Nambu, A., Tokuno, H. & Takada, M. (2002). Functional significance of the cortico-subthalamo-pallidal 'hyperdirect' pathway. *Neuroscience Research, 43*(2), 111–117.

Netuveli, G., Wiggins, R. D., Hildon, Z., Montgomery, S. M. & Blane, D. (2006). Quality of life at older ages: evidence from the English longitudinal study of aging (wave 1). *Journal of Epidemiology & Community Health, 60*(4), 357–363.

Onoda, K., Ishihara, M. & Yamaguchi, S. (2012). Decreased functional connectivity by aging is associated with cognitive decline. *Journal of Cognitive Neuroscience, 24*(11), 2186–2198.

Porges, E. C., Woods, A. J., Edden, R. A., Puts, N. A., Harris, A. D., Chen, H., . . . Williamson, J. B. (2017). Frontal gamma-aminobutyric acid concentrations are associated with cognitive performance in older adults. *Biological Psychiatry: Cognitive Neuroscience and Neuroimaging, 2*(1), 38–44.

Price, J. L. & Morris, J. C. (1999). Tangles and plaques in nondemented aging and 'preclinical' Alzheimer's disease. *Annals of Neurology: Official Journal of the American Neurological Association and the Child Neurology Society, 45*(3), 358–368.

Prins, N. D. & Scheltens, P. (2015). White matter hyperintensities, cognitive impairment and dementia: an update. *Nature Reviews Neurology, 11*(3), 157.

Rajah, M. N. & D'esposito, M. (2005). Region-specific changes in prefrontal function with age: a review of PET and fMRI studies on working and episodic memory. *Brain, 128*(9), 1964–1983.

Ramnani, N. (2006). The primate cortico-cerebellar system: anatomy and function. *Nature Reviews Neuroscience, 7*(7), 511.

Raz, N., Gunning, F. M., Head, D., Dupuis, J. H., McQuain, J., Briggs, S. D., . . . Acker, J. D. (1997). Selective aging of the human cerebral cortex observed in vivo: differential vulnerability of the prefrontal gray matter. *Cerebral Cortex, 7*(3), 268–282.

Raz, N., Lindenberger, U., Rodrigue, K. M., Kennedy, K. M., Head, D., Williamson, A., . . . Acker, J. D. (2005). Regional brain changes in aging healthy adults: general trends, individual differences and modifiers. *Cerebral Cortex, 15*(11), 1676–1689.

Reeve, A., Simcox, E. & Turnbull, D. (2014). Ageing and Parkinson's disease: why is advancing age the biggest risk factor? *Ageing Research Reviews, 14*, 19–30.

Reeves, S., Bench, C. & Howard, R. (2002). Ageing and the nigrostriatal dopaminergic system. *International Journal of Geriatric Psychiatry, 17*(4), 359–370.

Reuter-Lorenz, P. A. & Cappell, K. A. (2008). Neurocognitive aging and the compensation hypothesis. *Current Directions in Psychological Science, 17*(3), 177–182.

Rönnlund, M., Nyberg, L., Bäckman, L. & Nilsson, L.-G. (2005). Stability, growth, and decline in adult life span development of declarative memory: cross-sectional and longitudinal data from a population-based study. *Psychology and Aging, 20*(1), 3.

Rosano, C., Aizenstein, H. J., Studenski, S. & Newman, A. B. (2007). A regions-of-interest volumetric analysis of mobility limitations in community-dwelling older adults. *The Journals of Gerontology Series A: Biological Sciences and Medical Sciences, 62*(9), 1048–1055.

Rudow, G., O'Brien, R., Savonenko, A. V., Resnick, S. M., Zonderman, A. B., Pletnikova, O., . . . West, M. J. (2008). Morphometry of the human substantia nigra in ageing and Parkinson's disease. *Acta Neuropathologica, 115*(4), 461.

Rugg, M. D. (2017). Intepreting age-related differences in memory-related neural activity. In R. Cabeza, L. Nyberg & D. C. Park (eds), *Cognitive Neuroscience of Ageing*. New York: Oxford University Press. doi: 10.1093/acprof:oso/9780199372935.001.0001

Safe, A., Cooper, S. & Windsor, A. (1992). Cerebellar ataxia in the elderly. *Journal of the Royal Society of Medicine, 85*(8), 449.

Salat, D. H., Buckner, R. L., Snyder, A. Z., Greve, D. N., Desikan, R. S., Busa, E., . . . Fischl, B. (2004). Thinning of the cerebral cortex in aging. *Cerebral Cortex, 14*(7), 721–730.

Salat, D. H., Greve, D. N., Pacheco, J. L., Quinn, B. T., Helmer, K. G., Buckner, R. L. & Fischl, B. (2009). Regional white matter volume differences in nondemented aging and Alzheimer's disease. *NeuroImage, 44*(4), 1247–1258.

Salthouse, T. (2010). Selective review of cognitive aging. *Journal of the International Neuropsychological Society, 16*(5), 754–760.

Salthouse, T. (2012). Consequences of age-related cognitive declines. *Annual Review of Psychology, 63*, 201–226.

Sambataro, F., Murty, V. P., Callicott, J. H., Tan, H.-Y., Das, S., Weinberger, D. R. & Mattay, V. S. (2010). Age-related alterations in default mode network: impact on working memory performance. *Neurobiology of Aging, 31*(5), 839–852.

Scahill, R. I., Frost, C., Jenkins, R., Whitwell, J. L., Rossor, M. N. & Fox, N. C. (2003). A longitudinal study of brain volume changes in normal aging using serial registered magnetic resonance imaging. *Archives of Neurology, 60*(7), 989–994.

Schmahmann, J. D. (1991). An emerging concept: the cerebellar contribution to higher function. *Archives of Neurology, 48*(11), 1178–1187.

Schmahmann, J. D. (2000). The role of the cerebellum in affect and psychosis. *Journal of Neurolinguistics, 13*(2–3), 189–214.

Schöll, M., Lockhart, S. N., Schonhaut, D. R., O'Neil, J. P., Janabi, M., Ossenkoppele, R., . . . Schwimmer, H. D. (2016). PET imaging of tau deposition in the aging human brain. *Neuron, 89*(5), 971–982.

Seidler, R. D., Bernard, J. A., Burutolu, T. B., Fling, B. W., Gordon, M. T., Gwin, J. T., . . . Lipps, D. B. (2010). Motor control and aging: links to age-related brain structural, functional, and biochemical effects. *Neuroscience & Biobehavioral Reviews, 34*(5), 721–733.

Sepulcre, J., Schultz, A. P., Sabuncu, M., Gomez-Isla, T., Chhatwal, J., Becker, A., . . . Johnson, K. A. (2016). In vivo tau, amyloid, and gray matter profiles in the aging brain. *Journal of Neuroscience, 36*(28), 7364–7374.

Severson, J., Marcusson, J., Winblad, B. & Finch, C. (1982). Age-correlated loss of dopaminergic binding sites in human basal ganglia. *Journal of Neurochemistry, 39*(6), 1623–1631.

Sheline, Y. I., Raichle, M. E., Snyder, A. Z., Morris, J. C., Head, D., Wang, S. & Mintun, M. A. (2010). Amyloid plaques disrupt resting state default mode network connectivity in cognitively normal elderly. *Biological Psychiatry, 67*(6), 584–587.

Shiloh, Y. & Lederman, H. M. (2017). Ataxia-telangiectasia (AT): an emerging dimension of premature ageing. *Ageing Research Reviews, 33*, 76–88.

Sokoloff, L. (1960). The metabolism of the central nervous system in vivo. *Handbook of Physiology, Section I, Neurophysiology, 3*, 1843–1864.

Solesio-Jofre, E., Serbruyns, L., Woolley, D. G., Mantini, D., Beets, I. A. & Swinnen, S. P. (2014). Aging effects on the resting state motor network and interlimb coordination. *Human Brain Mapping, 35*(8), 3945–3961.

Sperling, R. A., Aisen, P. S., Beckett, L. A., Bennett, D. A., Craft, S., Fagan, A. M., . . . Montine, T. J. (2011). Toward defining the preclinical stages of Alzheimer's disease: recommendations from the National Institute on Aging-Alzheimer's Association work-groups on diagnostic guidelines for Alzheimer's disease. *Alzheimer's and Dementia*, 7(3), 280–292.

Sporns, O. (2013). Network attributes for segregation and integration in the human brain. *Current Opinion in Neurobiology*, 23(2), 162–171.

Spreng, R. N., Stevens, W. D., Viviano, J. D. & Schacter, D. L. (2016). Attenuated anticor-relation between the default and dorsal attention networks with aging: evidence from task and rest. *Neurobiology of Aging*, 45, 149–160.

Su, L., Wang, L., Chen, F., Shen, H., Li, B. & Hu, D. (2012). Sparse representation of brain aging: extracting covariance patterns from structural MRI. *PloS One*, 7(5), e36147.

Sudarsky, L. & Ronthal, M. (1983). Gait disorders among elderly patients: a survey study of 50 patients. *Archives of Neurology*, 40(12), 740–743.

Svennerholm, L., Boström, K. & Jungbjer, B. (1997). Changes in weight and compositions of major membrane components of human brain during the span of adult human life of Swedes. *Acta Neuropathologica*, 94(4), 345–352.

Tang, Y., Whitman, G. T., Lopez, I. & Baloh, R. W. (2001). Brain volume changes on longitudinal magnetic resonance imaging in normal older people. *Journal of Neuroimaging*, 11(4), 393–400.

Taniwaki, T., Okayama, A., Yoshiura, T., Togao, O., Nakamura, Y., Yamasaki, T., . . . Kira, J.-i. (2007). Age-related alterations of the functional interactions within the basal ganglia and cerebellar motor loops in vivo. *NeuroImage*, 36(4), 1263–1276.

Tomasi, D. & Volkow, N. D. (2012). Aging and functional brain networks. *Molecular Psychiatry*, 17(5), 549.

Vernooij, M. W., Ikram, M. A., Tanghe, H. L., Vincent, A. J., Hofman, A., Krestin, G. P., . . . van der Lugt, A. (2007). Incidental findings on brain MRI in the general population. *New England Journal of Medicine*, 357(18), 1821–1828.

Villemagne, V. L., Fodero-Tavoletti, M. T., Masters, C. L. & Rowe, C. C. (2015). Tau imaging: early progress and future directions. *The Lancet Neurology*, 14(1), 114–124.

Walhovd, K. B., Johansen-Berg, H. & Karadottir, R. T. (2014). Unraveling the secrets of white matter–bridging the gap between cellular, animal and human imaging studies. *Neuroscience*, 276, 2–13.

Walhovd, K. B., Westlye, L. T., Amlien, I., Espeseth, T., Reinvang, I., Raz, N., . . . Fischl, B. (2011). Consistent neuroanatomical age-related volume differences across multiple samples. *Neurobiology of Aging*, 32(5), 916–932.

Wang, J., Zuo, X., He, Y. (2010). Graph-based network analysis of resting-state functional MRI. *Frontiers in Systems Neuroscience*, doi:10.3389/fnsys.2010.00016.

Ward, N. & Frackowiak, R. (2003). Age-related changes in the neural correlates of motor performance. *Brain*, 126(4), 873–888.

Wichmann, T. & DeLong, M. R. (2013). The basal ganglia. In E. Kandel, J. Schwartz, T. Jessell, S. Siegelbaum & A. Hudspeth (eds), *Principles of Neural Science* (pp. 982–999). New York: McGraw Hill.

Wong, D. F., Wagner, H. N., Dannals, R. F., Links, J. M., Frost, J. J., Ravert, H. T., . . . Douglass, K. H. (1984). Effects of age on dopamine and serotonin receptors measured by positron tomography in the living human brain. *Science*, 226(4681), 1393–1396.

Woodruff-Pak, D. S., Vogel III, R. W., Ewers, M., Coffey, J., Boyko, O. B. & Lemieux, S. K. (2001). MRI-assessed volume of cerebellum correlates with associative learning. *Neurobiology of Learning and Memory*, 76(3), 342–357.

Wu, T., Zang, Y., Wang, L., Long, X., Hallett, M., Chen, Y., . . . Chan, P. (2007). Aging influence on functional connectivity of the motor network in the resting state. *Neuroscience Letters*, *422*(3), 164–168.

Yamamoto, M., Suhara, T., Okubo, Y., Ichimiya, T., Sudo, Y., Inoue, M., . . . Tanada, S. (2002). Age-related decline of serotonin transporters in living human brain of healthy males. *Life Sciences*, *71*(7), 751–757.

Yin, F., Sancheti, H., Patil, I. & Cadenas, E. (2016). Energy metabolism and inflammation in brain aging and Alzheimer's disease. *Free Radical Biology and Medicine*, *100*, 108–122.

Young, V. G., Halliday, G. M. & Kril, J. J. (2008). Neuropathologic correlates of white matter hyperintensities. *Neurology*, *71*(11), 804–811.

Zhang, H.-Y., Chen, W.-X., Jiao, Y., Xu, Y., Zhang, X.-R. & Wu, J.-T. (2014). Selective vulnerability related to aging in large-scale resting brain networks. *PloS One*, *9*(10), e108807.

2

ALZHEIMER'S DISEASE

Prodromal stages and dementia

Kerryn Pike and Glynda Kinsella

Introduction

Dementia afflicts almost 50 million worldwide (Prince et al., 2015), is the greatest cause of disability in people aged over 65 (Australian Institute of Health and Welfare, 2012), and a leading cause of death in Western countries (Australian Bureau of Statistics, 2016). It substantially impacts family and caregivers, and has a vast economic impact (e.g. > US $950 billion worldwide in 2015; Jia et al., 2018). Yet, it is likely to become an even bigger issue, with prevalence anticipated to nearly triple by 2050 (Prince et al., 2015), as survival age increases worldwide. Despite this, dementia remains the only disease within the ten most prevalent causes of death without a reliable method of prevention or cure (Alzheimer's Association, 2017).

Alzheimer's disease (AD) is the most common cause of dementia (60–80%; Alzheimer's Association, 2017); and, with the advent of reliable biomarkers, it is clear that AD starts long before dementia is diagnosed. Indeed, AD is now considered a continuum with dementia as the end stage (Jack et al., 2018). Therefore, we will consider the spectrum of AD presentations, from preclinical stages (including subjective cognitive decline, SCD), through the prodromal mild cognitive impairment (MCI) stage, and finally the dementia stage (Figure 2.1).

After briefly highlighting AD's origins as a pathological diagnosis, AD dementia, MCI, and preclinical AD (including SCD) are discussed, followed by review of key neuropathology and biomarkers. We then consider prevalence and onset, focusing on risk factors. Clinical issues are reviewed in the neuropsychology section, and in the final section current and potential future options for treatment and management are considered.

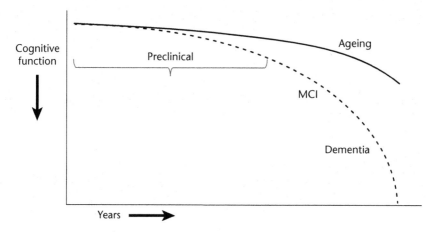

FIGURE 2.1 The continuum of Alzheimer's disease.

Diagnostic considerations

AD is named after Alois Alzheimer, a German neuropathologist and psychiatrist, who described the first case of AD dementia in 1906. The 'AD' stands for Auguste Deter, a 51-year-old woman who demonstrated cognitive and neuropsychiatric disturbances, and pronounced psychosocial impairment (Maurer, Volk & Gerbaldo, 1997). After her death, Alzheimer studied her brain's histopathology, reporting what is now considered the hallmark pathology of AD – beta-amyloid (Aβ) plaques and neurofibrillary tangles (ibid.).

For many years, the most common criteria in clinical and research settings used clinical symptoms to diagnose possible or probable AD dementia, with diagnosis of definite AD reliant on pathological confirmation through biopsy or autopsy (McKhann et al., 1984). These criteria were reasonably sensitive; 70–87% of people diagnosed with probable or possible AD demonstrated pathological AD at autopsy (Beach, Monsell, Phillips & Kukull, 2012). In 2010, with growing understanding that AD has a long preclinical and prodromal process, workgroups convened by the National Institute on Aging (NIA) and the Alzheimer's Association (AA) updated criteria for dementia due to AD, as well as creating criteria for the symptomatic predementia phase of AD, and the asymptomatic preclinical phase (Jack et al., 2011). The updated criteria also explicitly covered atypical presentations of AD dementia.

For AD dementia (McKhann et al., 2011), firstly dementia must be established, defined as cognitive or behavioural symptoms in at least two domains, interfering with function at work or usual activities, representing decline from previous levels, and not due to delirium or psychiatric disorder; and onset is typically insidious.

These criteria are largely similar to the *Diagnostic and Statistical Manual of Mental Disorders* (fifth edition) (DSM-V) criteria for Major Neurocognitive Disorder (American Psychiatric Association, 2013). An amnestic presentation is most common, involving prominent early deficits in learning and recall of new information. Atypical presentations of AD dementia may demonstrate prominent early deficits in language (Gorno-Tempini et al., 2011); visuospatial skills (Crutch et al., 2017); or behaviour and executive function (Ossenkoppele et al., 2015). Other causes must be excluded, including evidence for another dementia, or other disease or medication substantially impacting cognition. Diagnostic certainty is increased by documented cognitive decline over time or evidence of a causative genetic mutation. Pathophysiologically proved AD dementia requires evidence of AD neuropathology; whereas, possible AD dementia reflects an atypical course – for example, sudden onset – or an etiologically mixed presentation.

In the last 20 years, MCI has become the preferred term for patients in the prodromal stage of AD. The NIA-AA workgroup (Albert et al., 2011) diagnostic criteria are the first specifically referring to MCI due to AD (i.e. excluding alternative causes of MCI). The core clinical and cognitive criteria are essentially the same as those developed by Petersen et al. (1999); they focused on amnestic MCI, and broadened to include non-amnestic MCI by Winblad et al. (2004). They require: (a) concern regarding cognitive change; (b) objective cognitive impairment; (c) relatively preserved independence in functional activities; (d) not demented. Note that the DSM-V criteria for Mild Neurocognitive Disorder (American Psychiatric Association, 2013) were largely derived from these (Stokin, Krell-Roesch, Petersen & Geda, 2015). Greater likelihood that MCI is due to AD arises with exclusion of other causes, evidence of longitudinal decline, and, if relevant, history consistent with AD genetic factors. MCI is primarily a clinical judgement, and no specific guidance is provided regarding test selection, cut-off, or consistency of impairment. This imprecision is not so problematic in clinical settings, but does impact MCI research – creating difficulties aggregating data from different groups, and requiring care in generalising research findings.

The third set of criteria created by NIA-AA working groups were for the asymptomatic, preclinical stage of AD (Sperling et al., 2011). Since their publication, there has been an explosion in research on preclinical AD, resulting in a new NIA-AA updated research framework (Jack et al., 2018). These new guidelines, designed for research and not clinical practice at this stage, define and stage across the entire AD spectrum, treating AD as a continuum, rather than three separate stages. AD is defined by the underlying pathophysiological processes (identified by biomarkers or post-mortem examination) alone, i.e. the clinical consequences of AD are not required for diagnosis, which is a similar premise to the current International Working Group (IWG) criteria (Dubois et al., 2014, 2016). Three categories of biomarkers: Aβ, tau (relating to neurofibrillary tangles), and neurodegeneration, are used to determine a biomarker profile or category. A separate process is used to stage the severity of cognitive symptoms. Within the AD continuum, numeric clinical staging is used, encompassing categories very similar to past classifications. Stage 1 indicates no cognitive impairment, Stage 2 is transitional cognitive decline, Stage 3 reflects MCI, and Stages 4–6 represent mild, moderate, and severe dementia respectively (Jack et al., 2018).

Stage 2 recognises a transitional period for individuals with preclinical AD, between being completely cognitively normal, and meeting MCI criteria. During this period, individuals experience decline from their previous level of cognitive function, but continue performing within normative range on neuropsychological tests. This may be evident through subjective report of cognitive decline (SCD), or subtle evidence of decline on longitudinal testing (although performance is still within normative limits), or both (Jack et al., 2018). Recent evidence suggests that the presence of SCD doubles the risk of developing dementia (Mitchell, Beaumont, Ferguson, Yadegarfar & Stubbs, 2014).

To further consensus in use of the term SCD, a conceptual framework and research criteria were created by an international working-group (Jessen et al., 2014), requiring: (1) self-experienced persistent cognitive decline compared with a previously normal status and unrelated to an acute event, (2) normal demographic-adjusted performance on standardised cognitive tests, (3) exclusion of MCI or dementia, and (4) symptoms cannot be explained by another disorder (including psychiatric, neurological, medical, medication, or substance use). Features established to increase the likelihood that individuals with SCD have underlying AD include subjective memory decline (rather than other cognitive domains), age of onset after 60 and within the last 5 years, concern about the SCD, and self-report of poorer cognition than peers (ibid.).

Neuropathology and biomarkers

The three key biomarkers incorporated within the latest diagnostic criteria (Jack et al., 2018) reflect the key neuropathological features of AD: Aβ, tau, and neurodegeneration. Although AD is a complex disease with many influences, one of the fundamental early changes is a gradual, chronic imbalance in the production and clearance of Aβ, which leads to its accumulation and deposition in the brain (Aβ-plaques), and also triggers other processes that can result in neurodegeneration and dementia (Hardy & Higgins, 1992; Masters & Beyreuther, 2006; Selkoe, 1991, 2000).

Aβ is produced from cleavage of the amyloid-β precursor protein (APP) by the β-site APP cleaving enzyme 1 (BACE1) and γ-secretase enzymes (Hane, Lee & Leonenko, 2017). AD occurs when abnormal cleavage results in a higher than normal ratio of the toxic Aβ_{42} isoform compared to the more abundant Aβ_{40} (ibid.). In healthy people, excess Aβ is cleared from the brain, but in people with AD, Aβ misfolds, aggregates, and becomes neurotoxic, particularly in oligomer (soluble) form (ibid.; Klein, 2006; Masters & Beyreuther, 2006; Selkoe, 2000). Many possible mechanisms for Aβ's neurotoxicity have been identified including inflammation, oxidative stress, disruption of mitochondrial function, changes to the cell membrane, and modification of DNA structure, but the processes between

Aβ accumulation and neurodegeneration are not yet fully elucidated (Hane et al., 2017). Despite cleavage of Aβ throughout the brain, deposition begins in the default mode network as well as the hippocampal formation (Bero et al., 2011), but exactly what or how these regions regulate Aβ cleavage or clearance is undetermined (ibid.; Hane et al., 2017).

Current reliable Aβ biomarkers include low cerebrospinal fluid (CSF) Aβ$_{42}$ and high ligand retention on amyloid positron emission tomography (PET) imaging (Jack et al., 2016, 2018). The advent of amyloid imaging (Klunk et al., 2004) revolutionised AD research, particularly by enabling recognition of the continuum of AD. A number of different Aβ-radiotracers are now in use (Figure 2.2; see also Plate 2 in the colour section), and PET scans using any of these demonstrate a similar typical distribution in people with AD dementia. Increased uptake is observed in the precuneus, posterior cingulate, frontal cortex, and caudate nuclei, followed by lateral temporal and parietal cortex (e.g. Rowe et al., 2007; Villemagne et al., 2017), the same regions where Aβ is typically distributed post-mortem (Braak & Braak, 1997). Moreover, Aβ-imaging with post-mortem studies confirm radiotracer distribution matches histopathology (Clark et al., 2012; Ikonomovic et al., 2008; Seo et al., 2017).

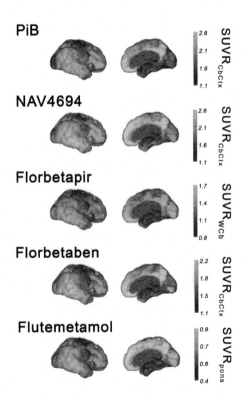

FIGURE 2.2 Surface projection of PET images of patients with Alzheimer's disease obtained with different Aβ imaging radiotracers.

Presently, it is unclear whether the development of neurofibrillary tangles – intraneuronal inclusions composed of hyperphosphorylated tau protein – is a direct consequence of excess Aβ, is independent of Aβ, or whether there are interdependent pathways (Hane et al., 2017; Jack et al., 2016). The presence of both Aβ plaques and neurofibrillary tangles is required for a diagnosis of AD (Jack et al., 2018). Tau alone, however, is implicated in a number of other neurodegenerative diseases (Hane et al., 2017). Tau is a microtubule-associated protein, expressed by the microtubule-associated protein-tau (MAPT), which misfolds in AD and aggregates in paired helical fragments and neurofibrillary tangles (ibid.). Which form of tau is most neurotoxic is currently unclear, with proposed mechanisms of toxicity which include altered microtubule stability and regulation of neuronal activity (ibid.). Neurofibrillary tangles are found throughout the cortex in AD dementia, but initial cortical location is within the transentorhinal region of the medial temporal lobe before encroaching on the entorhinal cortex, hippocampus, and finally the neocortex (Braak, Thal, Ghebremedhin & Del Tredici, 2011). Biomarkers of tau pathology are elevated CSF phosphorylated tau (p-tau) and the recently developed tau PET (Jack et al., 2016, 2018; Villemagne, Fodero-Tavoletti, Masters & Rowe, 2015).

The third type of biomarkers in the new criteria are those of neurodegeneration or neural injury, including elevated CSF total tau (t-tau), [18F]-fluorodeoxyglucose (FDG)-PET hypometabolism, and atrophy on magnetic resonance imaging (MRI; Jack et al., 2016, 2018). FDG-PET in typical AD is characterised by early and most severe hypometabolism in the parieto-temporal regions, posterior cingulate cortex, and medial temporal lobe (Mosconi et al., 2010). Atrophy on MRI appears initially and most severely in the medial temporal lobe (entorhinal cortex and hippocampus; Frisoni, Fox, Jack, Scheltens & Thompson, 2010). Although these biomarkers are recognised to occur later in the pathological process of AD, they are the least specific to AD, occurring in many other conditions (Jack et al., 2016, 2018).

Prevalence and risk factors

Dementia affects almost 50 million people worldwide, with even distribution throughout different regions and countries, and approximately 9.9 million new cases each year (Prince et al., 2015). Our understanding of factors increasing the risk of dementia – both modifiable and non-modifiable – has grown substantially in recent times. Age is the strongest risk factor, and associated with an exponential increase in the incidence of dementia – doubling every 6 years or so from an incidence of 4 per 1000 person-years at age 60 years to 105 per 1000 person-years at 90+ (ibid.). There appears, however, to be an inflection point around age 85, and studies disagree on whether incidence continues to increase but at a lower rate, plateaus, or declines (Robinson, Lee & Hane, 2017).

Family history is the second greatest risk factor, with a first degree relative with dementia conferring 3.5 times the chance of developing AD dementia (van Duijn & Hofman, 1992). Family history risk relates to shared genetic and environmental factors. Regarding genetics, mutations in three different genes have been linked to autosomal dominant AD: APP on chromosome 21 (51 known mutations to date), Presenilin 1 (PSEN1) on chromosome 14, (219 mutations to date), and Presenilin 2 (PSEN2) on chromosome 1 (16 mutations to date; www.molgen. vib-ua.be/ADMutations; Cruts, Theuns & Van Broeckhoven, 2012). All result in an altered rate of APP secretase cleavage, resulting in increased release of the toxic $A\beta_{42}$ peptide (Tanzi & Bertram, 2005). These genes are only related to early-onset (< 65 years) AD dementia, however, and only explain 5–10% of early-onset cases (Cacace, Sleegers & Van Broeckhoven, 2016).

The strongest genetic risk factor for late-onset AD is carriage of the ε4 allele of apolipoprotein E (APOE; Harold et al., 2009; Saunders et al., 1993), which contributes 7% to overall dementia incidence (Livingston et al., 2017). The APOE gene (chromosome 19) has three main polymorphic alleles (ε2, ε3, ε4). ε4 is neither necessary nor sufficient for AD dementia, but the ε4 allele is associated with increased prevalence of AD and lowered onset age, whereas the ε2 allele appears to have a protective effect (Corder et al., 1993). The APOE gene codes for a lipoprotein (APOE) involved in lipid transport. Although the exact mechanisms remain unclear, ε4 increases AD risk through both Aβ-dependent and Aβ-independent pathways, including neuronal cholesterol transport and peripheral cholesterol metabolism (Liu, Kanekiyo, Xu & Bu, 2013).

Technological advances have substantially advanced knowledge regarding genetic factors underlying late-onset AD, particularly genome-wide association studies (GWAS). GWAS have enabled identification of genetic variations and loci enriched in people with AD, finding 30 genes (27 loci) distributed across 14 chromosomes to date, and implicating additional biological pathways in AD pathogenesis including immune system, cholesterol metabolism, and endosomal-vesicle recycling (Nacmias, Bagnoli, Piaceri & Sorbi, 2018; Scheltens et al., 2016). Some of the major genetic risk factors associated with AD include BIN1, PICALM, and TREM2, and the interested reader should refer to Robinson et al. (2017), for a more comprehensive discussion than can be included in this overview chapter. Furthermore, there is growing evidence for epigenetic changes (changes in gene expression that do not alter deoxyribonucleic acid (DNA) sequence, e.g. activating or silencing genes) in AD including changes in micro-RNA, DNA methylation, and histone acetylation (Fenoglio, Scarpini, Serpente & Galimberti, 2018; Robinson et al., 2017).

The final major non-modifiable risk factor is gender, with more women than men afflicted by AD, even when accounting for longevity (Mazure & Swendsen, 2016; Mielke, Vemuri & Rocca, 2014). This factor has not received much research attention to date, but both biological and social impacts may confer greater risk in women (Mielke et al., 2014). Suggested social explanations include the different educational and job opportunities available for women who are now in their seventies and above (ibid.), and leads us to consider modifiable risk factors.

Management of modifiable risk factors may prevent 35% of dementia cases (Livingston et al., 2017). Cardiovascular risk factors, including mid-life hypertension and obesity, and later-life smoking, diabetes, and physical inactivity, account for a number of the modifiable risk factors, whose management reduces dementia risk via decreased risk of vascular lesions, atrophy, and neurodegeneration (Livingston et al., 2017; Norton, Matthews, Barnes, Yaffe & Brayne, 2014). Low educational attainment (no secondary schooling) and mid-life hearing loss are both thought to impact dementia risk through reduction of brain cognitive reserve (Livingston et al., 2017; Valenzuela & Sachdev, 2006). Higher education appears to delay the appearance of cognitive decline (Karr, Graham, Hofer & Muniz-Terrera, 2018). Hearing loss may additionally increase cognitive load on an already vulnerable brain (McCoy et al., 2005), or may lead to social isolation and depression (Gopinath et al., 2009; Huang, Dong, Lu, Yue & Liu, 2010) – which in themselves increase dementia risk. Depression is postulated to increase risk through its impact on stress hormones, neuronal growth factors, and hippocampal volume (Alexopoulos, 2003). Other factors mooted to increase risk for dementia, but for which the evidence is less clear, include anxiety (Gulpers et al., 2016), traumatic brain injuries (Mendez, 2017; Perry et al., 2016), sleep disorders (Ju, Lucey & Holtzman, 2014; Spira, Chen-Edinboro, Wu & Yaffe, 2014), and environmental risk factors (Killin, Starr, Shiue & Russ, 2016), including dwelling near major roads (Chen et al., 2017).

Like dementia, prevalence of MCI increases with age, being present in 6.7% of 60–64-year-olds, increasing to 25.2% of 80–84-year-olds (Petersen et al., 2018). Lower education level is also associated with a higher prevalence of MCI, but any gender differences are still debated (ibid.). MCI is associated with a cumulative incidence, ~15% of developing dementia within 2 years, approximately triple the risk of developing AD dementia within 2–5 years compared to older adults without MCI (ibid.). Those who do not develop dementia can remain stable or revert to normal cognition; however, even those who revert to normal are at increased risk of eventually developing dementia, compared to people never diagnosed with MCI (Lopez et al., 2012; Roberts et al., 2014). Factors influencing the rate of progression to dementia include setting (memory clinic has greater rate of progression than epidemiological studies; Petersen et al., 2009) and type of MCI (amnestic MCI has a greater rate of conversion than nonamnestic MCI; Busse, Hensel, Gühne, Angermeyer & Riedel-Heller, 2006; Yaffe, Petersen, Lindquist, Kramer & Miller, 2006). Predictors of conversion from MCI to AD include the degree of memory impairment, presence of APOE ε4 genotype, and positive AD biomarkers (CSF, Aβ imaging, FDG-PET, MRI; Petersen et al., 2009).

To date, there are no epidemiological studies to determine an accurate incidence and prevalence of preclinical AD in the general community, although imaging studies find approximately 30–40% of apparently healthy older adults are Aβ-positive (e.g. Jack et al., 2018; Pike et al., 2011), consistent with autopsy studies (Bennett et al., 2006; Knopman et al., 2003). The prevalence of SCD varies widely, depending on the definition and base population, but impacts at least a third of older adults from the general community (Jonker, Geerlings & Schmand, 2000; Mewton, Sachdev, Anderson, Sunderland & Andrews, 2014), with some studies finding up to 95% report at least one symptom (Slavin et al., 2010).

A number of studies have demonstrated biological changes in SCD consistent with AD, including Aβ-imaging, atrophy, microstructural changes, and functional activation (Chételat et al., 2010; Erk et al., 2011; Jessen et al., 2006; Meiberth et al., 2015; Rodda, Dannhauser, Cutinha, Shergill & Walker, 2009; Ryu et al., 2017). Most compellingly, a meta-analysis found that SCD approximately doubles the chance of developing dementia (Mitchell et al., 2014). Nevertheless, it is unclear which factors impact the progression from SCD to dementia, providing an area of active research.

Clinical vignette

Phyllis (77 years), who had lived on her own for several years, was becoming reluctant to leave her house. Her family started to notice that she was refusing to attend family gatherings and avoiding the company of friends. In conversation with her niece, Phyllis confided that she was worried about being unable to remember the names of members in her water aerobics class and had forgotten where she had parked her car after her last visit to the aquatic centre. She also commented that her hearing was poor, but she was reluctant to talk to her local doctor about her hearing loss, anticipating that she would find the technology of a hearing aid difficult to learn. Phyllis also revealed she was worried about becoming unable to continue to live alone.

With some persuasion from her family, Phyllis agreed to visit her local doctor. He conducted routine blood tests, which all came back normal, and recommended that she should attend a memory clinic where she could be assessed by a specialist health team, including a clinical neuropsychologist. He also referred Phyllis to an audiologist to determine the level of her hearing loss. The audiologist recommended a hearing aid but it was only after a close friend spent several weeks teaching Phyllis, through repeated practice, how she could easily adjust the hearing aid through her mobile phone, that Phyllis found self-confidence to wear the aid and started to enjoy family gatherings again.

The memory clinic team organised for Phyllis to have an MRI scan, which revealed mild bilateral hippocampal atrophy, and patchy white matter ischaemic change. Following an assessment, the neuropsychologist confirmed that Phyllis's memory and learning were impaired and that the profile was consistent with Alzheimer's disease (AD). As Phyllis could still independently manage most of her everyday activities, and her difficulties were confined to memory-related situations, the memory clinic team decided that Phyllis was presenting with the early stages of the disease – mild cognitive impairment (MCI) likely to be due to AD. A feedback session with Phyllis and her family provided psychoeducation about the diagnosis, links to support services, and organisation of a follow-up review to monitor cognitive capacity.

The neuropsychologist recommended that Phyllis join a memory group that was being run through the memory clinic. Within the group program, Phyllis learnt strategies to compensate for her everyday memory difficulties, including how to manage her anxiety in situations that challenged her memory. Of particular importance, Phyllis was taught a simple strategy for remembering names by actively retrieving them over increasing intervals (spaced retrieval). By using this technique with the help of her niece, Phyllis was able to learn the names of most of the regular attendees at her water aerobics class and happily started attending the sessions again. Phyllis's niece also attended the memory group sessions and learnt several practical skills that she could use to help her aunt maintain her independence in her home environment.

Neuropsychology

Neuropsychological assessment includes the history (directly from the patient, an informant whenever possible, and medical file), behavioural presentation, as well as qualitative and quantitative aspects of test performance. In the context of AD, neuropsychological assessment is key in establishing the stage of AD, along with differential diagnosis from other forms of dementia, medical, or psychiatric conditions, to inform diagnosis and management.

AD is characterised by insidious onset and gradual decline, and usually (but not invariably) the most prominent symptom is impaired episodic memory and learning (Bäckman, Jones, Berger, Laukka & Small, 2005; Collie & Maruff, 2000; Twamley, Ropacki & Bondi, 2006). Subtle changes in memory can be evident up to 10 years prior to diagnosis of dementia (Amieva et al., 2005; Karr et al., 2018), and biomarker studies demonstrate worse memory (e.g. Pike et al., 2011, 2007) and greater memory decline in people who have high levels of Aβ (e.g. Villemagne et al., 2011; see Baker et al., 2017; Hedden et al., 2013 for review). Early episodic learning and memory changes are consistent with observed early neuropathology of medial temporal lobe structures responsible for encoding and consolidation of new information (Eichenbaum, Yonelinas & Ranganath, 2007). People with AD dementia have difficulty in acquisition of new information, with flattened learning curves, reduced primacy effect, and fragile encoding and consolidation, evident in difficulty remembering information after a delay (Salmon & Bondi, 2009; Storey, Kinsella & Slavin, 2001). Typically, little benefit is received from recognition cues (Delis et al., 1991; Pike & Savage, 2008), but this is not always the case (Pike, Rowe, Moss & Savage, 2008). Difficulty utilising semantic encoding strategies is reported (Bäckman, 1998; Buschke, Sliwinski, Kuslansky & Lipton, 1997), which is also evident in MCI (Hutchens et al., 2012), and even SCD in some instances (Pike, Zeneli, Ong, Price & Kinsella, 2015), but not others (Pike, Ong, Clare & Kinsella, 2017). A temporal memory gradient is described, with better recall of distant past than recent memories (Müller et al., 2014; Sagar, Cohen, Sullivan, Corkin & Growdon, 1988).

A special type of episodic memory, prospective memory, refers to the ability to remember intentions, or things one wants to do. It is a complex cognitive action, relying on both episodic memory (to recall the task) and executive function (to plan, monitor, and execute at the appropriate time; McDaniel & Einstein, 2011).

Substantial prospective memory impairment is observed for people with AD dementia (van den Berg, Kant & Postma, 2012), and MCI (Delprado, Kinsella, Ong & Pike, 2013; Delprado et al., 2012; for review see Kinsella, Pike, Cavuoto & Lee, 2018). Indeed, prospective memory tasks may be sensitive to the subtle memory changes reported in SCD (Lee, Ong, Pike & Kinsella, 2018), which is an important area for future research, particularly given the association with everyday function (Beaver & Schmitter-Edgecombe, 2017) and independent living (Woods, Weinborn, Velnoweth, Rooney & Bucks, 2012).

There is also evidence for preclinical decline, of small magnitude, in other cognitive domains, including executive function, processing speed, visuospatial ability, and attention (Bäckman et al., 2005; Baker et al., 2017; Hedden et al., 2013; Twamley et al., 2006). These changes reflect neuropathology, even at the MCI stage, spreading beyond the medial temporal lobe (Haroutunian, Hoffman & Beeri, 2009; Libon et al., 2010). There is considerable variation regarding which domain is affected after memory (e.g. Karr et al., 2018), however executive functions and semantic memory are often affected early; followed by difficulty with attention, working memory, and remote memory; visuospatial and perceptual deficits occurring a little later in the disease course; and impairments in praxis and phonological and syntactical aspects of language by the moderate stage of dementia (Hodges, 2006; Salmon & Bondi, 2009; Storey et al., 2001). By the stage of severe dementia, global cognitive impairment is evident.

The course described above illustrates the most common amnestic presentation, but atypical presentations of AD dementia are well recognised. Logopenic primary progressive aphasia presents with initial impairment in word finding, confrontational naming, and sentence and phrase repetition, reflecting reduced phonological working memory (Gorno-Tempini et al., 2011). Phonological speech errors may be present, but semantics and motor speech are spared, and there is no frank agrammatism. Autopsy (ibid.; Grossman, 2010) and biomarker studies (Leyton et al., 2011; Wolk et al., 2012) often demonstrate AD pathology.

Neuropathology in posterior cortical atrophy is similarly often, but not always, underlying AD (Crutch et al., 2017). It presents with initial visual and other posterior cognitive impairments, including visuospatial and visuoperceptual disorders, alexia, and features of Gerstmann's syndrome (acalculia, agraphia, finger agnosia, left/right disorientation) and Balint's syndrome (simultanagnosia, oculomotor apraxia, optic ataxia, environmental agnosia; ibid.). Memory, language, and executive functions are relatively intact early, and neuroimaging demonstrates prominent occipto-parietal or occipto-temporal atrophy, hypometabolism, and hypoperfusion (ibid.).

AD may also present with predominant behavioural features (apathy, loss of empathy, and disinhibition more common than perseveration and hyperorality) and/or difficulties with executive functions – the so-called 'frontal variant of AD', perhaps more aptly named the behavioural/dysexecutive variant (Ossenkoppele et al., 2015). This tends to be early-onset (under 65 years), with a predominantly behavioural or dysexecutive presentation, although first symptoms are usually cognitive (ibid.). In the behavioural variant, memory, executive function, and behaviour are all impaired early, whereas in the dysexecutive variant, only executive function is impaired, with memory and behaviour relatively spared (ibid.).

Neuropsychiatric and behavioural symptoms are common in AD, experienced by up to 90% of patients with AD dementia, including psychosis (delusions, hallucinations, sleep disorder), affective symptoms (depression, anxiety), apathy (apathy, appetite disorder), and hyperactivity (agitation, aggression, wandering; Aalten et al., 2007; Tible, Riese, Savaskan & von Gunten, 2017; van der Linde, Stephan, Savva, Dening & Brayne, 2012). These symptoms are associated with decreased quality of life, more rapid cognitive decline, poorer prognosis, increased functional impairment and caregiver burden, earlier institutionalisation, and increased direct care costs (Tible et al., 2017; van der Linde et al., 2012). Neuropsychiatric symptoms, particularly apathy, depression and anxiety, are also common in people with mild cognitive impairment, and similarly associated with more rapid cognitive decline (Gallagher, Fischer & Iaboni, 2017; Yates, Clare & Woods, 2013). They have also been identified before the onset of cognitive decline, with the presence of apathy and depression predicting the onset of future MCI (Geda et al., 2014; Yates et al., 2013).

This typical cognitive and behavioural course described for AD dementia is used to help differentiate it from other conditions (Salmon & Bondi, 2009; Storey et al., 2001). For example, in addition to the presence of parkinsonism, fluctuating alertness and attention, and visual hallucinations, dementia with Lewy bodies tends to present prominent visuospatial/constructional difficulties, impaired attention and working memory, psychomotor slowing, and less severe impairment on delayed recall tasks than AD (Boeve, 2004; McKeith et al., 2017). Vascular cognitive disorder is associated with cerebrovascular disease, and often gait disturbance, urinary symptoms, and personality or mood changes, with cognitive symptoms predominantly reduced processing speed, working memory, and executive functions (including set-shifting), while memory recall difficulties tend to be due to difficulties with retrieval rather than retention (Sachdev et al., 2014). The behavioural variant of frontotemporal dementia can be differentiated based on the primacy of personality and behavioural changes, and executive dysfunction, but otherwise relatively preserved cognition (Rascovsky et al., 2011). Depression may be indicated by more acute onset, cognitive concerns out of proportion to performance, dysphoric mood and loss of self-esteem, along with a cognitive profile of difficulties with effortful processing, diminished effort, reduced processing speed, attention, and executive functions, and a retrieval memory profile (Bieliauskas & Drag, 2013).

In clinical practice, however, pathology often co-occurs, with Lewy bodies and vascular lesions commonly co-existing with AD (Schneider, Arvanitakis, Bang & Bennett, 2007; White et al., 2002), and varied comorbidities, including depression, that can affect the neuropsychological profile. Hence, neuropsychological assessment is important to identify not only the hallmark features of AD, but also additional causes of cognitive impairment, and factors that may exacerbate poor functioning and could be better managed. Therapeutically, the assessment can provide the patient and family with appropriate psychoeducation about the likely disease course, prognosis, and management.

Treatment and management

Currently, there is no cure for AD. Nevertheless, medications, behavioural strategies, and risk factor reduction can be used to optimally manage disease symptoms and improve quality of life. Although there is overlap, different management options are more or less applicable depending on broad disease stage. Patient-centred approaches are fundamental, considering the most important symptoms to the patient, co-morbid illnesses, current living situation and support network, and situation evolution.

Five medications (3 cholinesterase inhibitors, 1 N-methyl-D-aspartate [NMDA] antagonist, 1 combined cholinesterase inhibitor/NMDA antagonist) are currently approved to improve cognition in AD dementia. The cholinesterase inhibitors are donepezil (Aricept), rivastigmine (Exelon) and galantamine (Reminyl, Razadyne); these prevent acetylcholine breakdown, resulting in more available neurotransmitter. They are not effective for all patients, have a moderate therapeutic effect, slow – rather than reverse – decline, with mostly gastrointestinal adverse effects (nausea, vomiting, diarrhoea; Birks, 2006). Memantine (Namenda, Ebixa) is an NMDA antagonist, blocking pathological activation of NMDA receptors to prevent excitatory effects of excess glutamate implicated in AD (Farlow, 2004). It is used in moderate-severe AD dementia, providing mild improvements in cognition, clinical impression, and daily function, with few side effects (McShane, Areosa Sastre & Minakaran, 2006).

Pharmacological agents may also assist neuropsychiatric symptoms in AD, including antipsychotics (psychosis; agitation), and antidepressants (depression), although careful consideration and monitoring is needed given the potentially serious side effects (Dyer, Harrison, Laver, Whitehead & Crotty, 2018; Livingston et al., 2017). These concerns suggest nonpharmacological interventions should be the first line of intervention (Dyer et al., 2018; Livingston et al., 2017). At diagnosis, psychoeducation for client and family regarding the condition, prognosis, future planning, and access to support services is important. Tailored interventions including education and skills training for caregivers regarding behavioural symptom management, activity planning and environmental modification, and enhanced caregiver support and self-care can improve neuropsychiatric symptoms and caregivers' reactions to the behaviours, with similar effect size to medications, but no adverse effects (Brodaty & Arasaratnam, 2012). Functional analysis, considering a specific behaviour's purpose, antecedents, and consequences, is particularly helpful to develop individualised interventions (Moniz Cook et al., 2012). Modified psychotherapeutic approaches for the patient (therapeutic conversation, counselling, or cognitive behavioural therapy), demonstrate benefit in improving depression and clinician-rated (though not self- or carer-rated) anxiety (Orgeta,

Spector & Orrell, 2011). Finally, given the high number of people with dementia in nursing homes, consideration should be given to environmental design, including unobtrusive safety measures, varied ambience, single rooms, and controlled stimulation levels (Fleming & Purandare, 2010). The ultimate environmental modification is the notion of 'dementia villages', with one implemented at Hogeweyk in the Netherlands, and others planned in Australia, the United Kingdom, and the United States of America.

Nonpharmacological options for improving cognition in AD dementia can be broadly considered in terms of cognitive stimulation, cognitive training, cognitive rehabilitation, and physical activity. Cognitive stimulation therapy, usually involving engagement in group activities with non-specific cognitive stimulation (e.g. reality orientation, reminiscence/music/art/validation therapy), appears effective for people with mild-moderate dementia, and is often implemented in nursing homes (Huntley, Gould, Liu, Smith & Howard, 2015; Woods, Aguirre, Spector & Orrell, 2012). It has a modest effect on cognition and self-reported quality of life, but not activities of daily living (Huntley et al., 2015; Woods, Aguirre, et al., 2012). Strength of the evidence regarding its effectiveness is limited, however, by the lack of active control groups, follow-up studies, and rater blinding (Huntley et al., 2015; Woods, Aguirre, et al., 2012).

Cognitive training involves guided practice on tasks reflecting particular cognitive domains (e.g. memory, attention, processing speed; Bahar-Fuchs, Clare & Woods, 2013; Clare, 2008). In high-quality randomised controlled trials, there appear to be no significant positive effects of cognitive training on global cognition, mood, or activities of daily living for people with dementia (Bahar-Fuchs et al., 2013). A more recent systematic review, however, found 21/31 randomised controlled trials reported a positive cognitive training effect on at least one cognitive outcome – usually global cognition or training-specific tasks (Kallio, Öhman, Kautiainen, Hietanen & Pitkälä, 2017). Positive effects were more likely with more intense training (24+ sessions) and greater frequency (>1 per week), but there was little evidence that the effort expended translated to benefit in everyday function (Kallio et al., 2017).

In contrast, cognitive rehabilitation involves an individualised approach whereby the person with dementia (and potentially their family) works with clinicians to identify and develop strategies for personally relevant goals (Bahar-Fuchs et al., 2013; Clare, 2008). There have only been a few cognitive rehabilitation studies in dementia; however, these demonstrate improved goal performance and satisfaction – for both the person with dementia and their family carers (Clare et al., in press; Clare et al., 2010), and reduced functional decline 2 years later (Amieva et al., 2016). Effective strategies for people with dementia that can be incorporated into cognitive rehabilitation include procedural memory training (Eslinger & Damasio, 1986; Sabe, Jason, Juejati, Leiguarda & Starkstein, 1995), dual cognitive support (support at both encoding and retrieval of information e.g. Bäckman, 1998; Kinsella, Ong, Storey, Wallace & Hester, 2007), and spaced retrieval (Camp, 2001; Clare, Wilson, Carter, Roth & Hodges, 2002; Creighton, van der Ploeg & O'Connor, 2013).

Increased physical activity is also suggested to improve cognition in dementia, but there are few randomised controlled trials, with mixed results. Groot et al. (2016) and Farina, Rusted, and Tabet (2014) reported positive effects, although a Cochrane review (Forbes, Forbes, Blake, Thiessen & Forbes, 2015) failed to support this view, but did find improved activities of daily living. Despite the unclear cognitive benefits of exercise in dementia, it is recommended as it improves cardiovascular and cerebrovascular health, and is tolerated and feasible for people with mild-moderate dementia (Livingston et al., 2017).

Technological advances offer new methods for supporting people with dementia to manage memory problems, minimise safety risks, and improve quality of life, including electronic pill dispenser boxes, electronic diaries, wearable cameras (e.g. Silva, Pinho, Macedo & Moulin, 2017), interactive 'pet' robots (e.g. Moyle et al., 2017), tracking devices, and fall sensors. Although these methods are promising, most existing studies are limited by small samples, unreliable technology, conduct outside the home environment, and outcomes unrelated to everyday function and quality of life (Fleming & Sum, 2014; King & Dwan, 2017; van der Roest, Wenborn, Pastink, Dröes & Orrell, 2017).

Given the substantial pathology and cognitive decline present by the dementia stage of AD, there has been much interest in treatments targeted at the earlier MCI and preclinical stages. Delaying disease onset by 5 years is estimated to produce ~40% reduction in disease frequency (Alzheimer's Association, 2015). Clinical trials of the cholinesterase inhibitors, however, demonstrated insufficient treatment effect in people with MCI (Doody et al., 2009; Feldman et al., 2007; Petersen et al., 2005; Salloway et al., 2004; Winblad et al., 2008), and there are currently no specific cognitive enhancing drugs available for MCI or preclinical AD. There are, however, over 100 agents listed in current clinical trials, consisting of 70% disease modifying therapies, 14% cognitive enhancers, 13% neuropsychiatric treatments, and the remainder undisclosed (Cummings, Lee, Mortsdorf, Ritter & Zhong, 2017; Fillit, Friedman, Hara, Koemeter-Cox & McKeehan, 2017).

With the lack of current pharmacological options in MCI and preclinical AD, the focus is on nonpharmacological options, particularly cognitive training and rehabilitation. Given more intact residual cognitive resources and insight, people with MCI may have greater capacity to benefit from cognitive interventions than people with dementia. Moreover, early intervention provides the family with training in strategies they can adopt or modify over time, should cognition and function deteriorate further. These principles are particularly salient for cognitively intact older adults with preclinical AD or at increased risk of developing AD, such as SCD, and match consumer expectation that disclosure of preclinical AD status would be associated with access to risk reduction strategies and follow-up monitoring and care (Milne et al., 2018; Stites, 2018).

Understandably, therefore, there has been a veritable explosion in cognitive intervention studies for MCI and cognitively intact older adults. Many studies have mixed samples, thus we will discuss the findings together, highlighting any group differences. Indeed, a recent meta-analysis found no difference in the effect size of cognitive interventions between people with MCI and cognitively intact older adults (Mewborn, Lindbergh & Miller, 2017). Despite this, within individual studies, people with MCI do not always demonstrate the same benefit, for example Kinsella et al. (2016) reported smaller gains in strategy knowledge, strategy use, and contentment, and less retention of benefits in MCI at follow-up compared with cognitively intact older adults.

Approaches to cognitive interventions in these groups are highly variable, offering clinicians the opportunity to tailor an intervention to their client's particular needs; however, it also highlights the difficulty in evaluating outcomes across various intervention studies. The evidence to date is mixed regarding the efficacy of cognitive interventions in both MCI and cognitively intact older adults, with benefits generally found but varying in terms of the effect size and measure (Hill et al., 2016; Jean, Bergeron, Thivierge & Simard, 2010; Kelly et al., 2014; Martin, Clare, Altgassen, Cameron & Zehnder, 2011; Reijnders, van Heugten & van Boxtel, 2013). Heterogeneity is evident in methodological quality, outcome measures, intervention and participant characteristics, and presence or type of controls. A recent large meta-analysis suggests small overall effect sizes compared to active control groups, with training in working memory, memory, processing speed, or multimodal producing cognitive test improvement (Mewborn et al., 2017). Shorter sessions (< 0.5 hours), occurring 1–2 times per week, with overall more than 20 sessions, appears most effective for improving cognitive outcomes, with no impact of demographic (age, education) factors (ibid.). Future modifications may include online interventions, which will improve access, but must ensure sufficient clinician input (Lampit, Hallock & Valenzuela, 2014; Pike et al., 2018).

When examining discrete cognitive outcomes, individual training might be more effective, although benefits are still obtained in groups (Mewborn et al., 2017). But a major issue with contemporary studies is focusing on test performance, rather than everyday outcomes, despite participants valuing improved self-efficacy over performance (Barrios et al., 2016). Many group benefits (e.g. normalisation, improved memory contentment, self-efficacy) are not measured by cognitive test performance (Kinsella et al., 2016). Furthermore, for older adults with SCD, expectancy-modification is an important component of cognitive interventions (Metternich, Kosch, Kriston, Härter & Hüll, 2010), which may be most effectively achieved in a group enabling peer-to-peer support in boosting self-efficacy (West, Bagwell & Dark-Freudeman, 2008). A recent meta-analysis specifically examined the everyday impact of cognitive interventions for MCI (Chandler, Parks, Marsiske, Rotblatt & Smith, 2016), finding small, but significant, overall effects for activities of daily living, mood, and metacognitive outcomes, but not for quality of life. Similarly, studies with mixed older adult samples report small to moderate improvements in everyday functioning five (Willis et al., 2006) and ten years (Rebok et al., 2014) post-intervention.

Regarding SCD, using the current definition involving exclusion of objective cognitive impairment, there are few studies examining cognitive interventions.

The studies reported suggest that people with SCD benefit from memory training (Pike et al., 2015); in some cases to the same extent as older adults without SCD (Engvig et al., 2014; Pike et al., 2017).

Almost no studies to date have been designed with sufficient longitudinal follow-up to determine if the intervention prevents future cognitive decline and dementia. One exception is the ACTIVE study, recently reporting that after 10 years, speed of processing training resulted in a 29% reduction in dementia risk compared to an untreated control group (Edwards et al., 2017). Given the substantial impact of modifiable factors on development of dementia (Livingston et al., 2017; Norton et al., 2014), interventions targeting general lifestyle, especially in mid-life, hold great promise. Research suggests exercise improves cognition for older adults with MCI (Fiatarone Singh et al., 2014; Rodakowski, Saghafi, Butters & Skidmore, 2015; Wang et al., 2014) and without cognitive impairment (Colcombe & Kramer, 2003; Etnier, Nowell, Landers & Sibley, 2006; Etnier et al., 1997; Smith et al., 2010; van Uffelen, Paw, Hopman-Rock & van Mechelen, 2008). There is also evidence that diets – such as the Mediterranean diet – that focus on vegetables, legumes, fruits, and wholegrains support cognition (Barnard et al., 2014; Hardman, Kennedy, Macpherson, Scholey & Pipingas, 2016; Valls-Pedret et al., 2015). There are currently a number of large intervention studies combining cognitive interventions with other lifestyle interventions, such as the FINGER (Finnish Geriatric Intervention Study to Prevent Cognitive Impairment and Disability) trial (Ngandu et al., 2015), the MAPT trial (Andrieu et al., 2017), and the preDIVA trial (van Charante et al., 2016). None of these intensive RCTs have had impacts on dementia risk in 2–3 years, although FINGER did find small but significant changes in executive functions and processing speed. Longer follow-up may be necessary.

Concluding remarks

AD and resulting cognitive decline presents one of the largest contemporary health issues and will become even larger in response to ageing populations worldwide. With the development of reliable biomarkers of $A\beta$, tau, and neurodegeneration, the long preclinical stage of AD has been confirmed, and the latest research criteria describe a continuum from preclinical stages without cognitive impairment, transitional cognitive decline (including SCD), mild cognitive impairment, through to dementia. AD dementia typically presents with early prominent memory impairment, which is also evident in the preclinical stages. Even then, though, there are often subtle cognitive changes in additional cognitive domains. Neuropsychiatric changes are also common throughout the continuum, and need addressing in individualised treatment plans. Despite there being no current prevention or cure, cognitive and behavioural changes can be addressed through a variety of treatment and management techniques, which can be individually tailored to optimally manage AD symptoms throughout the continuum. Importantly, increasing public awareness and knowledge regarding modifiable factors that can reduce risk of developing dementia, has potential to significantly reduce the burden of the disease within the community.

Abbreviations

AA	Alzheimer's Association
Aβ	beta-amyloid
AD	Alzheimer's disease
APOE	apolipoprotein E
CSF	cerebrospinal fluid
DNA	deoxyribonucleic acid
FDG	fluorodeoxyglucose
GWAS	genome-wide association studies
IWG	International Working Group
MCI	mild cognitive impairment
MRI	magnetic resonance imaging
NIA	National Institute on Aging
NMDA	N-methyl-D-aspartate
PET	positron emission tomography
SCD	subjective cognitive decline

Further reading

Clare, L. (2008). *Neuropsychological Rehabilitation and People with Dementia*. Hove: Psychology Press.

Jack, C. R., Bennett, D. A., Blennow, K., Carrillo, M. C., Dunn, B., Haeberlein, S. B., . . . Sperling, R. (2018). NIA-AA Research Framework: Toward a biological definition of Alzheimer's disease. *Alzheimer's & Dementia, 14*(4), 535–562. doi:10.1016/j.jalz.2018.02.018

Livingston, G., Sommerlad, A., Orgeta, V., Costafreda, S. G., Huntley, J., Ames, D., . . . Mukadam, N. (2017). Dementia prevention, intervention, and care. *The Lancet, 390*(10113), 2673–2734. doi:10.1016/S0140-6736(17)31363-6

Salmon, D. P. & Bondi, M. W. (2009). Neuropsychological assessment of dementia. *Annual Review of Psychology, 60*, 257–282.

References

Aalten, P., Verhey, F. R., Boziki, M., Bullock, R., Byrne, E. J., Camus, V., . . . Robert, P. H. (2007). Neuropsychiatric syndromes in dementia. Results from the European Alzheimer Disease Consortium: Part I. *Dementia and Geriatric Cognitive Disorders, 24*(6), 457–463. doi:10.1159/000110738

Albert, M. S., DeKosky, S. T., Dickson, D., Dubois, B., Feldman, H. H., Fox, N. C., . . . Phelps, C. H. (2011). The diagnosis of mild cognitive impairment due to Alzheimer's disease: Recommendations from the National Institute on Aging-Alzheimer's Association workgroups on diagnostic guidelines for Alzheimer's disease. *Alzheimer's & Dementia, 7*(3), 270–279. doi:10.1016/j.jalz.2011.03.008

Alexopoulos, G. S. (2003). Vascular disease, depression, and dementia. *Journal of the American Geriatrics Society, 51*(8), 1178–1180. doi:10.1046/j.1532-5415.2003.51373.x

Alzheimer's Association. (2015). *Changing the Trajectory of Alzheimer's Disease: How a Treatment by 2025 Saves Lives and Dollars*. Chicago, IL: Alzheimer's Association. Retrieved from www.alz.org/documents_custom/trajectory.pdf

Alzheimer's Association. (2017). *2017 Alzheimer's Disease Facts and Figures*. Chicago, IL: Alzheimer's Association. Retrieved from www.alz.org/documents_custom/2017-facts-and-figures.pdf

American Psychiatric Association. (2013). *Diagnostic and Statistical Manual of Mental Disorders* (5th ed.). Washington, DC: American Psychiatric Association.

Amieva, H., Jacqmin-Gadda, H., Orgogozo, J.-M., Le Carret, N., Helmer, C., Letenneur, L., . . . Dartigues, J.-F. (2005). The 9 year cognitive decline before dementia of the Alzheimer type: A prospective population-based study. *Brain, 128*(5), 1093–1101. doi:10.1093/brain/awh451

Amieva, H., Robert, P. H., Grandoulier, A.-S., Meillon, C., De Rotrou, J., Andrieu, S., . . . Dartigues, J.-F. (2016). Group and individual cognitive therapies in Alzheimer's disease: The ETNA3 randomized trial. *International Psychogeriatrics, 28*(5), 707–717. doi:10.1017/S1041610215001830

Andrieu, S., Guyonnet, S., Coley, N., Cantet, C., Bonnefoy, M., Bordes, S., . . . Vellas, B. (2017). Effect of long-term omega 3 polyunsaturated fatty acid supplementation with or without multidomain intervention on cognitive function in elderly adults with memory complaints (MAPT): A randomised, placebo-controlled trial. *The Lancet Neurology, 16*(5), 377–389. doi:10.1016/S1474-4422(17)30040-6

Australian Bureau of Statistics. (2016). Causes of death, Australia, 2015. Retrieved from www.abs.gov.au/ausstats/abs@.nsf/mf/3303.0

Australian Institute of Health and Welfare. (2012). Dementia in Australia. Retrieved from www.aihw.gov.au/WorkArea/DownloadAsset.aspx?id=10737422943

Bäckman, L. (1998). The link between knowledge and remembering in Alzheimer's disease. *Scandinavian Journal of Psychology, 39*(3), 131–139. doi:10.1111/1467-9450.393067

Bäckman, L., Jones, S., Berger, A.-K., Laukka, E. J. & Small, B. J. (2005). Cognitive impairment in preclinical Alzheimer's disease: A meta-analysis. *Neuropsychology, 19*(4), 520–531. doi:10.1037/0894-4105.19.4.520

Bahar-Fuchs, A., Clare, L. & Woods, B. (2013). Cognitive training and cognitive rehabilitation for persons with mild to moderate dementia of the Alzheimer's or vascular type: A review. *Alzheimer's Research & Therapy, 5*(4), 35–48. doi:10.1186/alzrt189

Baker, J. E., Lim, Y. Y., Pietrzak, R. H., Hassenstab, J., Snyder, P. J., Masters, C. L. & Maruff, P. (2017). Cognitive impairment and decline in cognitively normal older adults with high amyloid-β: A meta-analysis. *Alzheimer's & Dementia: Diagnosis, Assessment & Disease Monitoring, 6*, 108–121. doi:10.1016/j.dadm.2016.09.002

Barnard, N. D., Bush, A. I., Ceccarelli, A., Cooper, J., de Jager, C. A., Erickson, K. I., . . . Squitti, R. (2014). Dietary and lifestyle guidelines for the prevention of Alzheimer's disease. *Neurobiology of Aging, 35 Suppl 2*, S74–S78. doi:10.1016/j.neurobiolaging.2014.03.033

Barrios, P. G., González, R. P., Hanna, S. M., Lunde, A. M., Fields, J. A., Locke, D. E. & Smith, G. E. (2016). Priority of treatment outcomes for caregivers and patients with mild cognitive impairment: Preliminary analyses. *Neurology and Therapy, 5*(2), 1–10. doi:10.1007/s40120-016-0049-1

Beach, T. G., Monsell, S. E., Phillips, L. E. & Kukull, W. (2012). Accuracy of the clinical diagnosis of Alzheimer disease at National Institute on Aging Alzheimer Disease

Centers, 2005–2010. *Journal of Neuropathology and Experimental Neurology*, *71*(4), 266–273. doi:10.1097/NEN.0b013e31824b211b

Beaver, J. & Schmitter-Edgecombe, M. (2017). Multiple types of memory and everyday functional assessment in older adults. *Archives of Clinical Neuropsychology*, *32*(4), 413–426. doi:10.1093/arclin/acx016

Bennett, D. A., Schneider, J. A., Arvanitakis, Z., Kelly, J. F., Aggarwal, N. T., Shah, R. C. & Wilson, R. S. (2006). Neuropathology of older persons without cognitive impairment from two community-based studies. *Neurology*, *66*(12), 1837–1844. doi: 10.1212/01. wnl.0000219668.47116.e6

Bero, A. W., Yan, P., Roh, J. H., Cirrito, J. R., Stewart, F. R., Raichle, M. E., . . . Holtzman, D. M. (2011). Neuronal activity regulates the regional vulnerability to amyloid-β deposition. *Nature Neuroscience*, *14*(6), 750–756. doi:10.1038/nn.2801

Bieliauskas, L. A. & Drag, L. L. (2013). Differential diagnosis of depression and dementia. In L. D. Ravdin & H. L. Katzen (Eds.), *Handbook on the Neuropsychology of Aging and Dementia* (pp. 257–270). New York: Springer.

Birks, J. S. (2006). Cholinesterase inhibitors for Alzheimer's disease. *Cochrane Database of Systematic Reviews*, Issue 1. Art. No.:CD005593. doi:10.1002/14651858.CD005593

Boeve, B. F. (2004). Dementia with Lewy bodies. *Continuum: Lifelong Learning in Neurology*, *10*(1), 81–112. doi:10.1212/01.CON.0000293548.24436.f7

Braak, H. & Braak, E. (1997). Frequency of stages of Alzheimer-related lesions in different age categories. *Neurobiology of Aging*, *18*(4), 351–357. doi:10.1016/S0197–4580(97)00056-0

Braak, H., Thal, D. R., Ghebremedhin, E. & Del Tredici, K. (2011). Stages of the pathologic process in Alzheimer disease: Age categories from 1 to 100 years. *Journal of Neuropathology & Experimental Neurology*, *70*(11), 960–969. doi:10.1097/NEN.0b013e318232a379

Brodaty, H. & Arasaratnam, C. (2012). Meta-analysis of nonpharmacological interventions for neuropsychiatric symptoms of dementia. *American Journal of Psychiatry*, *169*(9), 946–953. doi: 10.1176/appi.ajp.2012.11101529

Buschke, H., Sliwinski, M. J., Kuslansky, G. & Lipton, R. B. (1997). Diagnosis of early dementia by the double memory test encoding specificity improves diagnostic sensitivity and specificity. *Neurology*, *48*(4), 989–996. doi:10.1212/WNL.48.4.989

Busse, A., Hensel, A., Gühne, U., Angermeyer, M. & Riedel-Heller, S. (2006). Mild cognitive impairment long-term course of four clinical subtypes. *Neurology*, *67*(12), 2176–2185. doi:10.1212/01.wnl.0000249117.23318.e1

Cacace, R., Sleegers, K. & Van Broeckhoven, C. (2016). Molecular genetics of early-onset Alzheimer's disease revisited. *Alzheimer's & Dementia*, *12*(6), 733–748. doi:10.1016/j. jalz.2016.01.012

Camp, C. J. (2001). From efficacy to effectiveness to diffusion: Making the transitions in dementia intervention research. *Neuropsychological Rehabilitation*, *11*(3–4), 495–517. doi:10.1080/09602010042000079

Chandler, M. J., Parks, A. C., Marsiske, M., Rotblatt, L. J. & Smith, G. E. (2016). Everyday impact of cognitive interventions in mild cognitive impairment: A systematic review and meta-analysis. *Neuropsychology Review*, *26*(3), 225–251. doi:10.1007/s11065-016-9330-4

Chen, H., Kwong, J. C., Copes, R., Tu, K., Villeneuve, P. J., van Donkelaar, A., . . . Burnett, R. T. (2017). Living near major roads and the incidence of dementia, Parkinson's disease, and multiple sclerosis: A population-based cohort study. *The Lancet*, *389*(10070), 718–726. doi:10.1016/S0140-6736(16)32399-6

Chételat, G., Villemagne, V. L., Bourgeat, P., Pike, K. E., Jones, G., Ames, D., . . . Rowe, C. C. (2010). Relationship between atrophy and β-amyloid deposition in Alzheimer disease. *Annals of Neurology*, *67*(3), 317–324. doi:10.1002/ana.21955

Clare, L. (2008). *Neuropsychological Rehabilitation and People with Dementia*. Hove, East Sussex: Psychology Press.

Clare, L., Kudlicka, A., Oyebode, J. R., Jones, R. W., Bayer, A., Leroi, I., . . . Woods, R. T. (in press). Goal-oriented cognitive rehabilitation in early-stage Alzheimer's and related dementias: A multi-centre single-blind randomised controlled trial (GREAT). *Health Technology Assessment*.

Clare, L., Linden, D. E. J., Woods, R. T., Whitaker, R., Evans, S. J., Parkinson, C. H., . . . Rugg, M. D. (2010). Goal-oriented cognitive rehabilitation for people with early-stage Alzheimer disease: A single-blind randomized controlled trial of clinical efficacy. *The American Journal of Geriatric Psychiatry*, *18*(10), 928–939. doi:10.1097/JGP.0b013e3181d5792a

Clare, L., Wilson, B. A., Carter, G., Roth, I. & Hodges, J. R. (2002). Relearning face-name associations in early Alzheimer's disease. *Neuropsychology*, *16*(4), 538. doi:10.1037//0894-4105.16.4.538

Clark, C. M., Pontecorvo, M. J., Beach, T. G., Bedell, B. J., Coleman, R. E., Doraiswamy, P. M., . . . Skovronsky, D. M. (2012). Cerebral PET with florbetapir compared with neuropathology at autopsy for detection of neuritic amyloid-β plaques: A prospective cohort study. *The Lancet Neurology*, *11*(8), 669–678. doi:10.1016/S1474-4422(12)70142-4

Colcombe, S. & Kramer, A. F. (2003). Fitness effects on the cognitive function of older adults: A meta-analytic study. *Psychological Science*, *14*(2), 125–130. doi:10.1111/1467-9280.t01-1-01430

Collie, A. & Maruff, P. (2000). The neuropsychology of preclinical Alzheimer's disease and mild cognitive impairment. *Neuroscience & Biobehavioral Reviews*, *24*(3), 365–374. doi:10.1016/S0149-7634(00)00012-9

Corder, E. H., Saunders, A. M., Strittmatter, W. J., Schmechel, D. E., Gaskell, P. C., Small, G., . . . Pericak-Vance, M. A. (1993). Gene dose of apolipoprotein E type 4 allele and the risk of Alzheimer's disease in late onset families. *Science*, *261*(5123), 921–923. doi:10.1126/science.8346443

Creighton, A. S., van der Ploeg, E. S. & O'Connor, D. W. (2013). A literature review of spaced-retrieval interventions: A direct memory intervention for people with dementia. *International Psychogeriatrics*, *25*(11), 1743–1763. doi:10.1017/S1041610213001233

Crutch, S. J., Lehmann, M., Schott, J. M., Rabinovici, G. D., Rossor, M. N. & Fox, N. C. (2012). Posterior cortical atrophy. *The Lancet Neurology*, *11*(2), 170–178. doi:10.1016/S1474-4422(11)70289-7

Crutch, S. J., Schott, J. M., Rabinovici, G. D., Murray, M., Snowden, J. S., van der Flier, W. M., . . . Fox, N. C. (2017). Consensus classification of posterior cortical atrophy. *Alzheimer's & Dementia*, *13*(8), 870–884. doi:10.1016/j.jalz.2017.01.014

Cruts, M., Theuns, J. & Van Broeckhoven, C. (2012). Locus-specific mutation databases for neurodegenerative brain diseases. *Human Mutation*, *33*(9), 1340–1344. doi:10.1002/humu.22117

Cummings, J., Lee, G., Mortsdorf, T., Ritter, A. & Zhong, K. (2017). Alzheimer's disease drug development pipeline: 2017. *Alzheimer's & Dementia: Translational Research & Clinical Interventions*, *3*(3), 367–384. doi:10.1016/j.trci.2017.05.002

Delis, D. C., Massman, P. J., Butters, N., Salmon, D. P., Cermak, L. S. & Kramer, J. H. (1991). Profiles of demented and amnesic patients on the California Verbal Learning Test: Implications for the assessment of memory disorders. *Psychological Assessment: A Journal of Consulting and Clinical Psychology*, *3*(1), 19–26. doi:10.1037/1040-3590.3.1.19

Delprado, J., Kinsella, G., Ong, B. & Pike, K. (2013). Naturalistic measures of prospective memory in amnestic mild cognitive impairment. *Psychology and Aging*, *28*(2), 322–332. doi:10.1037/a0029785

Delprado, J., Kinsella, G., Ong, B., Pike, K., Ames, D., Storey, E., . . . Rand, E. (2012). Clinical measures of prospective memory in amnestic mild cognitive impairment. *Journal of the International Neuropsychological Society*, *18*(02), 295–304. doi:10.1017/S135561771100172X

Doody, R. S., Ferris, S. H., Salloway, S., Sun, Y., Goldman, R., Watkins, W. E., . . . Murthy, A. K. (2009). Donepezil treatment of patients with MCI: A 48-week randomized, placebo-controlled trial. *Neurology*, *72*(18), 1555–1561. doi:10.1212/01.wnl. 0000344650.95823.03

Dubois, B., Feldman, H. H., Jacova, C., Hampel, H., Molinuevo, J. L., Blennow, K., . . . Cummings, J. L. (2014). Advancing research diagnostic criteria for Alzheimer's disease: The IWG-2 criteria. *The Lancet Neurology*, *13*(6), 614–629. doi:10.1016/S1474-4422(14)70090-0

Dubois, B., Hampel, H., Feldman, H. H., Scheltens, P., Aisen, P., Andrieu, S., . . . Jack, C. R. (2016). Preclinical Alzheimer's disease: Definition, natural history, and diagnostic criteria. *Alzheimer's & Dementia*, *12*(3), 292–323. doi:10.1016/j.jalz.2016.02.002

Dyer, S. M., Harrison, S. L., Laver, K., Whitehead, C. & Crotty, M. (2018). An overview of systematic reviews of pharmacological and non-pharmacological interventions for the treatment of behavioral and psychological symptoms of dementia. *International Psychogeriatrics*, *30*(3), 295–309. doi:10.1017/S1041610217002344

Edwards, J. D., Xu, H., Clark, D. O., Guey, L. T., Ross, L. A. & Unverzagt, F. W. (2017). Speed of processing training results in lower risk of dementia. *Alzheimer's & Dementia: Translational Research & Clinical Interventions*, *3*(4), 603–611. doi:10.1016/j. trci.2017.09.002

Eichenbaum, H., Yonelinas, A. P. & Ranganath, C. (2007). The medial temporal lobe and recognition memory. *Annual Review of Neuroscience*, *30*(1), 123–152. doi:10.1146/ annurev.neuro.30.051606.094328

Engvig, A., Fjell, A. M., Westlye, L. T., Skaane, N. V., Dale, A. M., Holland, D., . . . Walhovd, K. B. (2014). Effects of cognitive training on gray matter volumes in memory clinic patients with subjective memory impairment. *Journal of Alzheimer's Disease*, *41*(3), 779–791. doi:10.3233/JAD-131889

Erk, S., Spottke, A., Meisen, A., Wagner, M., Walter, H. & Jessen, F. (2011). Evidence of neuronal compensation during episodic memory in subjective memory impairment. *Archives of General Psychiatry*, *68*(8), 845–852. doi:10.1001/archgenpsychiatry. 2011.80

Eslinger, P. J. & Damasio, A. R. (1986). Preserved motor learning in Alzheimer's disease: Implications for anatomy and behavior. *Journal of Neuroscience*, *6*(10), 3006–3009. doi:10.1523/JNEUROSCI.06-10-03006.1986

Etnier, J. L., Nowell, P. M., Landers, D. M. & Sibley, B. A. (2006). A meta-regression to examine the relationship between aerobic fitness and cognitive performance. *Brain Research Reviews*, *52*(1), 119–130. doi:10.1016/j.brainresrev.2006.01.002

Etnier, J. L., Salazar, W., Landers, D. M., Petruzzello, S. J., Han, M. & Nowell, P. (1997). The influence of physical fitness and exercise upon cognitive functioning: A meta-analysis. *Journal of Sport and Exercise Psychology*, *19*(3), 249–277. doi:10.1123/jsep.19.3.249

Farina, N., Rusted, J. & Tabet, N. (2014). The effect of exercise interventions on cognitive outcome in Alzheimer's disease: A systematic review. *International Psychogeriatrics*, *26*(1), 9–18. doi:10.1017/S1041610213001385

Farlow, M. R. (2004). NMDA receptor antagonists: A new therapeutic approach for Alzheimer's disease. *Geriatrics*, *59*(6), 22–27. Retrieved from http://link.galegroup. com.ez.library.latrobe.edu.au/apps/doc/A120045376/EAIM?u=latrobe&sid=EAIM&x id=31c3c867

Feldman, H. H., Ferris, S., Winblad, B., Sfikas, N., Mancione, L., He, Y., . . . Lane, R. (2007). Effect of rivastigmine on delay to diagnosis of Alzheimer's disease from mild cognitive impairment: The InDDEx study. *The Lancet Neurology, 6*(6), 501–512. doi:10.1016/S1474-4422(07)70109-6

Fenoglio, C., Scarpini, E., Serpente, M. & Galimberti, D. (2018). Role of genetics and epigenetics in the pathogenesis of alzheimer's disease and frontotemporal dementia. *Journal of Alzheimer's Disease, 62*(3), 913–932. doi:10.3233/JAD-170702

Fiatarone Singh, M. A., Gates, N., Saigal, N., Wilson, G. C., Meiklejohn, J., Brodaty, H., . . . Valenzuela, M. (2014). The Study of Mental and Resistance Training (SMART) study – resistance training and/or cognitive training in mild cognitive impairment: A randomized, double-blind, double-sham controlled trial. *Journal of the American Medical Directors Association, 15*(12), 873–880. doi:10.1016/j.jamda.2014.09.010

Fillit, H., Friedman, L., Hara, Y., Koemeter-Cox, A. & McKeehan, N. (2017). *Closing in on a Cure: 2017 Alzheimer's Clinical Trials Report.* New York: Alzheimer's Drug Discovery Foundation. Retrieved from www.alzdiscovery.org/assets/content/static/ADDF-2017-Alzheimers-Clinical-Trials-Report.pdf

Fleming, R. & Purandare, N. (2010). Long-term care for people with dementia: Environmental design guidelines. *International Psychogeriatrics, 22*(7), 1084–1096. doi:10.1017/S1041610210000438

Fleming, R. & Sum, S. (2014). Empirical studies on the effectiveness of assistive technology in the care of people with dementia: A systematic review. *Journal of Assistive Technologies, 8*(1), 14–34. doi:10.1108/JAT-09-2012-0021

Forbes, D., Forbes, S. C., Blake, C. M., Thiessen, E. J. & Forbes, S. (2015). Exercise programs for people with dementia. *Cochrane Database of Systematic Reviews, 4,* article CD006489. doi:10.1002/14651858.CD006489.pub4

Frisoni, G. B., Fox, N. C., Jack, C. R., Scheltens, P. & Thompson, P. M. (2010). The clinical use of structural MRI in Alzheimer disease. *Nature Reviews Neurology, 6*(2), 67–77. doi:10.1038/nrneurol.2009.215

Gallagher, D., Fischer, C. E. & Iaboni, A. (2017). Neuropsychiatric symptoms in mild cognitive impairment: An update on prevalence, mechanisms, and clinical significance. *The Canadian Journal of Psychiatry, 62*(3), 161–169. doi:10.1177/0706743716648296

Geda, Y. E., Roberts, R. O., Mielke, M. M., Knopman, D. S., Christianson, T. J., Pankratz, V. S., . . . Rocca, W. A. (2014). Baseline neuropsychiatric symptoms and the risk of incident mild cognitive impairment: A population-based study. *American Journal of Psychiatry, 171*(5), 572–581. doi:10.1176/appi.ajp.2014.13060821

Gopinath, B., Wang, J. J., Schneider, J., Burlutsky, G., Snowdon, J., McMahon, C. M., . . . Mitchell, P. (2009). Depressive symptoms in older adults with hearing impairments: The Blue Mountains Study. *Journal of the American Geriatrics Society, 57*(7), 1306–1308. doi: 10.1111/j.1532-5415.2009.02317.x

Gorno-Tempini, M. L., Hillis, A. E., Weintraub, S., Kertesz, A., Mendez, M., Cappa, S. F., . . . Grossman, M. (2011). Classification of primary progressive aphasia and its variants. *Neurology, 76*(11), 1006–1014. doi:10.1212/WNL.0b013e31821103e6

Groot, C., Hooghiemstra, A. M., Raijmakers, P. G. H. M., van Berckel, B. N. M., Scheltens, P., Scherder, E. J. A., . . . Ossenkoppele, R. (2016). The effect of physical activity on cognitive function in patients with dementia: A meta-analysis of randomized control trials. *Ageing Research Reviews, 25,* 13–23. doi:10.1016/j.arr.2015.11.005

Grossman, M. (2010). Primary progressive aphasia: Clinicopathological correlations. *Nature Reviews Neurology, 6*(2), 88–97. doi:10.1038/nrneurol.2009.216

Gulpers, B., Ramakers, I., Hamel, R., Köhler, S., Voshaar, R. O. & Verhey, F. (2016). Anxiety as a predictor for cognitive decline and dementia: A systematic review and meta-analysis. *The American Journal of Geriatric Psychiatry, 24*(10), 823–842. doi:10.1016/j. jagp.2016.05.015

Hane, F. T., Lee, B. Y. & Leonenko, Z. (2017). Recent progress in Alzheimer's disease research, Part 1: Pathology. *Journal of Alzheimer's Disease, 57*(1), 1–28. doi:10.3233/ JAD-160882

Hardman, R. J., Kennedy, G., Macpherson, H., Scholey, A. B. & Pipingas, A. (2016). Adherence to a Mediterranean-style diet and effects on cognition in adults: A qualitative evaluation and systematic review of longitudinal and prospective trials. *Frontiers in Nutrition, 3*, 22–34. doi:10.3389/fnut.2016.00022

Hardy, J. A. & Higgins, G. A. (1992). Alzheimer's disease: The amyloid cascade hypothesis. *Science, 256*(5054), 184–185. Retrieved from http://ez.library.latrobe.edu.au/login?url= https://search-proquest-com.ez.library.latrobe.edu.au/docview/213544666?accoun tid=12001

Harold, D., Abraham, R., Hollingworth, P., Sims, R., Gerrish, A., Hamshere, M. L., . . . Williams, J. (2009). Genome-wide association study identifies variants at CLU and PICALM associated with Alzheimer's disease. *Nature Genetics, 41*(10), 1088–1093. doi:10.1038/ng.440

Haroutunian, V., Hoffman, L. B. & Beeri, M. S. (2009). Is there a neuropathology difference between mild cognitive impairment and dementia? *Dialogues in Clinical Neuroscience, 11*(2), 171–179. Retrieved from www.ncbi.nlm.nih.gov/pmc/articles/ mid/NIHMS267057/

Hedden, T., Oh, H., Younger, A. P. & Patel, T. A. (2013). Meta-analysis of amyloid-cognition relations in cognitively normal older adults. *Neurology, 80*(14), 1341–1348. doi:10.1212/WNL.0b013e31828ab35d

Hill, N. T. M., Mowszowski, L., Naismith, S. L., Chadwick, V. L., Valenzuela, M. & Lampit, A. (2016). Computerized cognitive training in older adults with mild cognitive impairment or dementia: A systematic review and meta-analysis. *American Journal of Psychiatry, 174*(4), 329–340. doi:10.1176/appi.ajp.2016.16030360

Hodges, J. R. (2006). Alzheimer's centennial legacy: Origins, landmarks and the current status of knowledge concerning cognitive aspects. *Brain, 129*(11), 2811–2822. doi:10.1093/ brain/awl275

Huang, C. Q., Dong, B. R., Lu, Z. C., Yue, J. R. & Liu, Q. X. (2010). Chronic diseases and risk for depression in old age: A meta-analysis of published literature. *Ageing Research Reviews, 9*(2), 131–141. doi:10.1016/j.arr.2009.05.005

Huntley, J. D., Gould, R. L., Liu, K., Smith, M. & Howard, R. J. (2015). Do cognitive interventions improve general cognition in dementia? A meta-analysis and meta-regression. *BMJ Open, 5*(4), 1–12. doi:10.1136/bmjopen-2014-005247

Hutchens, R. L., Kinsella, G. J., Ong, B., Pike, K. E., Parsons, S., Storey, E., . . . Clare, L. (2012). Knowledge and use of memory strategies in amnestic mild cognitive impairment. *Psychology and Aging, 27*(3), 768–777. doi:10.1037/a0026256

Ikonomovic, M. D., Klunk, W. E., Abrahamson, E. E., Mathis, C. A., Price, J. C., Tsopelas, N. D., . . . DeKosky, S. T. (2008). Post-mortem correlates of in vivo PiB-PET amyloid imaging in a typical case of Alzheimer's disease. *Brain, 131*(6), 1630–1645. doi:10.1093/brain/awn016

Jack, C. R., Albert, M. S., Knopman, D. S., McKhann, G. M., Sperling, R. A., Carrillo, M. C., . . . Phelps, C. H. (2011). Introduction to the recommendations from the National Institute on Aging-Alzheimer's Association workgroups on diagnostic guidelines for Alzheimer's disease. *Alzheimer's & Dementia, 7*(3), 257–262. doi:10.1016/j.jalz.2011.03.004

Jack, C. R., Bennett, D. A., Blennow, K., Carrillo, M. C., Dunn, B., Haeberlein, S. B., . . . Sperling, R. (2018). NIA-AA Research Framework: Toward a biological definition of Alzheimer's disease. *Alzheimer's & Dementia, 14*(4), 535–562. doi:10.1016/j. jalz.2018.02.018

Jack, C. R., Bennett, D. A., Blennow, K., Carrillo, M. C., Feldman, H. H., Frisoni, G. B., . . . Dubois, B. (2016). A/T/N: An unbiased descriptive classification scheme for Alzheimer disease biomarkers. *Neurology, 87*(5), 539–547. doi:10.1212/WNL.0000000 000002923

Jean, L., Bergeron, M.-È., Thivierge, S. & Simard, M. (2010). Cognitive intervention programs for individuals with mild cognitive impairment: Systematic review of the literature. *The American Journal of Geriatric Psychiatry, 18*(4), 281–296. doi:10.1097/ JGP.0b013e3181c37ce9

Jessen, F., Amariglio, R. E., Van Boxtel, M., Breteler, M., Ceccaldi, M., Chételat, G., . . . Wagner, M. (2014). A conceptual framework for research on subjective cognitive decline in preclinical Alzheimer's disease. *Alzheimer's & Dementia, 10*(6), 844–852. doi:10.1016/j.jalz.2014.01.001

Jessen, F., Feyen, L., Freymann, K., Tepest, R., Maier, W., Heun, R., . . . Scheef, L. (2006). Volume reduction of the entorhinal cortex in subjective memory impairment. *Neurobiology of Aging, 27*(12), 1751–1756. doi:10.1016/j.neurobiolaging.2005. 10.010

Jia, J., Wei, C., Chen, S., Li, F., Tang, Y., Qin, W., . . . Gauthier, S. (2018). The cost of Alzheimer's disease in China and re-estimation of costs worldwide. *Alzheimer's & Dementia, 14*(4), 483–491. doi:10.1016/j.jalz.2017.12.006

Jonker, C., Geerlings, M. I. & Schmand, B. (2000). Are memory complaints predictive for dementia? A review of clinical and population-based studies. *International Journal of Geriatric Psychiatry, 15*(11), 983–991. doi:10.1002/1099-1166(200011)15:11%3C983::AID-GPS 238%3E3.0.CO%3B2–5

Ju, Y.-E. S., Lucey, B. P. & Holtzman, D. M. (2014). Sleep and Alzheimer disease pathology: A bidirectional relationship. *Nature Reviews Neurology, 10*(2), 115–119. doi:10.1038/ nrneurol.2013.269

Kallio, E.-L., Öhman, H., Kautiainen, H., Hietanen, M. & Pitkälä, K. (2017). Cognitive training interventions for patients with Alzheimer's disease: A systematic review. *Journal of Alzheimer's Disease, 56*(4), 1349–1372. doi:10.3233/JAD-160810

Karr, J. E., Graham, R. B., Hofer, S. M. & Muniz-Terrera, G. (2018). When does cognitive decline begin? A systematic review of change point studies on accelerated decline in cognitive and neurological outcomes preceding mild cognitive impairment, dementia, and death. *Psychology and Aging, 33*(2), 195–218. doi:10.1037/pag0000236

Kelly, M. E., Loughrey, D., Lawlor, B. A., Robertson, I. H., Walsh, C. & Brennan, S. (2014). The impact of cognitive training and mental stimulation on cognitive and everyday functioning of healthy older adults: A systematic review and meta-analysis. *Ageing Research Reviews, 15*, 28–43. doi:10.1016/j.arr.2014.02.004

Killin, L. O. J., Starr, J. M., Shiue, I. J. & Russ, T. C. (2016). Environmental risk factors for dementia: A systematic review. *BMC Geriatrics, 16*(1), 175–202. doi:10.1186/s12877- 016-0342-y

King, A. C. & Dwan, C. (2017). Electronic memory aids for people with dementia experiencing prospective memory loss: A review of empirical studies. *Dementia: The International Journal of Social Research and Practice.* doi:10.1177/1471301217735180

Kinsella, G. J., Ames, D., Storey, E., Ong, B., Pike, K. E., Saling, M. M., . . . Rand, E. (2016). Strategies for improving memory: A randomized trial of memory groups for older people, including those with mild cognitive impairment. *Journal of Alzheimer's Disease, 49*(1), 31–43. doi:10.3233/JAD-150378

Kinsella, G. J., Ong, B., Storey, E., Wallace, J. & Hester, R. (2007). Elaborated spaced-retrieval and prospective memory in mild Alzheimer's disease. *Neuropsychological Rehabilitation, 17*(6), 688–706. doi:10.1080/09602010600892824

Kinsella, G. J., Pike, K. E., Cavuoto, M. G. & Lee, S. D. (2018). Mild cognitive impairment and prospective memory: Translating the evidence into neuropsychological practice. *The Clinical Neuropsychologist.* doi: 10.1080/13854046.2018.1468926

Klein, W. L. (2006). Synaptic targeting by Aβ oligomers (ADDLS) as a basis for memory loss in early Alzheimer's disease. *Alzheimer's & Dementia, 2*(1), 43–55. doi:10.1016/j.jalz.2005.11.003

Klunk, W. E., Engler, H., Nordberg, A., Wang, Y., Blomqvist, G., Holt, D. P., . . . Långström, B. (2004). Imaging brain amyloid in Alzheimer's disease with Pittsburgh Compound-B. *Annals of Neurology, 55*(3), 306–319. doi:10.1002/ana.20009

Knopman, D. S., Parisi, J. E., Salviati, A., Floriach-Robert, M., Boeve, B. F., Ivnik, R. J., . . . Petersen, R. C. (2003). Neuropathology of cognitively normal elderly. *Journal of Neuropathology & Experimental Neurology, 62*(11), 1087–1095. doi:10.1093/jnen/62.11.1087

Lampit, A., Hallock, H. & Valenzuela, M. (2014). Computerized cognitive training in cognitively healthy older adults: A systematic review and meta-analysis of effect modifiers. *PLoS Medicine, 11*(11), e1001756. doi:10.1371/journal.pmed.1001756

Lee, S. D., Ong, B., Pike, K. E. & Kinsella, G. J. (2018). Prospective memory and subjective memory decline: A neuropsychological indicator of memory difficulties in community-dwelling older people. *Journal of Clinical and Experimental Neuropsychology, 40*(2), 183–197. doi:10.1080/13803395.2017.1326465

Leyton, C. E., Villemagne, V. L., Savage, S., Pike, K. E., Ballard, K. J., Piguet, O., . . . Hodges, J. R. (2011). Subtypes of progressive aphasia: Application of the international consensus criteria and validation using β-amyloid imaging. *Brain, 134*(10), 3030–3043. doi:10.1093/brain/awr216

Libon, D. J., Xie, S. X., Eppig, J., Wicas, G., Lamar, M., Lippa, C., . . . Wambach, D. M. (2010). The heterogeneity of mild cognitive impairment: A neuropsychological analysis. *Journal of the International Neuropsychological Society, 16*(1), 84–93. doi:10.1017/S1355617709990993

Liu, C. C., Kanekiyo, T., Xu, H. & Bu, G. (2013). Apolipoprotein E and Alzheimer disease: Risk, mechanisms and therapy. *Nature Reviews Neurology, 9*(2), 106–118. doi:10.1038/nrneurol.2012.263

Livingston, G., Sommerlad, A., Orgeta, V., Costafreda, S. G., Huntley, J., Ames, D., . . . Mukadam, N. (2017). Dementia prevention, intervention, and care. *The Lancet, 390*(10113), 2673–2734. doi:10.1016/S0140-6736(17)31363-6

Lopez, O. L., Becker, J. T., Chang, Y.-F., Sweet, R. A., DeKosky, S. T., Gach, M. H., . . . Kuller, L. H. (2012). Incidence of mild cognitive impairment in the Pittsburgh Cardiovascular Health Study–Cognition Study. *Neurology, 79*(15), 1599–1606. doi:10.1212/WNL.0b013e31826e25f0

Martin, M., Clare, L., Altgassen, A. M., Cameron, M. H. & Zehnder, F. (2011). Cognition-based interventions for healthy older people and people with mild cognitive impairment. *Cochrane Database of Systematic Reviews 2011,* 1, article CD006220. doi:10.1002/14651858.CD006220.pub2

Masters, C. L. & Beyreuther, K. (2006). Alzheimer's centennial legacy: Prospects for rational therapeutic intervention targeting the Aβ amyloid pathway. *Brain, 129*(11), 2823–2839. doi:10.1093/brain/awl251

Maurer, K., Volk, S. & Gerbaldo, H. (1997). Auguste D and Alzheimer's disease. *The Lancet, 349*(9064), 1546–1549. doi:10.1016/S0140-6736(96)10203-8

Mazure, C. M. & Swendsen, J. (2016). Sex differences in Alzheimer's disease and other dementias. *The Lancet Neurology, 15*(5), 451–452. doi:10.1016/S1474-4422(16)00067-3

McCoy, S. L., Tun, P. A., Cox, L. C., Colangelo, M., Stewart, R. A. & Wingfield, A. (2005). Hearing loss and perceptual effort: Downstream effects on older adults' memory for speech. *The Quarterly Journal of Experimental Psychology Section A, 58*(1), 22–33. doi:10.1080/02724980443000151

McDaniel, M. A. & Einstein, G. O. (2011). The neuropsychology of prospective memory in normal aging: A componential approach. *Neuropsychologia, 49*(8), 2147–2155. doi:10.1016/j.neuropsychologia.2010.12.029

McKeith, I. G., Boeve, B. F., Dickson, D. W., Halliday, G., Taylor, J.-P., Weintraub, D., . . . Iranzo, A. (2017). Diagnosis and management of dementia with Lewy bodies: Fourth consensus report of the DLB Consortium. *Neurology, 89*(1), 88–100. doi:10.1212/WNL.0000000000004058

McKhann, G., Drachman, D., Folstein, M., Katzman, R., Price, D. & Stadlan, E. M. (1984). Clinical diagnosis of Alzheimer's disease: Report of the NINCDS-ADRDA Work Group under the auspices of Department of Health and Human Services Task Force on Alzheimer's Disease. *Neurology, 34*(7), 939. doi:10.1212/WNL.34.7.939

McKhann, G., Knopman, D. S., Chertkow, H., Hyman, B. T., Jack, C. R., Kawas, C. H., . . . Phelps, C. H. (2011). The diagnosis of dementia due to Alzheimer's disease: Recommendations from the National Institute on Aging-Alzheimer's Association workgroups on diagnostic guidelines for Alzheimer's disease. *Alzheimer's & Dementia, 7*(3), 263–269. doi:10.1016/j.jalz.2011.03.005

McShane, R., Areosa Sastre, A. & Minakaran, N. (2006). Memantine for dementia. *Cochrane Database of Systematic Reviews, 2*, article CD003154. doi:10.1002/14651858.CD003154.pub5

Meiberth, D., Scheef, L., Wolfsgruber, S., Boecker, H., Block, W., Träber, F., . . . Jessen, F. (2015). Cortical thinning in individuals with subjective memory impairment. *Journal of Alzheimer's Disease, 45*(1), 139–146. doi:10.3233/JAD-142322

Mendez, M. F. (2017). What is the relationship of traumatic brain injury to dementia? *Journal of Alzheimer's Disease, 57*(3), 667–681. doi:10.3233/JAD-161002

Metternich, B., Kosch, D., Kriston, L., Härter, M. & Hüll, M. (2010). The effects of nonpharmacological interventions on subjective memory complaints: A systematic review and meta-analysis. *Psychotherapy and Psychosomatics, 79*(1), 6–19. doi:10.1159/000254901

Mewborn, C. M., Lindbergh, C. A. & Miller, L. S. (2017). Cognitive interventions for cognitively healthy, mildly impaired, and mixed samples of older adults: A systematic review and meta-analysis of randomized-controlled trials. *Neuropsychology Review, 27*(4), 403–439. doi:10.1007/s11065-017-9350-8

Mewton, L., Sachdev, P., Anderson, T., Sunderland, M. & Andrews, G. (2014). Demographic, clinical, and lifestyle correlates of subjective memory complaints in the Australian population. *The American Journal of Geriatric Psychiatry, 22*(11), 1222–1232. doi:10.1016/j.jagp.2013.04.004

Mielke, M. M., Vemuri, P. & Rocca, W. A. (2014). Clinical epidemiology of Alzheimer's disease: Assessing sex and gender differences. *Clinical Epidemiology, 6*, 37–48. doi:10.2147/CLEP.S37929

Milne, R., Bunnik, E., Diaz, A., Richard, E., Badger, S., Gove, D., . . . Brayne, C. (2018). Perspectives on communicating biomarker-based assessments of Alzheimer's disease to cognitively healthy individuals. *Journal of Alzheimer's Disease, 62*(2), 487–498. doi:10.3233/JAD-170813

Mitchell, A., Beaumont, H., Ferguson, D., Yadegarfar, M. & Stubbs, B. (2014). Risk of dementia and mild cognitive impairment in older people with subjective memory complaints: Meta-analysis. *Acta Psychiatrica Scandinavica, 130*(6), 439–451. doi:10.1111/acps.12336

Moniz Cook, E. D., Swift, K., James, I., Malouf, R., De Vugt, M. & Verhey, F. (2012). Functional analysis-based interventions for challenging behaviour in dementia. *Cochrane Database of Systematic Reviews*, 2, article CD006929. doi:10.1002/14651858.CD006929.pub2

Mosconi, L., Berti, V., Glodzik, L., Pupi, A., De Santi, S. & de Leon, M. J. (2010). Pre-clinical detection of Alzheimer's disease using FDG-PET, with or without amyloid imaging. *Journal of Alzheimer's Disease, 20*(3), 843–854. doi:10.3233/JAD-2010-091504

Moyle, W., Jones, C. J., Murfield, J. E., Thalib, L., Beattie, E. R., Shum, D. K., . . . Draper, B. M. (2017). Use of a robotic seal as a therapeutic tool to improve dementia symptoms: A cluster-randomized controlled trial. *Journal of the American Medical Directors Association, 18*(9), 766–773. doi:10.1016/j.jamda.2017.03.018

Müller, S., Mychajliw, C., Hautzinger, M., Fallgatter, A. J., Saur, R. & Leyhe, T. (2014). Memory for past public events depends on retrieval frequency but not memory age in Alzheimer's disease. *Journal of Alzheimer's Disease, 38*(2), 379–390. doi:10.3233/JAD-130923

Nacmias, B., Bagnoli, S., Piaceri, I. & Sorbi, S. (2018). Genetic heterogeneity of Alzheimer's disease: Embracing research partnerships. *Journal of Alzheimer's Disease, 62* (3), 903–911. doi:10.3233/JAD-170570

Ngandu, T., Lehtisalo, J., Solomon, A., Levälahti, E., Ahtiluoto, S., Antikainen, R., . . . Kivipelto, M. (2015). A 2 year multidomain intervention of diet, exercise, cognitive training, and vascular risk monitoring versus control to prevent cognitive decline in at-risk elderly people (FINGER): A randomised controlled trial. *The Lancet, 385*(9984), 2255–2263. doi:10.1016/S0140-6736(15)60461-5

Norton, S., Matthews, F. E., Barnes, D. E., Yaffe, K. & Brayne, C. (2014). Potential for primary prevention of Alzheimer's disease: An analysis of population-based data. *The Lancet Neurology, 13*(8), 788–794. doi:10.1016/S1474-4422(14)70136-X

Orgeta, V., Spector, A. & Orrell, M. (2011). Psychological treatments for depression and anxiety in dementia and mild cognitive impairment. *Cochrane Database of Systematic Reviews*, 1, article CD009125. doi:10.1002/14651858.CD009125.pub2.

Ossenkoppele, R., Pijnenburg, Y. A., Perry, D. C., Cohn-Sheehy, B. I., Scheltens, N. M., Vogel, J. W., . . . Rabinovici, G. D. (2015). The behavioural/dysexecutive variant of Alzheimer's disease: Clinical, neuroimaging and pathological features. *Brain, 138*(9), 2732–2749. doi:10.1093/brain/awv191

Perry, D. C., Sturm, V. E., Peterson, M. J., Pieper, C. F., Bullock, T., Boeve, B. F., . . . Welsh-Bohmer, K. A. (2016). Association of traumatic brain injury with subsequent neurological and psychiatric disease: A meta-analysis. *Journal of Neurosurgery, 124*(2), 511–526. doi:10.3171/2015.2.JNS14503

Petersen, R. C., Lopez, O., Armstrong, M. J., Getchius, T. S., Ganguli, M., Gloss, D., . . . Rae-Grant, A. (2018). Practice guideline update summary: Mild cognitive impairment. Report of the Guideline Development, Dissemination, and Implementation Sub-committee of the American Academy of Neurology. *Neurology, 90*(3), 126–135. doi:10.1212/WNL.0000000000004826

Petersen, R. C., Roberts, R. O., Knopman, D. S., Boeve, B. F., Geda, Y. E., Ivnik, R. J., . . . Jack, C. R. (2009). Mild cognitive impairment: Ten years later. *Archives of Neurology, 66*(12), 1447–1455. doi:10.1001/archneurol.2009.266

Petersen, R. C., Smith, G. E., Waring, S. C., Ivnik, R. J., Tangalos, E. G. & Kokmen, E. (1999). Mild cognitive impairment: Clinical characterization and outcome. *Archives of Neurology, 56*(3), 303–308. doi:10.1001/archneur.56.3.303

Petersen, R. C., Thomas, R. G., Grundman, M., Bennett, D., Doody, R., Ferris, S., . . . Thal, L. J. (2005). Vitamin E and donepezil for the treatment of mild cognitive impairment. *New England Journal of Medicine, 352*(23), 2379–2388. doi:10.1056/NEJMoa050151

Pike, K. E., Chong, M. S., Hume, C. H., Keech, B. J., Konjarski, M., Landoldt, K. A., . . . Kinsella, G. J. (2018). Providing online memory interventions for older adults: A critical review and recommendations for development. *Australian Psychologist.* doi:10.1111/ap.12339

Pike, K. E., Ellis, K. A., Villemagne, V. L., Good, N., Chételat, G., Ames, D., . . . Rowe, C. C. (2011). Cognition and beta-amyloid in preclinical Alzheimer's disease: Data from the AIBL study. *Neuropsychologia, 49*(9), 2384–2390. doi:10.1016/j.neuropsychologia.2011.04.012

Pike, K. E., Ong, B., Clare, L. & Kinsella, G. J. (2017). Face-name memory training in subjective memory decline: How does office-based training translate to everyday situations? *Aging, Neuropsychology, and Cognition.* doi:10.1080/13825585.2017.1366971

Pike, K. E., Rowe, C., Moss, S. & Savage, G. (2008). Memory profiling with paired associate learning in Alzheimer's disease, mild cognitive impairment, and healthy aging. *Neuropsychology, 22*(6), 718–728. doi:10.1037/a0013050

Pike, K. E. & Savage, G. (2008). Memory profiling in mild cognitive impairment: Can we determine risk for Alzheimer's disease? *Journal of Neuropsychology, 2*(2), 361–372. doi:10.1348/174866407X227015

Pike, K. E., Savage, G., Villemagne, V. L., Ng, S., Moss, S. A., Maruff, P., . . . Rowe, C. C. (2007). β-amyloid imaging and memory in non-demented individuals: Evidence for preclinical Alzheimer's disease. *Brain, 130*(11), 2837–2844. doi:10.1093/brain%7E2Fawm238

Pike, K. E., Zeneli, A., Ong, B., Price, S. & Kinsella, G. J. (2015). Reduced benefit of memory elaboration in older adults with subjective memory decline. *Journal of Alzheimer's Disease, 47*(3), 705–713. doi:10.3233/JAD-150062

Prince, M. J., Wimo, A., Guerchet, M., Ali, G.-C., Wu, Y.-T. & Prina, M. (2015). *World Alzheimer Report 2015. The Global Impact of Dementia: An Analysis of Prevalence, Incidence, Cost and Trends.* London: Alzheimer's Disease International. Retrieved from: www.alz.co.uk/research/WorldAlzheimerReport2015.pdf

Rascovsky, K., Hodges, J. R., Knopman, D., Mendez, M. F., Kramer, J. H., Neuhaus, J., . . . Miller, B. L. (2011). Sensitivity of revised diagnostic criteria for the behavioural variant of frontotemporal dementia. *Brain, 134*(9), 2456–2477. doi:10.1093/brain/awr179

Rebok, G. W., Ball, K., Guey, L. T., Jones, R. N., Kim, H. Y., King, J. W., . . . Willis, S. L. (2014). Ten-year effects of the advanced cognitive training for independent and vital elderly cognitive training trial on cognition and everyday functioning in older adults. *Journal of the American Geriatrics Society, 62*(1), 16–24. doi:10.1111/jgs.12607

Reijnders, J., van Heugten, C. & van Boxtel, M. (2013). Cognitive interventions in healthy older adults and people with mild cognitive impairment: A systematic review. *Ageing Research Reviews, 12*(1), 263–275. doi:10.1016/j.arr.2012.07.003

Roberts, R. O., Knopman, D. S., Mielke, M. M., Cha, R. H., Pankratz, V. S., Christianson, T. J. H., . . . Petersen, R. C. (2014). Higher risk of progression to dementia in mild cognitive impairment cases who revert to normal. *Neurology, 82*(4), 317–325. doi:10.1212/WNL.0000000000000055

Robinson, M., Lee, B. Y. & Hane, F. T. (2017). Recent progress in Alzheimer's disease research, Part 2: Genetics and epidemiology. *Journal of Alzheimer's Disease, 57*(2), 317–330. doi:10.3233/JAD-161149

Rodakowski, J., Saghafi, E., Butters, M. A. & Skidmore, E. R. (2015). Non-pharmacological interventions for adults with mild cognitive impairment and early stage dementia: An updated scoping review. *Molecular Aspects of Medicine, 43*, 38–53. doi:10.1016/j.mam.2015.06.003

Rodda, J. E., Dannhauser, T. M., Cutinha, D. J., Shergill, S. S. & Walker, Z. (2009). Subjective cognitive impairment: Increased prefrontal cortex activation compared to controls during an encoding task. *International Journal of Geriatric Psychiatry, 24*(8), 865–874. doi:10.1002/gps.2207

Rowe, C. C., Ng, S., Ackermann, U., Gong, S. J., Pike, K., Savage, G., . . . Villemagne, V. L. (2007). Imaging β-amyloid burden in aging and dementia. *Neurology, 68*(20), 1718–1725. doi:10.1212/01.wnl.0000261919.22630.ea

Ryu, S. Y., Lim, E. Y., Na, S., Shim, Y. S., Cho, J. H., Yoon, B., . . . Yang, D. W. (2017). Hippocampal and entorhinal structures in subjective memory impairment: A combined MRI volumetric and DTI study. *International Psychogeriatrics, 29*(5), 785–792. doi:10.1017/S1041610216002349

Sabe, L., Jason, L., Juejati, M., Leiguarda, R. & Starkstein, S. E. (1995). Dissociation between declarative and procedural learning in dementia and depression. *Journal of Clinical and Experimental Neuropsychology, 17*(6), 841–848. doi:10.1080/01688639508402433

Sachdev, P., Kalaria, R., O'Brien, J., Skoog, I., Alladi, S., Black, S. E., . . . Scheltens, P. (2014). Diagnostic criteria for vascular cognitive disorders: A VASCOG statement. *Alzheimer Disease and Associated Disorders, 28*(3), 206–218. doi:10.1097/WAD.0000 000000000034

Sagar, H. J., Cohen, N. J., Sullivan, E. V., Corkin, S. & Growdon, J. H. (1988). Remote memory function in Alzheimer's disease and Parkinson's disease. *Brain, 111*(1), 185–206. doi: 10.1093/brain/111.1.185

Salloway, S., Ferris, S., Kluger, A., Goldman, R., Griesing, T., Kumar, D. & Richardson, S. (2004). Efficacy of donepezil in mild cognitive impairment: A randomized placebo-controlled trial. *Neurology, 63*(4), 651–657. doi:10.1212/01.WNL.0000134664.80320.92

Salmon, D. P. & Bondi, M. W. (2009). Neuropsychological assessment of dementia. *Annual Review of Psychology, 60*, 257–282. doi:10.1146/annurev.psych.57.102904.190024

Saunders, A. M., Strittmatter, W. J., Schmechel, D., George-Hyslop, P. S., Pericak-Vance, M., Joo, S., . . . Roses, A. D. (1993). Association of apolipoprotein E allele ε4 with late-onset familial and sporadic Alzheimer's disease. *Neurology, 43*(8), 1467–1467. doi:10.1212/WNL.43.8.1467

Scheltens, P., Blennow, K., Breteler, M. M. B., de Strooper, B., Frisoni, G. B., Salloway, S. & Van der Flier, W. M. (2016). Alzheimer's disease. *The Lancet, 388*, 505–517. doi:10.1016/S0140-6736(15)01124-1

Schneider, J. A., Arvanitakis, Z., Bang, W. & Bennett, D. A. (2007). Mixed brain pathologies account for most dementia cases in community-dwelling older persons. *Neurology, 69*(24), 2197–2204. doi:10.1212/01.wnl.0000271090.28148.24

Selkoe, D. J. (1991). The molecular pathology of Alzheimer's disease. *Neuron, 6*(4), 487–498. doi:10.1016/0896-6273(91)90052-2

Selkoe, D. J. (2000). Toward a comprehensive theory for Alzheimer's disease. Hypothesis: Alzheimer's disease is caused by the cerebral accumulation and cytotoxicity of amyloid β-protein. *Annals of the New York Academy of Sciences, 924*(1), 17–25. doi:10.1111/j.1749-6632.2000.tb05554.x

Seo, S. W., Ayakta, N., Grinberg, L. T., Villeneuve, S., Lehmann, M., Reed, B., . . . Rabinovici, G. D. (2017). Regional correlations between [11C] PIB PET and post-mortem burden of amyloid-beta pathology in a diverse neuropathological cohort. *NeuroImage: Clinical, 13*, 130–137. doi:10.1016/j.nicl.2016.11.008

Silva, A. R., Pinho, M. S., Macedo, L. & Moulin, C. J. A. (2017). The cognitive effects of wearable cameras in mild Alzheimer disease: An experimental study. *Current Alzheimer Research, 14*(12), 1270–1282. doi:10.2174/1567205014666170531083015

Slavin, M. J., Brodaty, H., Kochan, N. A., Crawford, J. D., Trollor, J. N., Draper, B. & Sachdev, P. S. (2010). Prevalence and predictors of 'subjective cognitive complaints' in the Sydney Memory and Ageing Study. *The American Journal of Geriatric Psychiatry, 18*(8), 701–710. doi:10.1097/JGP.0b013e3181df49fb

Smith, P. J., Blumenthal, J. A., Hoffman, B. M., Cooper, H., Strauman, T. A., Welsh-Bohmer, K., . . . Sherwood, A. (2010). Aerobic exercise and neurocognitive performance: A meta-analytic review of randomized controlled trials. *Psychosomatic Medicine, 72*(3), 239–252. doi:10.1097/PSY.0b013e3181d14633

Sperling, R. A., Aisen, P. S., Beckett, L. A., Bennett, D. A., Craft, S., Fagan, A. M., . . . Phelps, C.H. (2011). Toward defining the preclinical stages of Alzheimer's disease: Recommendations from the National Institute on Aging-Alzheimer's Association workgroups on diagnostic guidelines for Alzheimer's disease. *Alzheimer's & Dementia, 7*(3), 280–292. doi:10.1016/j.jalz.2011.03.003

Spira, A. P., Chen-Edinboro, L. P., Wu, M. N. & Yaffe, K. (2014). Impact of sleep on the risk of cognitive decline and dementia. *Current Opinion in Psychiatry, 27*(6), 478. doi:10.1097/YCO.0000000000000106.

Stites, S. D. (2018). Cognitively healthy individuals want to know their risk for Alzheimer's disease: What should we do? *Journal of Alzheimer's Disease, 62*(2), 499–502. doi:10.3233/JAD-171089

Stokin, G. B., Krell-Roesch, J., Petersen, R. C. & Geda, Y. E. (2015). Mild neurocognitive disorder: An old wine in a new bottle. *Harvard Review of Psychiatry, 23*(5), 368–376. doi:10.1097/HRP.0000000000000084

Storey, E., Kinsella, G. J. & Slavin, M. J. (2001). The neuropsychological diagnosis of Alzheimer's disease. *Journal of Alzheimer's Disease, 3*(3), 261–285. doi:10.3233/JAD-2001-3302

Tanzi, R. E. & Bertram, L. (2005). Twenty years of the Alzheimer's disease amyloid hypothesis: A genetic perspective. *Cell, 120*(4), 545–555. doi:10.1016/j.cell.2005.02.008

Tible, O. P., Riese, F., Savaskan, E. & von Gunten, A. (2017). Best practice in the management of behavioural and psychological symptoms of dementia. *Therapeutic Advances in Neurological Disorders, 10*(8), 297–309. doi:10.1177/1756285617712979

Twamley, E. W., Ropacki, S. A. L. & Bondi, M. W. (2006). Neuropsychological and neuroimaging changes in preclinical Alzheimer's disease. *Journal of the International Neuropsychological Society, 12*(5), 707–735. doi:10.1017/S1355617706060863

Valenzuela, M. J. & Sachdev, P. (2006). Brain reserve and dementia: A systematic review. *Psychological Medicine, 36*(4), 441–454. doi:10.1017/S0033291705006264

Valls-Pedret, C., Sala-Vila, A., Serra-Mir, M., Corella, D., De la Torre, R., Martínez-González, M. Á., . . . Ros, E. (2015). Mediterranean diet and age-related cognitive decline: A randomized clinical trial. *JAMA Internal Medicine, 175*(7), 1094–1103. doi:10.1001/jamainternmed.2015.1668

Van Charante, E. P. M., Richard, E., Eurelings, L. S., van Dalen, J.-W., Ligthart, S. A., Van Bussel, E. F., . . . van Gool, W. A. (2016). Effectiveness of a 6-year multidomain vascular care intervention to prevent dementia (preDIVA): A cluster-randomised controlled trial. *The Lancet, 388*(10046), 797–805. doi:10.1016/S0140-6736(16)30950-3

Van den Berg, E., Kant, N. & Postma, A. (2012). Remember to buy milk on the way home! A meta-analytic review of prospective memory in mild cognitive impairment and dementia. *Journal of the International Neuropsychological Society, 18*(4), 706–716. doi:10.1017/S1355617712000331

Van der Linde, R. M., Stephan, B. C., Savva, G. M., Dening, T. & Brayne, C. (2012). Systematic reviews on behavioural and psychological symptoms in the older or demented population. *Alzheimer's Research & Therapy, 4*(4), 28. doi:10.1186/alzrt131

Van der Roest, H. G., Wenborn, J., Pastink, C., Dröes, R. M. & Orrell, M. (2017). Assistive technology for memory support in dementia. *Cochrane Database of Systematic Reviews, 6,* article CD009627. doi:10.1002/14651858.CD009627.pub2

Van Duijn, C. M. & Hofman, A. (1992). Risk factors for Alzheimer's disease: The EURODEM collaborative re-analysis of case-control studies. *Neuroepidemiology, 11*(Suppl. 1), 106–113. doi:10.1159/000111000

Van Uffelen, J. G., Paw, M. J. C. A., Hopman-Rock, M. & van Mechelen, W. (2008). The effects of exercise on cognition in older adults with and without cognitive decline: A systematic review. *Clinical Journal of Sport Medicine, 18*(6), 486–500. doi:10.1097/JSM.0b013e3181845f0b

Villemagne, V. L., Doré, V., Bourgeat, P., Burnham, S. C., Laws, S., Salvado, O., . . . Rowe, C. C. (2017). Aβ-amyloid and tau imaging in dementia. *Seminars in Nuclear Medicine, 47*(1), 75–88. doi:10.1053/j.semnuclmed.2016.09.006

Villemagne, V. L., Fodero-Tavoletti, M. T., Masters, C. L. & Rowe, C. C. (2015). Tau imaging: Early progress and future directions. *The Lancet Neurology, 14*(1), 114–124. doi:10.1016/S1474-4422(14)70252-2

Villemagne, V. L., Pike, K. E., Chételat, G., Ellis, K. A., Mulligan, R. S., Bourgeat, P., . . . Rowe, C. C. (2011). Longitudinal assessment of Aβ and cognition in aging and Alzheimer disease. *Annals of Neurology, 69*(1), 181–192. doi:10.1002/ana.22248

Wang, C., Yu, J. T., Wang, H. F., Tan, C. C., Meng, X. F. & Tan, L. (2014). Non-pharmacological interventions for patients with mild cognitive impairment: A meta-analysis of randomized controlled trials of cognition-based and exercise interventions. *Journal of Alzheimer's Disease, 42*(2), 663–678. doi:10.3233/JAD-140660

West, R. L., Bagwell, D. K. & Dark-Freudeman, A. (2008). Self-efficacy and memory aging: The impact of a memory intervention based on self-efficacy. *Aging, Neuropsychology, and Cognition, 15*(3), 302–329. doi:10.1080/13825580701440510

White, L. O. N., Petrovitch, H., Hardman, J., Nelson, J., Davis, D. G., Ross, G. W., . . . Markesbery, W. R. (2002). Cerebrovascular pathology and dementia in autopsied Honolulu-Asia Aging Study participants. *Annals of the New York Academy of Sciences, 977*(1), 9–23. doi:10.1111/j.1749-6632.2002.tb04794.x

Willis, S. L., Tennstedt, S. L., Marsiske, M., Ball, K., Elias, J., Koepke, K. M., . . . Wright, E. (2006). Long-term effects of cognitive training on everyday functional outcomes in older adults. *JAMA, 296*(23), 2805–2814. doi:10.1001/jama.296.23.2805

Winblad, B., Gauthier, S., Scinto, L., Feldman, H., Wilcock, G. K., Truyen, L., . . . Nye, J. S. (2008). Safety and efficacy of galantamine in subjects with mild cognitive impairment. *Neurology, 70*(22), 2024–2035. doi:10.1212/01.wnl.0000303815.69777.26

Winblad, B., Palmer, K., Kivipelto, M., Jelic, V., Fratiglioni, L., Wahlund, L. O., . . . Petersen, R. C. (2004). Mild cognitive impairment – beyond controversies, towards a consensus: Report of the International Working Group on Mild Cognitive Impairment. *Journal of Internal Medicine, 256*(3), 240–246. doi:10.1111/j.1365-2796.2004.01380.x

Wolk, D. A., Price, J. C., Madeira, C., Saxton, J. A., Snitz, B. E., Lopez, O. L., . . . DeKosky, S. T. (2012). Amyloid imaging in dementias with atypical presentation. *Alzheimer's & Dementia, 8*(5), 389–398. doi:10.1016/j.jalz.2011.07.003

Woods, B., Aguirre, E., Spector, A. E. & Orrell, M. (2012). Cognitive stimulation to improve cognitive functioning in people with dementia. *Cochrane Database of Systematic Reviews*, 2, article CD005562. doi:10.1002/14651858.CD005562.pub2.

Woods, S. P., Weinborn, M., Velnoweth, A., Rooney, A. & Bucks, R. S. (2012). Memory for intentions is uniquely associated with instrumental activities of daily living in healthy older adults. *Journal of the International Neuropsychological Society*, *18*(1), 134–138. doi:10.1017/S1355617711001263

Yaffe, K., Petersen, R. C., Lindquist, K., Kramer, J. & Miller, B. (2006). Subtype of mild cognitive impairment and progression to dementia and death. *Dementia and Geriatric Cognitive Disorders*, *22*(4), 312–319. doi:10.1159/000095427

Yates, J. A., Clare, L. & Woods, R. T. (2013). Mild cognitive impairment and mood: A systematic review. *Reviews in Clinical Gerontology*, *23*(4), 317–356. doi:10.1017/S0959259813000129

3

PARKINSON'S DISEASE

Robert Iansek and Mary Danoudis

Introduction

Parkinson's disease (PD) is considered to be a very complex illness, with symptomatology extending beyond the well-known motor disturbances (Chaudhuri, Odin, Antonini & Martinez-Martin, 2011). Furthermore, its pathogenesis is such that it is almost life-long in its presence, making the overall clinical burden increasingly extensive, particularly given the ongoing lack of a known disease modifying agent or process (Salat, Noyce, Schrag & Tolosa, 2016). Symptomatic treatment for motor disturbances has become quite refined but is still basically focused on levodopa (L-Dopa) replacement or L-Dopa substitutes (Williams et al., 2017). Non-motor symptoms represent major management dilemmas. It is generally accepted that multidisciplinary team care is required in one form or another to cope with this complexity and cumulative morbidity, but the exact service delivery model is still to be determined (van der Marck et al., 2013).

A recent review of the definition of PD was in response to a clearer understanding of the pathology of the disorder, the recognition that early non-motor signs do not fit in with accepted diagnostic criteria, the advancement in genetics, the concerted effort to identify bio-markers and the availability of reliably effective therapies (Berg et al., 2014). Bayesian diagnostic approaches have been proposed by the Movement Disorder Society (MDS) to standardise the process of clinically separating PD from Parkinson-related disorders (Postuma et al., 2015). In addition the same approach has been suggested in the pre-diagnostic identification of future PD patients based on prior probabilities of known risk factors (Berg et al., 2015). Such diagnostic approaches have been designed to facilitate future trials of disease modifying agents or processes.

The onset of PD can be years, maybe decades, before the cardinal signs of the disorder manifest. The challenge is to identify early features and factors that can be used to identify those at risk of developing PD in this prediagnostic stage of the disorder. Age of onset seems to be a major risk factor for PD as numerous trials have consistently demonstrated the higher prevalence and incidence rates in the elderly age groups (Collier, Kanaan & Kordower, 2017). How age-related changes are intertwined with the more recently proposed pathogenic mechanisms are yet to be elucidated. Numerous genetic abnormalities, both monogenic forms and genetic risk factors, have been identified as predisposing to PD (Klein & Westenberger, 2012). The identified disturbances in proteins and cellular processes have focused on transmitter packaging, release and reuptake, mitochondrial turnover, control and degradation, cellular mechanisms involved in abnormal protein clearance as well as inflammatory mechanisms. Numerous possible intervention options have been identified from such knowledge, but as yet none have been validated. Overall the possible prion type transmission of an insoluble form of alpha synuclein (ASN) has been generally accepted as the pathological basis of PD but how that concept relates to the demonstrated genetic associated disturbances has not been clarified and the multifactorial options for the transition of normal to abnormal ASN still remain an enigma (Dehay et al., 2015).

An understanding of basal ganglia (BG) function and how malfunction may lead to the vast symptomatology in PD is of paramount importance in regard to management approaches. While unravelling its role has been difficult, this difficulty has stemmed from a number of misconceptions, the major of which is to micro analyse its structure to infer function rather than look at it as a 'black box' and to use clinical observation to infer function of this 'black box'. The use of this latter approach then suggests that the BG have only one function but directed to a variety of domains that include movement, behaviour, cognition and mood (Middleton & Strick, 2000). That function is to enable the performance of tasks in all those domains in an automatic manner that does not require attention resources (Wu, Kansaku & Hallet, 2004). Attention control mechanisms can override or run in parallel to automatic control. Automatic control requires task selection, task maintenance and sequential management of the task (Wu, Chan & Hallet, 2010). To perform these parallel tasks the BG have a large functional reserve, which is available to most brain components, much like the random access memory of a computer.

In PD the ability to automate becomes disrupted due to dopamine loss in the striatum and its associated and progressive denervation changes (Cunnington, Bradshaw & Iansek, 1996). The manifestations of disrupted automation vary according to the domain served by the different anatomically connected components of the striatum (Wu et al., 2010). In addition there occurs a shift to attention control as a compensatory mechanism, however attention can only manage one or two tasks at a time and as a result there is a shrinking of the large functional reserve normally available through the BG, leaving attention control to try and cope with multiple demands (Yogev-Seligmann, Hausdorff & Giladi, 2008). In the motor domain automatic movement plans may not be selected; if selected, they may not be maintained till conclusion; or if maintained, the selected amplitude maybe reduced and the sequential maintenance may degrade (Iansek, Huxham & McGinley, 2006; Morris, Iansek, McGinley, Matyas & Huxham, 2005). This results in akinesia, hypokinesia and the sequence effect. In the non-motor domains, these same changes may lead to disturbance in a variety of instrumental activities of daily living, such as holding a conversation, driving a motor vehicle, shopping, handyman jobs, cooking and medication compliance (Iansek, Danoudis & Bradfield, 2013). In addition, the inability to perform these automatic tasks, when previously they were very easily performed, leads to anxiety, depression, social withdrawal and non-participation in normal domestic, social and community events. This chapter will address these points in more detail to enable the reader to be aware of the current knowledge on all these fronts.

Preliminary considerations

It is now generally accepted that the well-known motor features of PD are a late manifestation of the underlying pathological process. The finding of a monogenetic form of autosomal dominant PD laid the foundation for this understanding (Polymeropoulos et al., 1997). The abnormal protein in this genetic abnormality, ASN, was subsequently found to be a major component of the Lewy body, the pathological hallmark of PD. In the Lewy body, the ASN is composed of filamentous sheets, which are non-degradable by the cell. However, ASN can occur in differing soluble forms, which are necessary for neurotransmitter functions and non-filamentous pathological forms can be found in neurites (Dehay et al., 2015).

Studies by Braak and his colleagues, which utilised antibodies to this form of ASN, found that its initial presence was in the dorsal motor nucleus of the vagus nerve and the olfactory bulb (Braak, Del Tredici et al., 2003). The presence of ASN in neurites was found to ascend the brainstem and it was not till much later that it was present in the mid brain and substantia nigra (SN). It subsequently spread to the diencephalon and cortex. A correlation was found between ASN location and clinical severity of PD (Braak, Rub, Gai & Del Tredici, 2003). The implication that this is an infective type process has subsequently been confirmed in numerous animal studies demonstrating transfer of pathological ASN from one animal to another (Luk et al., 2012) and from human to animal (Recasens & Dehay, 2014) as well as human to human (Kordower & Brundin, 2016). These findings have raised the prospect that ASN in its pathological form behaves in a prion-like manner. The origins of the transformation of ASN to its pathological form are unknown but its presence in enteric gut neurons raise that prospect of its origins, as the gut is innervated by the vagus nerve (Svensson et al., 2015).

The Braak findings also suggest that pre-motor symptoms may exist due to lower brainstem involvement (Braak, Rub et al., 2003). In fact a number of large cohort studies have confirmed the presence of constipation, sleep disorders, cardiac arrhythmias, anosmia and mood disorders in asymptomatic subjects who subsequently develop PD (Morens et al., 1996). The lead time from pre-motor symptoms and motor PD varies from 5 to 15 years. The Braak findings also lay the foundation for the clinical basis of the complexity and cumulative morbidity of PD.

In concert with these concepts of pathogenesis, numerous studies have examined how ASN is regulated in normal cellular processes and how its disturbance may lead to accumulation in the cell and eventually cell death (Uchihara & Giasson, 2016). The protein (Parkin) of another identified monogenic form of PD suggested that degradation of ASN in the proteasome pathway would be impaired, either by the altered structure of ASN in the genetic form, or by transformational change or by lack of a binding protein (Parkin) to enable the entry into the proteasome for digestion (Shimura et al., 2001). The other degradation pathway in the lysosome has also been investigated extensively and abnormal ASN may affect lysosome function. The misfolded ASN can interact with plasma membranes and interfere with basic neuronal processes, such as endothelial reticulum Golgi trafficking, mitochondrial activity and neurotransmission (Volta, Milnerwood & Farrer, 2015).

Clinical vignette

A 52-year-old male was referred to the Kingston Centre Movement Disorders Clinic in 2015. He had Parkinson's disease for 7 years and was diagnosed and managed by an external neurologist. At the time of referral he was in supervised care. He experienced motor fluctuations resulting in severe slow periods ('off' times) where his walking was compromised by festination and motor blocks. The 'off' times were associated with anxiety, pain in the legs and depressed mood. This was in the context of longstanding depression, anxiety and alcoholism, for which he had been under psychiatric care. He had put on a lot of weight due to binge eating.

During his initial assessment he very quickly changed motor states from normal ('on' period) to marked inability to walk, asymmetric tremor, impaired balance and very slow bed mobility ('off' period). He was on a complex regime of medication that consisted of frequent dosing of L-Dopa with a COMT (catecholmethyltransferase) inhibitor, high doses of both a dopamine agonist and an anticholinergic agent. He was also on an atypical antidepressant, agomelatine. Admission to the Kingston Centre Movement Disorder ward was arranged, to (1) reduce dopamine agonists, (2) introduce a major tranquilliser (quetiapine), which has minimal hypokinetic effects, to reduce impulse control disorder (ICD) and (3) re-titrate L-Dopa to minimise 'off' times, and (4) for psychiatry review.

Following adjustments to his PD medications, he was discharged back to his facility with improved behaviour and more consistent mobility. At his follow-up review as an outpatient, the family reported ongoing excessive alcohol intake and binge eating. The tranquilliser was increased and an urgent psychiatry referral again was made, which he failed to attend. Neuropsychological evaluation was performed in 2017 as a prelude to a new psychiatry attendance and this confirmed his pre-existing impulse control disorder (ICD) with prior binge eating and alcohol in late teens and early twenties. Over the previous twelve months the family confirmed cognitive decline in organisation, planning and judgement with behavioural disinhibition including being socially and sexually inappropriate, easily angered and having little insight. The neuropsychological report demonstrated severe executive dysfunction, rigidity of thinking, impulsivity, reduced attention span, slow processing speed and reductions in new learning and memory. He had limited insight into his deficits. Psychiatry review was consistently refused.

In 2018, the residential facility had reached a crisis point due to the escalating behavioural and psychotic disturbance. The subject was given an ultimatum of eviction within a week. Urgent review was sought in the clinic and with a community psychiatrist. To minimise the neuropsychiatric side-effects of his Parkinson's medications, the dopamine agonist and COMT inhibitor were ceased, the anticholinergic agent was weaned and L-Dopa was only administered in the earlier part of the day. Admission to the ward resulted in further increases in tranquilliser medication (quetiapine), additional serotonin reuptake inhibitor was added for depression, as well as clonazepam for rapid eye movement behaviour disturbance (RBD). The diagnosis of PD-related dementia was reconfirmed. A urinary tract infection identified during this in-patient admission, was treated. These collective interventions resulted in the settling of the psychosis and behaviour. Mobility was impaired overnight and early morning, due to the reduction in his PD medications, but generally the subject was able to manage with minor assistance. He was discharged back to another facility with experience in dementia care.

This case report illustrates the interaction between pre-existing personality traits, the complexity of the underlying disease and the impact of the medication, with both positive and negative outcomes. This case presentation also demonstrates some of the typical motor and non-motor symptoms experienced by people with young onset PD. Here we see advancing putamen denervation with severe motor 'off' times, but also caudate involvement with profound executive dysfunction. In contrast there appears to be nucleus accumbens overactivity with ICD-related to the long acting dopamine agonist causing the equivalent of 'behavioural dystonia'. We also have multiple non motor symptoms (pain, anxiety, transient mood changes) and extra basal ganglia involvement manifesting dementia, depression and RBD. Management of such scenarios involves a comprehensive care approach by multidisciplinary teams whose providers have appropriate training, knowledge and experience to optimise function and yet minimise side effects for the patient, the family and the facilities providing care.

Diagnostic considerations

The UK Parkinson's Disease Society Brain Bank Clinical Diagnostic Criteria have been used universally by movement disorders specialists, and in research, in the diagnosis of PD (Hughes, Daniel, Kilford & Lees, 1992). The criteria include the presence of the cardinal motor symptom of rigidity and at least one of the following: bradykinesia, rest tremor and postural instability. No reliable biomarkers have been identified to date that can replace the process of diagnosis using these cardinal clinical criteria.

A task force established by the International Parkinson and Movement Disorder Society recently reviewed these diagnostic criteria, along with several others, and subsequently published revised criteria (Postuma et al., 2015). The revision was in response to advances in the understanding of the pathophysiology of PD and the growing recognition that non-motor symptoms can precede the onset of the typical motor symptoms by years (Berg et al., 2014). The Movement Disorder Society for Parkinson's disease (MDS-PD) criteria are largely intended for use in research, but they are also seen as being clinically useful to assist in the diagnosis of PD and Parkinson-related conditions. The aim of the new criteria is to improve accuracy of diagnosis, in particular among less experienced clinicians, and to increase reliability between testers and centres when conducting research with participants who have PD.

The MDS criteria for diagnosis of PD are based on the presence of cardinal motor symptoms, absolute exclusion criteria (e.g. vertical gaze palsy), 'red flags' (e.g. early bulbar dysfunction) and supportive criteria (e.g. positive motor response to L-Dopa) (Postuma et al., 2015). For the diagnosis of Parkinsonism, bradykinesia must be present, along with either rest tremor or rigidity or both. Once Parkinsonism is diagnosed, then the presence of any absolute exclusion criteria is determined as the diagnosis of PD is excluded if one or more exclusion criteria are found. If no exclusion criteria are found, then red flags are checked. If there are 'red flags', the diagnosis of PD cannot be established. The presence of at least two supportive criteria and no red flags, supports the diagnosis of established PD (90% specificity). Finally, a probable diagnosis of PD can be confirmed if the number of red flags is equal to the number of supportive criteria (80% specificity and sensitivity), as long as the number of red flags does not exceed two.

A similar Bayesian approach was used to predict the likelihood of developing PD based on prior probabilities of published risk factors for PD (Berg et al., 2015). This approach utilises the age adjusted prior probability and then adds likelihood ratios of published information on predictive data to provide a greater than 80% certainty of having prodromal PD. This diagnostic information combines estimates of background risk (from environmental risk factors and genetic findings) and results of diagnostic marker testing. Diagnostic markers had to have prospective evidence documenting ability to predict clinical PD. They include motor and non-motor clinical symptoms, clinical signs, and ancillary diagnostic tests. This predictive model was developed to simplify and standardise future trials of disease modifying agents and processes (Berg et al., 2015).

Subtypes

The variability in the symptoms and progression of this disorder has led investigators to hypothesise that there were distinct subgroups in PD that could help explain this variability (Fereshtehnejad, Zeighami, Dagher & Postuma, 2017; Lewis et al., 2005). Subtyping is seen as having the potential to lead to a better understanding of the underlying causes of this disorder, to predicting prognosis and to facilitating the design of tailored interventions. Subtyping also has important application in clinical trials where is it important to control for variability.

Studies have defined subtypes based on factors such as clinical features, motor severity, motor complications, some non-motor features and demographic characteristics (Erro et al., 2013; van Rooden et al., 2010). A common classification of subtypes has been according to age – old age at onset with associated rapid disease progression and young onset with slow progression (van Rooden et al., 2010). Clinical observations from large cohort studies have resulted in the identification of clusters of clinical features. An example is the early classification model that categorised PD into two motor subtypes: tremor dominant PD and postural instability and gait difficulty (PIGD) (Jankovic et al., 1990). These subtypes were identified from the individual's baseline clinical characteristics. Allocation to either subgroup was dependent on the ratio of the average global tremor score to that of the average PIGD score using the Unified Parkinson's Disease Rating Scale (ibid.). Characteristics such as younger age of onset and better cognition were associated with the tremor subgroup whereas the PIGD subtype was associated with greater bradykinesia and worse mentation (ibid.). Using these subgroups to stratify participants, one of the first large cohort longitudinal studies showed the PIGD group annual rate of decline was higher than that of the tremor-dominant group (Jankovic & Kapadia, 2001). These findings supported the hypothesis that the distinct subtypes have different rates of progression.

Later studies challenged these findings (Vu, Nutt & Holford, 2012). Vu and colleagues investigated the progression of the four key symptoms of PD (tremor, rigidity, bradykinesia and PIGD) prospectively over 8 years using data from the DATATOP cohort (ibid.). Using differing analysis to that used in the earlier analysis of the DATATOP study, the investigators showed that the person's classification as either a tremor dominant or PIGD subtype was not predictive of their rate of deterioration. Another finding was the conversion of many participants from the tremor dominant subgroup to PIGD, but not the other way around, over the period of the trial. It was suggested that these two subtypes reflect the stage of the person's disease rather than being distinct subgroups (ibid.).

Fereshtehnejad and colleagues prospectively followed a large cohort of people with PD and applied cluster analysis based on phenotyping and prospective testing of clinical subtypes (Fereshtehnejad et al., 2015). A broad range of motor function, neuropsychological function, sleep pattern and non-motor features were measured using a range of validated tools. They identified three subgroups with the most prominent baseline features and prognosis being: (1) *mainly motor*, with mild mood disturbance, moderate motor signs and slow progression; (2) *diffuse*, with severe motor symptoms, greater mood changes, orthostatic hypotension, mild cognitive impairment (MCI) and rapid progression; (3) and an intermediate group with orthostatic hypotension but no MCI, severe gait disturbance and high falls rate and moderate progression. Importantly disease duration did not differ between the groups, suggesting the subgroups were not a marker of stage.

It should be noted that there remains no consensus among leading Parkinson's groups on a universally accepted classification of PD subtypes (Postuma et al., 2016). Shortcomings in these past studies mean that their findings cannot be confidently generalised to the whole PD population. Further studies are required that incorporate variables such as biomarkers to advance the certainty in the identification of phenotypes.

Biomarkers

Since Parkinson first described PD in his essay on the 'shaking palsy', the clinical characterisation of PD has progressed but we are still left with the need to identify objective markers. Objective markers are important for the identification of those at risk of developing PD, for accurate diagnosis, for measuring changes over the duration of the disorder and for subtype classification. The development of biomarkers is not without its challenges, such as biomarker measurement reliability, standardisation of protocols, and for understanding the relationship between biomarkers and the pathophysiology of PD.

Biomarkers have been described as consisting of clinical, biochemical, genetic and imaging subgroups (Delenclos, Jones, McLean & Uitti, 2016). Alternatively biomarkers can be categorised as trait (risk of disease), state (diagnosis of disease) or rate markers (progress of disease) (Fox & Growdon, 2004). Potential biomarker sources include biological fluids, peripheral tissues, imaging, genetics and technology based motor testing (Delenclos et al., 2016). The main candidate for body fluid and skin biomarkers has been detection of ASN (Halliday, Del Tredici & Braak, 2006). Attempts at measurement have included CSF, blood, saliva and urine (Malek et al., 2014).

Antibodies to various forms of ASN exist but to date specificity has been low. Alternate candidates have been neurofilament light chain, as it is a marker of neuronal injury, but this also has been found to be nonspecific. Serum uric acid levels have some protective effects in development of PD but its usefulness in isolation is limited. Detection of ASN in skin, salivary glands and gut wall have all been demonstrated in PD as well as in prodromal PD, but issues relating to section staining and counting procedures have had limited usefulness so far (Delenclos et al., 2016).

Advances in genetic processing, analysis and ease of risk factor identification has resulted in a number of possible options which include: a genetic risk score which sums and weighs the risk count of 28 identified loci via the genome wide association studies, analysis of ribonucleic acid (RNA) transcription patterns and expression patterns of micro RNA panels (Nalls et al., 2015). Imaging biomarkers are still in the development phase as most modalities are nonspecific for PD and Parkinson-related conditions (Chahine & Stern, 2017).

Epidemiology

The Bayesian approach followed by the MDS in predicting prodromal PD, utilising the age specific occurrence in its prior probability, focuses the attention of age-related processes in its pathogenesis (Collier et al., 2017). Numerous studies have examined both the prevalence and incidence of PD world-wide and although there are numerous methodological problems with the techniques used in ascertainment, published meta-analyses, which have focused only on the more valid approaches, all confirm this association (Ascherio & Schwarzschild, 2016; Hirsch, Jette, Frolkis, Steeves & Pringsheim, 2016; Pringsheim, Jette, Frolkis & Steeves, 2014). In particular both the prevalence and incidence of PD increase from the age of 50 years to 80+ years from 0.1% to 4.5% (population) and from fewer than 10 to around 700 cases (100,000 person years) respectively. There continues to be variability in prevalence in relation to sex (male > female), to race (white > black) and to region (South America > Europe/North America/Australia > Asia).

The determination of risk factors for PD, as well as protective factors, has been based on longitudinal studies that have followed large cohorts of subjects from 10 to 40 years and have prospectively documented clinical features, anthropological measures, lifestyle, dietary intake as well as a variety of blood sampling. These studies have identified a number of possible risk factors, some of which may be better causally linked than others (Morens et al., 1996; Palacios et al., 2014).

Pesticide exposure has been associated with increased risk, particularly pesticides that impact on mitochondrial function (rotenone & paraquat) (Tanner et al., 2011). High intake of dairy products was associated with a higher risk, more in men than in women; however, the possibility of a pesticide as a contaminant could not be ruled out (Jiang, Ju, Jiang & Zhang, 2014). There appears to be an increased risk of PD in subjects with established melanoma and similarly early subjects with PD, not requiring medication, showed an increased risk of developing melanoma (Olsen, Friis & Frederiksen, 2006). The underlying cause of these associations is uncertain. Less clear associations relate to traumatic head injury, diabetes, lipid disturbances, alcohol, estrogen, vitamin intake or total fat intake (Ascherio & Schwarzschild, 2016).

Protective factors have been well documented and some are used in the development of a predictive score for prodromal PD. The use of tobacco has been repeatedly found to have a protective effect in the development of PD (Chen et al., 2010; Morens et al., 1996). Although the mechanism is unclear there is a suggestion it may relate to the neuroprotective effect of nicotine. Furthermore, studies have documented a change in the male to female ratio of prevalence influenced by changing smoking habits between males and females (Morozova, O'Reilly & Ascherio, 2008). This study found an overall reduction in PD of 74% in smokers. High levels of uric acid (highest quartile of plasma urate) have been shown to have a lower prevalence of PD (Weisskopf, O'Reilly, Chen, Schwarzschild & Ascherio, 2007). Studies have consistently shown that this benefit was not due to other associated lifestyle approaches such as age, smoking, physical activity and alcohol consumption. How high urate levels protect against PD is unclear, with suggestions being that it may have an antioxidant effect. Caffeine intake has been shown to also reduce the risk of PD, more so in males than females (Liu et al., 2012). Caffeine is an adenosine receptor antagonist and its benefit may be related to that effect within the internal striatal circuitry. An association has also been found between frequent moderate or vigorous physical activity with a 34% reduction in PD, particularly when performed at a younger age before the onset of PD (Yang et al., 2015). Possible mechanisms include increased urate and release of neurotrophic factors, and regulation of dopamine turnover. Ibuprofen has been the only non-steroidal anti-inflammatory agent to reduce the risk of PD, suggesting it may have specific neuroprotective properties in its own right (Gao, Chen, Schwarzschild & Ascherio, 2011).

The almost tenfold increase in the prevalence of PD between the 50- and 80-year age groups suggests that ageing and the pathogenesis of PD may share common mechanisms (Ascherio & Schwarzschild, 2016). Typically in PD the loss of substantia nigra (SN) neurons is patchy and located initially in the ventral tier. Prior studies had shown that ageing affected the dorsal tier neurons. These studies examined cell loss with now questionable counting approaches. More sophisticated methods now available have allowed the examination of cellular processes of the SN neurons in greater depth and have demonstrated that in aging primates changes occur in cellular processing known to be present in PD SN neurons and that these changes are specifically present in the ventral tier. These processes involve impaired proteasome and lysosome functions, oxidative and nitrative damage as well as inflammation. These processes were shown to worsen with increasing primate age. These findings suggest that aging creates a vulnerable pre-PD state, which may be destabilised by numerous other factors described previously (Collier et al., 2017).

Genetics

Parkinson's disease is a genetically very heterogeneous condition with approximately 28 different chromosome regions possibly involved in causation (Klein & Westenberger, 2012). To a large degree, this burgeoning of genetic information has occurred in the context of ever increasing sophistication in technical and computerised processing capacity. Current techniques, such as next generation sequencing, can describe the genome of an individual patient and identify known genetic abnormalities to assist in the classification and role of a possible genetic basis of the underlying PD phenotype (ibid.). In addition, the multitude of described genetic disturbances has resulted in a vast research spectrum examining the underlying pathogenic processes integrating with cellular research of protein mis-folding, protein trafficking, protein degradation, mitochondrial trafficking and proteasome/lysosome dysfunction (ibid.).

Six monogenic forms of PD, two dominant and four recessive forms, have been identified (Klein & Westenberger, 2012). In addition there are twelve genetic risk factors for PD. Generally, these account for 30% of familial PD and 3–5% of sporadic PD. In clinical practice identification of a possible genetic basis for PD is difficult because of reduced penetrance of genes (gene phenotype is not always present), variable expressivity of the gene (degree of phenotypic expression varies) and phenocopy phenomenon (phenotypic similarity but different gene or non-genetic basis). The first identified gene to cause autosomal dominant PD involved alteration to the ASN protein, with missense mutations, triplications or duplications of the gene (Polymeropoulos et al., 1997). It presents with a rapidly progressive form of early onset (< 50 years). It is interesting that the missense mutations change the configuration of the ASN to form toxic oligomers, protofibrils and fibrils. These entities are present in the Lewy bodies.

The most commonly encountered genetic autosomal dominant cause of late onset PD is leucine rich repeat kinase 2 (LRRK2) gene. The LRRK2 gene mutation is present in 2–40% of differing populations, being highest in Arab descent (40%) and Ashkanazi Jewish descent (20%) (Lesage et al., 2006). Approximately fifty missense and nonsense mutations have been described, and sixteen are pathogenic. The exact pathogenic mechanisms are unclear.

The first autosomal recessive identified gene was the Parkin gene, described in Japanese families (Klein & Lohmann-Hedrich, 2007). A large number of exon mutations and single nucleotide changes have been described, either deletions or duplications. Parkin gene mutations are the most common cause of juvenile PD (age < 21 years onset) (ibid.). Typically although there is SN nerve cell loss there are few Lewy bodies found at post-mortem. Parkin is an ubiquitin ligase, which binds to other proteins to facilitate entry to the proteasome for digestion and elimination. It has been suggested that normal ASN in this condition is unable to be regulated properly through the proteasome pathway leading to accumulation and subsequent cell death.

The second most common autosomal recessive gene mutation is phosphate induced kinase 1 (Pink1) (Healy et al., 2004). It is also responsible for juvenile onset PD and, like Parkin mutations, appears to interfere with the trafficking of damaged mitochondria for autophagic clearance in the lysosome (Youle & Narendra, 2011).

Ideally genetic testing should be easily available to specialist centres to assist with more accurate diagnosis, education and management. However, currently costs are a major problem and it has been recommended that testing should be considered in juvenile onset PD, early onset PD with atypical features or a positive family history and for late onset PD with a strong family history. Genetic testing should be carried out with counselling support.

Neuropsychology

In order to understand the neuropsychological consequences of PD, it is of first importance to understand BG function and how malfunction occurs in PD. Unfortunately, BG function has been neglected from a research perspective over the last 20 years and any relevant publications are all influenced by the same type of misconceptions that prevailed in earlier years (Crossman & Obeso, 2016; Giordano et al., 2018; Piron et al., 2016; Schechtman, Noblejas, Mizrahi, Dauber & Bergman, 2016). These misconceptions relate to: the micro-analysis of its structure to infer function rather than look at the BG as a 'black box' and to use clinical observations to infer function of this 'black box', the difficulty separating the basic problem from compensatory mechanisms, which occur as a result of the basic problem, and the failure to design paradigms that separate attention control from automatic control. Due to the complex neuronal involvement in PD outside of the BG, there must exist some framework that enables the separation of BG malfunction from malfunction outside the BG. In this account, we will use the 'black box' approach, focusing on the separation of the compensatory components from the actual function and demonstrating the complementary functions of attention and automation in the control of BG tasks (Iansek & Danoudis, 2017; Iansek et al., 2013).

In simple terms, the BG are arranged into two loops; an input loop, the striatum (caudate and putamen) and an output loop, the globus pallidus – subthalamic nucleus (Obeso et al., 2008). The input loop has connections with the motor cortical regions, the cortical association areas, the limbic cortex and the intralaminar nuclei of the thalamus. The output loop feeds back to the same input areas via the ventrolateral thalamic nuclei. Histologically all structures are homogeneous and so should undertake the same processing of information, and by consequence enable their functions to be underpinned by the same mechanisms, irrespective of their connectivity. Automatic motor control is the best understood and this will be used as the template for explaining function.

The BG automates movement (Marsden, 1982) or motor skills, enabling motor performance without the use of attention. To perform this function the BG interrelate with the motor cortical regions; the supplementary motor area (SMA) and the pre-supplementary motor area (PSMA) (Wu et al., 2010; Wu et al., 2004). The PSMA is involved with selection of movement plans and the SMA is involved in the maintenance of the plan and its sequential management. The BG enable these actions by maintaining both the selection and the plan in readiness as well as regulating its sequential management with the SMA in an online process (Wu et al., 2004). At a neuronal level, these functions are best seen in globus pallidus neuronal discharge patterns, which characteristically occur as tonic (sustained) and phasic (burst-like) type activity (Brotchie, Iansek & Horne, 1991). The former pattern is contributing to the maintenance tasks and the latter with the sequential management task. The phasic bursts are generated online as each sub-movement terminates. This burst then terminates the preparatory SMA activity for the next sub-movement, releasing the next movement and initiating the preparation for the next plus one sub-movement, much like a domino effect. This online process uses the end of the *past* sub-movement to trigger the release of the *current* sub-movement and to prepare for the *next* upcoming sub-movement (Brotchie et al., 1991). The preciseness of this interaction enables the speed and precision needed for motor skill performance. A change of intention terminates one plan and initiates another. In reality, multiple plans coexist and are thus automated simultaneously as the BG have a large functional reserve. Intentional control of movement utilises the premotor area, the cingulate gyrus and the cuneate gyrus, regulating movement by sensory feedback, predominantly visual in nature. It may work independently or in parallel to the automatic control and there is a constant transition from one control mechanism to the other depending on the circumstances prevailing at the time of the performance of the task.

In PD, the reduction of striatal dopamine interferes with the output to the motor cortical regions in two ways: disturbed maintenance of the selection and the plan, and disturbance in the sequential management of the plan (Iansek et al., 2006; Morris et al., 2005). The BG are somatotopically organised but the dopamine cell loss is patchy and initially affecting the ventral tier of the SN cell bodies, but eventually extending to other parts of the SN (Collier et al., 2017). Clinically, this results in variable involvement of motor control affecting arm and hand predominantly (compared to leg, foot, or bulbar involvement) and more in the SMA projections than the PSMA. These variations result in differing motor manifestations depending on initial location of SN loss, subsequent SN spread and severity of dopamine losses. The somatotopic areas involved will demonstrate a mismatch between the desired amplitude, or speed, that was required to be maintained and the actual amplitude or speed of the movement. This disparity is directly related to the degree of dopamine loss; the greater the dopamine loss the greater the disparity and the greater the reduction in overall amplitude of the plan. Movements thus become smaller and slower.

Superimposed on this deficit there may be disturbance in the sequential management of the task. Here the phasic bursts (timing cues) become corrupted resulting in a loss of preciseness in the concatenation of one sub-movement to the next (Cunnington et al., 1996). This manifests as an ever reducing amplitude (sequence effect) inevitably resulting in a motor block of the movement (Iansek et al., 2006). The smaller the background amplitude the more likely the sequence effect will dominate the movement (Chee, Murphy, Danoudis, Georgiou-Karistianis & Iansek, 2009). The inability to adequately maintain plan selection can result in failure of plan initiation. This deficit is clinically manifest for some plans and not others. For example, the subject may not be able to perform sit to stand, but may be able to fall forward to the knees and be able to stand from that position; or the subject may be able to initiate a walk backwards but not a walk forwards.

There is also a characteristic inability in PD subjects to appreciate the degree of their motor deficits (Ho, Iansek & Bradshaw, 1999). It is unclear whether this is a normal manifestation of automatic movement control that is only evident in PD subjects because of the motor mismatch, or whether it represents a deficit in the internal referencing of movement. In the latter case the sense of achieved movement must occur at the command level rather than at the executive level. This deficit implies that subjects with PD are unable to improve their motor mismatch voluntarily as they are unaware of the problem and its severity.

It is important to understand how attention control of movement interrelates with the impaired automatic control in PD. It appears that attention control assumes a more important role in PD subjects as a means to compensate for the deficit in automatic control. In this regard, if subjects concentrate on a movement task it can improve in amplitude, but it never normalises (Morris, Iansek, Matyas & Summers, 1994). Attention control appears to have the capacity to augment automatic control by changing the intention and consequently re-planning the task, rather than influencing the task directly. The new programming is still using the BG SMA control mechanisms and as such it results in an inadequate improvement in amplitude. This is readily seen by asking subjects to walk faster, write bigger or speak louder. This is easily done by the subject with improvement in amplitude, but the change never normalises the amplitude (Morris et al., 2005). To some degree most movements that are performed with such concentration are performed in an attentional compensatory manner. However, if attention is withdrawn the amplitude reduces back to the smaller uncompensated level. This change can be quite significant depending on the circumstance. If the person is walking and approaching a doorway or a distracting environment, the resultant decrease in attention may cause a sufficiently reduced step length to enable the sequence effect to manifest resulting in festination, a possible freezing episode and a fall (Iansek & Danoudis, 2017). This concept of compensated attention control in PD is rarely appreciated and typically not controlled in research paradigms.

It is possible to utilise attention control to normalise movement in subjects with PD by providing sensory feedback regarding normal movement amplitude. The most effective sensory feedback is usually visual, but can be priopioceptive or auditory (Morris, Iansek, Matyas & Summers, 1996). This immediate improvement and normalisation of amplitude is easily elicited by demonstrating the correct amplitude and asking subjects to concentrate on performing the movement with that size. Once the correct amplitude is seen, the subject can continue to perform the correct amplitude movement without the visual guide indefinitely as long as the subject is able to concentrate. If attention is diverted then the movement reverts back to the BG size (ibid.). This interaction between attention and automation occurs constantly and generally most subjects perform better, but not normally, when they concentrate.

The function of automating tasks, and its disturbance in PD, is also expected to occur in the non-motor domains. The caudate nucleus have broad connections with the association areas of the cerebral cortex and its role has been extensively reviewed previously (Obeso et al., 2008). Executive dysfunction has been identified as the most prominent cognitive deficit in PD and involves impairment of working memory, sequencing, planning, initiation, impulse inhibition, reasoning and set-shifting (Caccappolo & Marder, 2010).

In order to understand these deficits and to place them into the context of the functions and malfunctions previously described, it is best to examine deficits described by subjects with PD in instrumental activities of daily living. Driving a motor vehicle is a good example. This is an automatic cognitive task performed in addition to multiple automatic motor tasks, all of which are run through the BG SMA interaction (Stolwyk, Charlton, Triggs, Iansek & Bradshaw, 2006). The cognitive set (maintenance) is the destination and the preset of right and left turns to reach the destination is the sequence management component. With attention, subjects are able to manage the task but may possibly be impaired by motor disturbances (Stolwyk, Triggs, Charlton, Iansek & Bradshaw, 2005). If distracted, and attention is lost, then the subject may lose their way, take the wrong turn, or both (Stolwyk, Triggs, et al., 2006).

The ability to hold a conversation is another example. The difficulty in this context is due to the inability to maintain multiple cognitive tasks in readiness, in other words a shrinking of working memory (Baddeley, 1986) or of RAM memory as described above. The main complaints are loss of context, loss of intended reply, loss of previous comments in conversation, and inability to recall the correct word.

Shopping is a third example. This requires the maintenance of sequential cognitive sets, each with its own sequence of events management. In this context one may need to go to the butcher, the baker and the greengrocer, and each destination requires the purchase of a number of articles. If a list is kept of destination and purchases then the task is possible to complete, but this requires attention and visual feedback from the written list as a compensatory mechanism. These examples illustrate that the same functions and malfunctions that are present in the motor domain apply equally to the cognitive domain.

In the behavioural context subjects with PD demonstrate difficulties in self-directed and self-initiated planning of events. Typically if an external source, such as family member or friend, plans an event or events then the person with PD attends, participates and enjoys the encounter. However, if left to themselves, the person with PD is less likely to initiate involvement in these events. There is a general acceptance of the status quo without motivation, enquiry and in some cases the presence of apathy. This behaviour illustrates the paucity of selection and maintenance capacity to enable multiple options to remain in readiness, in an automatic sense to be able to subconsciously choose from options and progress with the chosen option.

In summary, the BG are involved with the automatic control of tasks in multiple domains. The automation involves selection of tasks, maintenance of tasks and the sequential management of each task. PD can result in inability to select some tasks, maintain tasks or sequence each task. The clinical manifestations depend on context and task, but in all situations attention acts in a compensatory mechanism and with appropriate feedback can at times normalise the task, but at a cost to normal flexibility and range of movement, cognition or behaviour.

Neuromodulation

New developments in the behaviour of BG neuroanatomical circuits, as revealed by recordings from target nuclei in deep brain stimulation (DBS) surgery, suggest that symptoms of PD may be underpinned by an altered electrical state and that resetting of this altered electrical state by high frequency stimulation (HFS) may correct electrical behaviour and function (Brown et al., 2001). DBS is now a well-established treatment of advanced PD. It is underpinned by the identification of the target nucleus with MRI stereo-tactic mechanisms and physiological recordings of single cell discharges performed in the awake state (Martinez-Ramirez, Hu, Bona, Okun & Wagle Shukla, 2015). Once identified HFS is applied to the nuclear structure to determine symptomatic improvements in tremor, rigidity and hypokinesia. If the improvement is considered appropriate and a large enough electrical window exists (> 4 milliamps) without side effects, then a quadripolar permanent electrode is positioned in the same area and secured to the skull. A subsequent procedure connects the electrode to the stimulator. The latter can be programmed to maximise benefits and minimise side effects. Quite commonly the electrode is not connected immediately to the stimulator and numerous studies have used the unconnected externalised scalp leads to record neuronal population activity in the nearby regions (field potentials) with the nucleus chosen, both in the 'off' state and when 'on' after medication as well as during actual stimulation of the nucleus at frequencies known to produce clinical benefit.

Electroencephalographic or magnetoencephalographic recordings from the scalp can also be recorded, providing a simultaneous deep nuclear and motor-cortical electrical picture of such clinical states (Oswal et al., 2016). These studies suggest that within the connections between the globus pallidus, sub-thalamic nucleus and the motor-cortical regions, the neuronal discharge tends to synchronise at different frequencies in rhythmic patterns. These synchonised rhythms are simultaneously evident in all three locations. In the 'off' state, the rhythm frequencies are in the low beta (11–14 hertz) and high beta (21–30 hertz) range. This beta range is associated with hypokinesia. With administration with medication, in the form of L-Dopa, the beta frequencies attenuate as hypokinesia and rigidity improve. In the 'on' state the resonant frequency is in the gamma range (70 hertz) (Williams et al., 2002). Stimulation of the STN (130 hertz) also attenuates the low beta frequencies and the reduced power in this frequency range also correlates with the clinical improvement in hypokinesia and rigidity. Furthermore, HFS of the STN results in attenuation of the broad beta band in the mesial cortex over the SMA but not the preSMA (Oswal et al., 2016). It was also possible to suggest that the mesial cortical areas were driving the STN through the direct cortical STN pathway in the hypokinetic state, and that DBS of the STN suppressed this drive. Overall, this novel concept of electrical rhythms subserving normal and symptomatic states and the capacity to reverse abnormal states with electrical stimulation, may provide explanations for some of the other BG conditions at the borderland of neurology and psychiatry.

Treatment

A detailed account of treatment options in PD is beyond the scope of this chapter; however, suffice to say that L-Dopa replacement therapy is still the mainstay of treatment as it is still the most potent dopaminergic agent available, it is cheap, easy to use and produces reliable benefits with dramatic improvements in hypokinesia and rigidity (Olanow, Stern & Sethi, 2009). It has been blamed for the development of motor fluctuations, but in reality these are due to the progressive striatal denervation that takes place over the many years of continual SN nerve cell loss (Schrag & Quinn, 2000). It is a potent drug so it is very effective at signaling the degree of denervation across the timeline of the illness; here it is the messenger of denervation not the cause. The dopaminergic agonist agents have weak dopaminergic effects and as such are incapable of adequately demonstrating the denervation changes as can be readily demonstrated with L-Dopa. Even in advanced PD, where oral L-Dopa effects become unpredictable, infusion of L-Dopa in a gel form into the jejunum (DuoDopa) results in very good motor outcomes with consistency of benefit and minimal dyskinesia (Williams et al., 2017). Such outcomes parallel those of DBS surgery of the STN. The major issues in relation to management relate to the vast variety of non-motor symptoms and the complexity associated with a lifelong illness occurring in an ageing individual. The provision of care has been underpinned by the Parkinson Charter. The Parkinson Charter was declared on 11 April 1997 (European Parkinson's Disease Association, undated). It was developed after a global client survey which revealed great concerns regarding the clinical services provided to people with Parkinson and their families (Findley, 2002). The Charter states that every person with Parkinson has a right to: an accurate diagnosis, access to a specialist in PD, access to allied health services, to continuity of care and to participate in making decisions about their care.

The best way to develop an appropriate service would be to use the charter as the template. In this context, the Comprehensive Parkinson Care program was developed (Morris & Iansek, 1997). It has a holistic approach, dealing with all aspects of the condition, its consequences, ramifications and associated conditions. It uses scientifically proven interventions which include medical, surgical, rehabilitative, educational, supportive and lifelong maintenance. It utilises multidisciplinary teams which consist of all relevant clinicians. The teams can have client contact in the clinic, home, as an inpatient or phone. It provides continuity of care; the client and family being able to access the program over the life of the individual irrespective of the severity of the condition and wherever they may reside. Finally, all team members possess extensive knowledge and experience and only see clients with Parkinson or related conditions. The supportive evidence for such an approach is patchy, as logistically it is difficult to control for the many variables that such a program entails. However, given the complexity of the condition, the cumulative comorbidities, the age-related comorbidities and the Parkinson Charter itself, it should be self-evident that such an approach satisfies the ideal care requirement.

Concluding remarks

The global knowledge of Parkinson's disease has exploded, due to the ever-increasing escalation of research into the many fronts of this condition. This chapter has focused on the more interesting and pertinent areas, and organised the information so that it is readily understood without making the content too complex, but with sufficient material to stimulate further interest in the reader. It is expected that the field will very quickly alter with the burgeoning amount of published information, but the general direction of the covered topics should enable the reader to progress any further interest from the foundations laid in place in this chapter.

Abbreviations

ASN	alpha synuclein
BG	basal ganglia
DBS	deep brain stimulation
HFS	high frequency stimulation
L–Dopa	levodopa
LRRK2	leucine rich repeat kinase 2
MCI	mild cognitive impairment
MDS	Movement Disorder Society
MRI	magnetic resonance imaging
PD	Parkinson's disease
PIGD	postural instability and gait difficulty
PSMA	pre-supplementary motor area
RNA	ribonucleic acid
SMA	supplementary motor area
SN	substantia nigra

Further reading

Domingo, A. & Klein, C. (2018). Genetics of Parkinson disease. *Handbook of Clinical Neurology, Part 1, 147* (3rd series), 211–227.

Maiti, P., Manna, J., & Dunbar, G. L. (2017). Current understanding of the molecular mechanisms in Parkinson's disease: targets for potential treatments. *Translational Neurodegeneration, 6,* 28.

Marsili, L., Rizzo, G. & Colosimo, C. (2018). Diagnostic criteria for Parkinson's disease: from James Parkinson to the concept of prodromal disease. *Frontiers in Neurology, 9,* 156.

Suarez-Cedeno, G., Suescun, J., & Schiess, M. C. (2017). Earlier intervention with deep brain stimulation for Parkinson's disease. *Parkinson's Disease, 2017,* article 9358153.

Titova, N., Padmakumar, C., Lewis, S. J. G., & Chaudhuri, K. R. (2017). Parkinson's: a syndrome rather than a disease? *Journal of Neural Transmission, 124,* 907–914.

Xu, L. & Pu, J. (2016). Alpha-synuclein in Parkinson's disease: from pathogenetic dysfunction to potential clinical application. *Parkinson's Disease, 2016,* article 1720621.

References

Ascherio, A. & Schwarzschild, M. A. (2016). The epidemiology of Parkinson's disease: risk factors and prevention. *Lancet Neurology, 15*(12), 1257–1272. doi:10.1016/S1474-4422(16)30230-7

Baddeley, A. (1986). *Working Memory.* Oxford: Oxford University Press.

Berg, D., Postuma, R. B., Adler, C. H., Bloem, B. R., Chan, P., Dubois, B., . . . Deuschl, G. (2015). MDS research criteria for prodromal Parkinson's disease. *Movement Disorders, 30*(12), 1600–1611. doi:10.1002/mds.26431

Berg, D., Postuma, R. B., Bloem, B., Chan, P., Dubois, B., Gasser, T., . . . Deuschl, G. (2014). Time to redefine PD? Introductory statement of the MDS Task Force on the definition of Parkinson's disease. *Movement Disorders, 29*(4), 454–462. doi:10.1002/mds.25844

Braak, H., Del Tredici, K., Rub, U., de Vos, R. A., Jansen Steur, E. N. & Braak, E. (2003). Staging of brain pathology related to sporadic Parkinson's disease. *Neurobiology of Aging,* *24*(2), 197–211.

Braak, H., Rub, U., Gai, W. P. & Del Tredici, K. (2003). Idiopathic Parkinson's disease: possible routes by which vulnerable neuronal types may be subject to neuroinvasion by an unknown pathogen. *Journal of Neural Transmission, 110*(5), 517–536. doi:10.1007/s00702-002-0808-2

Brotchie, P., Iansek, R. & Horne, M. K. (1991). Motor function of the monkey globus pallidus. 2. Cognitive aspects of movement and phasic neuronal activity. *Brain, 114* (Pt 4), 1685–1702.

Brown, P., Oliviero, A., Mazzone, P., Insola, A., Tonali, P. & Di Lazzaro, V. (2001). Dopamine dependency of oscillations between subthalamic nucleus and pallidum in Parkinson's disease. *Journal of Neuroscience, 21*(3), 1033–1038.

Caccappolo, E. & Marder, K. (2010). Cognitive impairment in non-demented patients with Parkinson's disease. In M. Emre (ed.), *Cognitive Impairment and Dementia in Parkinson's Disease.* (pp. 179–198). Oxford: Oxford University Press.

Chahine, L. M. & Stern, M. B. (2017). Parkinson's disease biomarkers: where are we and where do we go next? *Movement Disorders Clinical Practice, 4*(6), 796–805.

Chaudhuri, K. R., Odin, P., Antonini, A. & Martinez-Martin, P. (2011). Parkinson's disease: the non-motor issues. *Parkinsonism & Related Disorders, 17*(10), 717–723. doi:10.1016/j.parkreldis.2011.02.018

Chee, R., Murphy, A., Danoudis, M., Georgiou-Karistianis, N. & Iansek, R. (2009). Gait freezing in Parkinson's disease and the stride length sequence effect interaction. *Brain, 132*(Pt 8), 2151–2160. doi:10.1093/brain/awp053

Chen, H., Huang, X., Guo, X., Mailman, R. B., Park, Y., Kamel, F., . . . Blair, A. (2010). Smoking duration, intensity, and risk of Parkinson disease. *Neurology, 74*(11), 878–884. doi:10.1212/WNL.0b013e3181d55f38

Collier, T. J., Kanaan, N. M. & Kordower, J. H. (2017). Aging and Parkinson's disease: different sides of the same coin? *Movement Disorders, 32*(7), 983–990. doi:10.1002/mds.27037

Crossman, A. R. & Obeso, J. A. (2016). Functions of the basal ganglia-paradox or no paradox? *Movement Disorders, 31*(8), 1120–1121. doi:10.1002/mds.26745

Cunnington, R., Bradshaw, J. L. & Iansek, R. (1996). The role of the supplementary motor area in the control of voluntary movement. *Human Movement Science, 15,* 627–647.

Dehay, B., Bourdenx, M., Gorry, P., Przedborski, S., Vila, M., Hunot, S., . . . Meissner, W. G. (2015). Targeting alpha-synuclein for treatment of Parkinson's disease: mechanistic and therapeutic considerations. *Lancet Neurology, 14*(8), 855–866. doi:10.1016/S1474-4422(15)00006-X

Delenclos, M., Jones, D. R., McLean, P. J. & Uitti, R. J. (2016). Biomarkers in Parkinson's disease: advances and strategies. *Parkinsonism & Related Disorders, 22 Suppl 1,* S106–110. doi:10.1016/j.parkreldis.2015.09.048

Erro, R., Vitale, C., Amboni, M., Picillo, M., Moccia, M., Longo, K., . . . Barone, P. (2013). The heterogeneity of early Parkinson's disease: a cluster analysis on newly diagnosed untreated patients. *PloS One, 8*(8), e70244. doi:10.1371/journal.pone.0070244

European Parkinson's Disease Association (undated). EPDA Charter. Retrieved from www.epda.eu.com/en/projects/past-projects/charter/

Fereshtehnejad, S. M., Romenets, S. R., Anang, J. B., Latreille, V., Gagnon, J. F. & Postuma, R. B. (2015). New clinical subtypes of Parkinson disease and their longitudinal progression: a prospective cohort comparison with other phenotypes. *Journal of the American Medical Association, Neurology, 72*(8), 863–873. doi:10.1001/jamaneurol.2015.0703

Fereshtehnejad, S. M., Zeighami, Y., Dagher, A. & Postuma, R. B. (2017). Clinical criteria for subtyping Parkinson's disease: biomarkers and longitudinal progression. *Brain*, *140*(7), 1959–1976. doi:10.1093/brain/awx118

Findley, L. J. (2002). Factors impacting on quality of life in Parkinson's disease: results from an international survey. *Movement Disorders*, *17*(1), 60–67. doi:doi:10.1002/mds.10010

Fox, N. & Growdon, J. H. (2004). Biomarkers and surrogates. *NeuroRx*, *1*(2), 181.

Gao, X., Chen, H., Schwarzschild, M. A. & Ascherio, A. (2011). Use of ibuprofen and risk of Parkinson disease. *Neurology*, *76*(10), 863–869. doi:10.1212/WNL.0b013e31820f2d79

Giordano, N., Iemolo, A., Mancini, M., Cacace, F., De Risi, M., Latagliata, E. C., . . . De Leonibus, E. (2018). Motor learning and metaplasticity in striatal neurons: relevance for Parkinson's disease. *Brain*, *141*(2), 505–520. doi:10.1093/brain/awx351

Halliday, G. M., Del Tredici, K. & Braak, H. (2006). Critical appraisal of brain pathology staging related to presymptomatic and symptomatic cases of sporadic Parkinson's disease. *Journal of Neural Transmission, Supplementum* (70), 99–103.

Healy, D. G., Abou-Sleiman, P. M., Gibson, J. M., Ross, O. A., Jain, S., Gandhi, S., . . . Lynch, T. (2004). PINK1 (PARK6) associated Parkinson disease in Ireland. *Neurology*, *63*(8), 1486–1488.

Hirsch, L., Jette, N., Frolkis, A., Steeves, T. & Pringsheim, T. (2016). The incidence of Parkinson's disease: a systematic review and meta-analysis. *Neuroepidemiology*, *46*(4), 292–300. doi:10.1159/000445751

Ho, A. K., Iansek, R. & Bradshaw, J. L. (1999). Regulation of parkinsonian speech volume: the effect of interlocuter distance. *Journal of Neurology, Neurosurgery and Psychiatry*, *67*(2), 199–202.

Hughes, A. J., Daniel, S. E., Kilford, L. & Lees, A. J. (1992). Accuracy of clinical diagnosis of idiopathic Parkinson's disease: a clinico-pathological study of 100 cases. *Journal of Neurology, Neurosurgery and Psychiatry*, *55*(3), 181–184.

Iansek, R. & Danoudis, M. (2017). Freezing of gait in Parkinson's disease: its pathophysiology and pragmatic approaches to management. *Movement Disorders Clinical Practice*, *4*(3), 290–297. doi:10.1002/mdc3.12463

Iansek, R., Danoudis, M. & Bradfield, N. (2013). Gait and cognition in Parkinson's disease: implications for rehabilitation. *Reviews in the Neurosciences*, *24*(3), 293–300. doi:10.1515/revneuro-2013-0006

Iansek, R., Huxham, F. & McGinley, J. (2006). The sequence effect and gait festination in Parkinson disease: contributors to freezing of gait? *Movement Disorders*, *21*(9), 1419–1424. doi:10.1002/mds.20998

Jankovic, J. & Kapadia, A. S. (2001). Functional decline in Parkinson disease. *Archives of Neurology*, *58*(10), 1611–1615.

Jankovic, J., McDermott, M., Carter, J., Gauthier, S., Goetz, C., Golbe, L., . . . Weiner, W. (1990). Variable expression of Parkinson's disease: a base-line analysis of the DATATOP cohort. The Parkinson Study Group. *Neurology*, *40*(10), 1529–1534.

Jiang, W., Ju, C., Jiang, H. & Zhang, D. (2014). Dairy foods intake and risk of Parkinson's disease: a dose-response meta-analysis of prospective cohort studies. *European Journal of Epidemiology*, *29*(9), 613–619. doi:10.1007/s10654-014-9921-4

Klein, C. & Lohmann-Hedrich, K. (2007). Impact of recent genetic findings in Parkinson's disease. *Current Opinion in Neurology*, *20*(4), 453–464. doi:10.1097/WCO.0b013e3281e6692b

Klein, C. & Westenberger, A. (2012). Genetics of Parkinson's disease. *Cold Spring Harbor Perspectives in Medicine*, *2*(1), a008888. doi:10.1101/cshperspect.a008888

Kordower, J. H. & Brundin, P. (2016). Mechanisms for cell-to-cell propagation no longer lag behind. *Movement Disorders*, *31*(12), 1798–1799. doi:10.1002/mds.26879

Lesage, S., Durr, A., Tazir, M., Lohmann, E., Leutenegger, A. L., Janin, S., . . . French Parkinson's Disease Genetics Study Group (2006). LRRK2 G2019S as a cause of Parkinson's disease in North African Arabs. *New England Journal of Medicine, 354*(4), 422–423. doi:10.1056/NEJMc055540

Lewis, S. J., Foltynie, T., Blackwell, A. D., Robbins, T. W., Owen, A. M. & Barker, R. A. (2005). Heterogeneity of Parkinson's disease in the early clinical stages using a data driven approach. *Journal of Neurology, Neurosurgery and Psychiatry, 76*(3), 343–348. doi:10. 1136/jnnp.2003.033530

Liu, R., Guo, X., Park, Y., Huang, X., Sinha, R., Freedman, N. D., . . . Chen, H. (2012). Caffeine intake, smoking, and risk of Parkinson disease in men and women. *American Journal of Epidemiology, 175*(11), 1200–1207. doi:10.1093/aje/kwr451

Luk, K. C., Kehm, V., Carroll, J., Zhang, B., O'Brien, P., Trojanowski, J. Q. & Lee, V. M. (2012). Pathological alpha-synuclein transmission initiates Parkinson-like neurode-generation in nontransgenic mice. *Science, 338*(6109), 949–953. doi:10.1126/science. 1227157

Malek, N., Swallow, D., Grosset, K. A., Anichtchik, O., Spillantini, M. & Grosset, D. G. (2014). Alpha-synuclein in peripheral tissues and body fluids as a biomarker for Parkinson's disease: a systematic review. *Acta Neurologica Scandinavica, 130*(2), 59–72. doi:10.1111/ane.12247

Marsden, C. D. (1982). The mysterious motor function of the basal ganglia: The Robert Wartenberg Lecture. *Neurology, 32*(5), 514–539.

Martinez-Ramirez, D., Hu, W., Bona, A. R., Okun, M. S. & Wagle Shukla, A. (2015). Update on deep brain stimulation in Parkinson's disease. *Translational Neurodegeneration, 4*, 12. doi:10.1186/s40035-015-0034-0

Middleton, F. A. & Strick, P. L. (2000). Basal ganglia and cerebellar loops: motor and cognitive circuits. *Brain Research: Brain Research Reviews, 31*(2–3), 236–250.

Morens, D. M., Davis, J. W., Grandinetti, A., Ross, G. W., Popper, J. S. & White, L. R. (1996). Epidemiologic observations on Parkinson's disease: incidence and mortality in a prospective study of middle-aged men. *Neurology, 46*(4), 1044–1050.

Morozova, N., O'Reilly, E. J. & Ascherio, A. (2008). Variations in gender ratios support the connection between smoking and Parkinson's disease. *Movement Disorders, 23*(10), 1414–1419. doi:10.1002/mds.22045

Morris, M. & Iansek, R. (1997). *Parkinson's Disease: A Team Approach.* Cheltenham, Australia: Southern Health Care Network.

Morris, M., Iansek, R., McGinley, J., Matyas, T. & Huxham, F. (2005). Three-dimensional gait biomechanics in Parkinson's disease: evidence for a centrally mediated amplitude regulation disorder. *Movement Disorders, 20*(1), 40–50. doi:10.1002/mds.20278

Morris, M. E., Iansek, R., Matyas, T. A. & Summers, J. J. (1994). The pathogenesis of gait hypokinesia in Parkinson's disease. *Brain, 117*(Pt 5), 1169–1181.

Morris, M. E., Iansek, R., Matyas, T. A. & Summers, J. J. (1996). Stride length regulation in Parkinson's disease: normalization strategies and underlying mechanisms. *Brain, 119* (Pt 2), 551–568.

Nalls, M. A., McLean, C. Y., Rick, J., Eberly, S., Hutten, S. J., Gwinn, K., . . . Parkinson's Progression Marker Initiative investigators (2015). Diagnosis of Parkinson's disease on the basis of clinical and genetic classification: a population-based modelling study. *Lancet Neurology, 14*(10), 1002–1009. doi:10.1016/S1474-4422(15)00178-7

Obeso, J. A., Rodriguez-Oroz, M. C., Benitez-Temino, B., Blesa, F. J., Guridi, J., Marin, C. & Rodriguez, M. (2008). Functional organization of the basal ganglia: therapeutic implications for Parkinson's disease. *Movement Disorders, 23 Suppl 3*, S548–559. doi:10.1002/ mds.22062

Olanow, C. W., Stern, M. B. & Sethi, K. (2009). The scientific and clinical basis for the treatment of Parkinson disease (2009). *Neurology*, *72*(21 Suppl 4), S1–136. doi:10.1212/WNL.0b013e3181a1d44c

Olsen, J. H., Friis, S. & Frederiksen, K. (2006). Malignant melanoma and other types of cancer preceding Parkinson disease. *Epidemiology*, *17*(5), 582–587. doi:10.1097/01.ede.0000229445.90471.5e

Oswal, A., Beudel, M., Zrinzo, L., Limousin, P., Hariz, M., Foltynie, T., . . . Brown, P. (2016). Deep brain stimulation modulates synchrony within spatially and spectrally distinct resting state networks in Parkinson's disease. *Brain*, *139*(Pt 5), 1482–1496. doi:10.1093/brain/aww048

Palacios, N., Fitzgerald, K., Roberts, A. L., Hart, J. E., Weisskopf, M. G., Schwarzschild, M. A., . . . Laden, F. (2014). A prospective analysis of airborne metal exposures and risk of Parkinson disease in the nurses' health study cohort. *Environmental Health Perspectives*, *122*(9), 933–938.

Piron, C., Kase, D., Topalidou, M., Goillandeau, M., Orignac, H., N'Guyen, T. H., . . . Boraud, T. (2016). The globus pallidus pars interna in goal-oriented and routine behaviors: resolving a long-standing paradox. *Movement Disorders*, *31*(8), 1146–1154. doi:10.1002/mds.26542

Polymeropoulos, M. H., Lavedan, C., Leroy, E., Ide, S. E., Dehejia, A., Dutra, A., . . . Nussbaum, R. L. (1997). Mutation in the alpha-synuclein gene identified in families with Parkinson's disease. *Science*, *276*(5321), 2045–2047.

Postuma, R. B., Berg, D., Adler, C. H., Bloem, B. R., Chan, P., Deuschl, G., . . . Stern, M. (2016). The new definition and diagnostic criteria of Parkinson's disease. *Lancet Neurology*, *15*(6), 546–548. doi:10.1016/S1474-4422(16)00116-2

Postuma, R. B., Berg, D., Stern, M., Poewe, W., Olanow, C. W., Oertel, W., . . . Deuschl, G. (2015). MDS clinical diagnostic criteria for Parkinson's disease. *Movement Disorders*, *30*(12), 1591–1601. doi:10.1002/mds.26424

Pringsheim, T., Jette, N., Frolkis, A. & Steeves, T. D. (2014). The prevalence of Parkinson's disease: a systematic review and meta-analysis. *Movement Disorders*, *29*(13), 1583–1590. doi:10.1002/mds.25945

Recasens, A. & Dehay, B. (2014). Alpha-synuclein spreading in Parkinson's disease. *Frontiers in Neuroanatomy*, *8*, 159. doi:10.3389/fnana.2014.00159

Salat, D., Noyce, A. J., Schrag, A. & Tolosa, E. (2016). Challenges of modifying disease progression in prediagnostic Parkinson's disease. *Lancet Neurology*, *15*(6), 637–648. doi:10.1016/S1474-4422(16)00060-0

Schechtman, E., Noblejas, M. I., Mizrahi, A. D., Dauber, O. & Bergman, H. (2016). Pallidal spiking activity reflects learning dynamics and predicts performance. *Proceedings of the National Academy of Sciences of the United States of America*, *113*(41), E6281–E6289. doi:10.1073/pnas.1612392113

Schrag, A. & Quinn, N. (2000). Dyskinesias and motor fluctuations in Parkinson's disease: a community-based study. *Brain*, *123*(Pt 11), 2297–2305.

Shimura, H., Schlossmacher, M. G., Hattori, N., Frosch, M. P., Trockenbacher, A., Schneider, R., . . . Selkoe, D. J. (2001). Ubiquitination of a new form of alpha-synuclein by Parkin from human brain: implications for Parkinson's disease. *Science*, *293*(5528), 263–269. doi:10.1126/science.1060627

Stolwyk, R. J., Charlton, J. L., Triggs, T. J., Iansek, R. & Bradshaw, J. L. (2006). Neuropsychological function and driving ability in people with Parkinson's disease. *Journal of Clinical and Experimental Neuropsychology*, *28*(6), 898–913. doi:10.1080/13803390591000909

Stolwyk, R. J., Triggs, T. J., Charlton, J. L., Iansek, R. & Bradshaw, J. L. (2005). Impact of internal versus external cueing on driving performance in people with Parkinson's disease. *Movement Disorders, 20*(7), 846–857. doi:10.1002/mds.20420

Stolwyk, R. J., Triggs, T. J., Charlton, J. L., Moss, S., Iansek, R. & Bradshaw, J. L. (2006). Effect of a concurrent task on driving performance in people with Parkinson's disease. *Movement Disorders, 21*(12), 2096–2100. doi:10.1002/mds.21115

Svensson, E., Horvath-Puho, E., Thomsen, R. W., Djurhuus, J. C., Pedersen, L., Borghammer, P. & Sorensen, H. T. (2015). Vagotomy and subsequent risk of Parkinson's disease. *Annals of Neurology, 78*(4), 522–529. doi:10.1002/ana.24448

Tanner, C. M., Kamel, F., Ross, G. W., Hoppin, J. A., Goldman, S. M., Korell, M., . . . Langston, J. W. (2011). Rotenone, Paraquat, and Parkinson's disease. *Environmental Health Perspectives, 119*(6), 866–872.

Uchihara, T. & Giasson, B. I. (2016). Propagation of alpha-synuclein pathology: hypotheses, discoveries, and yet unresolved questions from experimental and human brain studies. *Acta Neuropathologica, 131*(1), 49–73. doi:10.1007/s00401-015-1485-1

Van der Marck, M. A., Bloem, B. R., Borm, G. F., Overeem, S., Munneke, M. & Guttman, M. (2013). Effectiveness of multidisciplinary care for Parkinson's disease: a randomized, controlled trial. *Movement Disorders, 28*(5), 605–611. doi:10.1002/mds.25194

Van Rooden, S. M., Heiser, W. J., Kok, J. N., Verbaan, D., van Hilten, J. J. & Marinus, J. (2010). The identification of Parkinson's disease subtypes using cluster analysis: a systematic review. *Movement Disorders, 25*(8), 969–978. doi:10.1002/mds.23116

Volta, M., Milnerwood, A. J. & Farrer, M. J. (2015). Insights from late-onset familial Parkinsonism on the pathogenesis of idiopathic Parkinson's disease. *Lancet Neurology, 14*(10), 1054–1064. doi:10.1016/S1474-4422(15)00186-6

Vu, T. C., Nutt, J. G. & Holford, N. H. (2012). Progression of motor and nonmotor features of Parkinson's disease and their response to treatment. *British Journal of Clinical Pharmacology, 74*(2), 267–283. doi:10.1111/j.1365-2125.2012.04192.x

Weisskopf, M. G., O'Reilly, E., Chen, H., Schwarzschild, M. A. & Ascherio, A. (2007). Plasma urate and risk of Parkinson's disease. *American Journal of Epidemiology, 166*(5), 561–567. doi:10.1093/aje/kwm127

Williams, D., Tijssen, M., Van Bruggen, G., Bosch, A., Insola, A., Di Lazzaro, V., . . . Brown, P. (2002). Dopamine-dependent changes in the functional connectivity between basal ganglia and cerebral cortex in humans. *Brain, 125*(Pt 7), 1558–1569.

Williams, D. R., Evans, A. H., Fung, V. S. C., Hayes, M., Iansek, R., Kimber, T., . . . Sue, C. M. (2017). Practical approaches to commencing device-assisted therapies for Parkinson disease in Australia. *Internal Medicine Journal, 47*(10), 1107–1113.

Wu, T., Chan, P. & Hallet, M. (2010). Effective connectivity of neural networks in automatic movements in Parkinson's disease. *Neuroimage, 49*, 2581–2587.

Wu, T., Kansaku, K. & Hallet, M. (2004). How self-initiated memorized movements become automatic: a functional MRI study. *Journal of Neurophysiology, 91*, 1690–1698.

Yang, F., Trolle Lagerros, Y., Bellocco, R., Adami, H. O., Fang, F., Pedersen, N. L. & Wirdefeldt, K. (2015). Physical activity and risk of Parkinson's disease in the Swedish National March Cohort. *Brain, 138*(Pt 2), 269–275. doi:10.1093/brain/awu323

Yogev-Seligmann, G., Hausdorff, J. M. & Giladi, N. (2008). The role of executive function and attention in gait. *Movement Disorders, 23*(3), 329–342; quiz 472. doi:10.1002/mds.21720

Youle, R. J. & Narendra, D. P. (2011). Mechanisms of mitophagy. *Nature Reviews: Molecular Cell Biology, 12*(1), 9–14. doi:10.1038/nrm3028

4

HUNTINGTON'S DISEASE

Aileen K. Ho

Introduction

Huntington's disease (HD), a rare and progressive inherited neurological disorder that manifests in the classic triad of motor, cognitive and neuropsychiatric features, usually strikes between the third and fifth decade of life. Remorselessly, over a period of approximately 15–20 years, motor impairment, cognitive loss and neuropsychiatric changes manifest in the patient so that virtually no aspect of life is left untouched by the ravages of this disease. There is currently no tangible evidence for disease-modifying treatment, nor is there any means of delaying disease onset or significantly ameliorating the course of the disease. Purely symptomatic treatment can be of some utility in this complex condition. The fear and stigma associated with HD poses an additional burden to patients and their wider family circle when faced with the spectre of this monogenetic disease that has an inevitably fatal prognosis.

Prevalence

HD occurs worldwide affecting between 4 and 8 people in every 100,000 in Western populations, with a lower prevalence rate in Asian and African ethnicities (Harper, 1992). With the identification of the HD gene in 1993 and hence the availability of genetic testing to determine the length of the causative CAG (cytosine-adenine-guanine) expansion, it has been possible to conclusively diagnose HD. This is particularly helpful in cases of *de novo* patients with no known family history, where there may have been previously unknown intermediate or low penetrance alleles. With the availability of genetic testing, and despite its low uptake by at risk individuals, there have since been indications of a rise in prevalence figures up to 13.7 per 100,000 (Fisher & Hayden, 2014); however, the pattern of Caucasian prominence remains.

Clinical vignette

This vignette follows the story of Mariella, who grew up knowing that her grandmother was always a bit different and had rather strange mannerisms. When she was in secondary school, Mariella's father's behaviour started to become rather uncharacteristic and erratic. He too became restless and clumsy, demonstrating odd jerks and twitches as he moved. This was when she learnt from her parents that her father and grandmother both had Huntington's disease, and that she had a 50% chance of inheriting the faulty HD gene. As Mariella started university it was clear that her grandmother's condition was deteriorating. Mariella grappled with whether or not to undergo genetic testing, and decided she did not want to know her status as there was no treatment available. Not knowing was better than facing the knowledge of an unfavourable test result. Instead, she concentrated on living her life as normally as she could. She embarked on a successful career in finance, working globally, and returned home to get married in her early thirties. By now her parents had separated, and her father was about to enter a care home as he was severely affected by HD. Mariella had always been open about being at risk for HD, and her husband had been aware of this for many years. As they were hoping to start a family, Mariella felt it was the right time to get tested, and they went for genetic counselling together. This was the same process her younger sister, who tested negative for the HD gene, had gone through several years previously. Mariella only found out about this recently at their grandmother's funeral. When her test results came, they revealed that Mariella did indeed carry the HD gene. She was rather taken aback by this bad news although she had understood there was an equal chance for either outcome. The reality of living with the knowledge of developing HD in the future affected her more than she had anticipated. She had chosen to be tested to find certainty, but was still riddled by (different) uncertainties and questions. She struggled to come to terms with living with her gene positive presymptomatic status and its future implications. Her mood was affected as she became increasingly withdrawn. She felt clumsier than usual and work was more of a struggle as she felt less sharp mentally. Sleep was difficult as many worrying thoughts charged through her mind as she wondered if she was starting to experience early signs and symptoms of HD. This persisted over several years and eventually she decided to stop working due to the stress of her demanding role. She had not told anyone about her genetic status apart from her husband, who was with her during the genetic testing process. Mariella did consider preimplantation genetic diagnosis and in vitro fertilisation to avoid passing on the HD mutation, but then fell pregnant naturally and gave birth to a baby boy. At that point, her father was no longer able to communicate clearly and relied on a feeding tube for nutrition.

The story pauses at Mariella's father's funeral where she is still feeling the weight of the multiple different roles the disease had enforced on her – a presymptomatic (or possibly prodromal) gene positive HD carrier, mother of a child who is at a 50% risk of the same disease, and as the daughter of a man who valiantly fought an all-consuming disease for two decades. As Mariella tripped slightly on the stairs at the event, she felt the collective gaze of the entire clan on her, magnifying her self-consciousness, as she navigated her way around the buffet table trying to balance her meal while making conversation. On reflection, her mind felt slow and foggy, a far cry from her former high-flying executive self of five years ago when she thrived on juggling multiple fast-moving tasks. In contrast, she often felt anxious and on edge, having lost the motivation to do all but what was absolutely necessary for her and her young family.

Diagnostic considerations

A diagnosis of HD is based on neurological presentation, and is confirmed after a positive genetic test for the presence of the CAG expansion in the huntingtin gene. This occurs in the context of a family history of HD, and also after excluding other possible causes. A firm diagnosis is currently made on the basis of the motor signs and symptoms (Reilmann, Leavitt & Ross, 2014), where extraneous involuntary movement is present, often together with slowed voluntary movement that may be reduced in range and/or fluency of execution. Before overt onset based on these motor changes, individuals do not have manifest disease and are not considered symptomatic. However, there is something of a false dichotomy here, as very gradual motor changes over a period of time mean that pinpointing an exact moment of onset is often not entirely feasible, and that onset may be a matter of degree and with an increasing level of confidence over time.

Discernible changes in cognitive function, mood, and/or behaviour may in fact predate motor onset. Often, these changes may manifest before clear motor signs and symptoms emerge. These cognitive and behavioural changes are less straightforward to interpret and to attribute directly to the disease, as they can be more subjective and also interact dynamically with the broader context of life. Nevertheless, there is a pathophysiological basis for these emotional, cognitive and behavioural changes in HD and they can have a substantial impact on individuals and their families many years prior to the motor symptoms that are a defining point for diagnosis.

Within the premanifest phase, a further distinction can be drawn using more sensitive ways of examining motoric and cognitive facets of behaviour. The advent of genetic testing – such as Predict-HD (Patrick, Curtis, Engelberg, Nielsen & McCown, 2003) and Track-HD (Tabrizi et al., 2012) – and cohorts of premanifest individuals who are amenable to neuroimaging research and more detailed behavioural studies, has shown that a transitory prodromal period exists before manifest disease can be detected. This period is marked by small changes in psychomotor tasks such as the Symbol Digit Modalities Test, the Stroop word-reading task, quantitative motor measures such as hand tap variability, in addition to structural brain imaging. These are subtle prodromal signs and symptoms that may not be detected in everyday life, nor may they hinder functional performance, but are early indicators of change that may be linked to under par performance.

Better understanding of the emergence of subtle non-motor changes has led to suggestions of more nuanced and expanded diagnostic criteria (Reilmann et al., 2014). Nevertheless, disease onset is currently defined by motor onset, and the presence of motor symptoms remains the basis for a diagnosis of clinically manifest disease.

The gradual unfolding of motor, cognitive and behavioural changes that culminate in manifest HD means that in reality, diagnosis and the communication of diagnosis is not clear cut (McCusker & Loy, 2017). The onset of HD, or indeed its progression across stages, occurs on a cumulative spectrum of confidence rather than manifesting as discrete events. This is usually reflected in clinical care where a considered approach is often taken reflecting the person's individual circumstances. Clinical assessment and discussions over several periodic consultations serve as a means for reflection and review, and allow individuals time and space to process and adjust to the conceptual and practical aspects of progression in HD. Therefore, a gradual process of disclosure of diagnosis and progression can be helpful in clinical management and care.

Genetics and gene testing

The cause of HD rests within a single gene. The huntingtin (HTT) gene on the short arm of chromosome 4p16.3 is aberrant due to a toxic gain-of-function CAG trinucleotide repeat mutation (MacDonald et al., 1993). This expanded HTT gene with the atypically long polyglutamine sequence is responsible for the over production of the protein huntingtin, which sets off a toxic chain of events that results in neuronal atrophy. While by no means the only region affected, the striatum is the epicentre of the pathological disease process. The expanded Huntingtin gene affects the medium spiny neurons involved in the indirect and also the direct pathway of the cortico-striato-pallido-thalamo-cortical loops that regulate motor, cognitive and behavioural function (Gusella & MacDonald, 2006).

As a polyglutamine disease, HD is autosomal dominant, and so each biological child of an affected parent has a 50% chance of inheriting the abnormal expansion and developing HD (MacDonald et al., 1993). It is also fully penetrant when the CAG repeat size is 40 or over, with the certainty of onset of the disease at some point within a normal life span. CAG repeat sizes of between 36 and 39 are rare and still in the disease range, but have reduced penetrance, and this is usually associated with later onset and/or a milder disease course (Quarrell et al., 2007). Intermediate alleles with 27 to 35 CAG repeats are also rare, and are not associated with features of HD per se. While these individuals will not develop symptoms themselves, they may have offspring who fall in the affected range of over 40 CAG repeats, resulting in de novo cases of HD. This scenario is more common if the father carries the intermediate allele, as paternal transmission is more susceptible to 'anticipation', where the CAG repeat size increases substantially when it is passed on due to greater instability in the development of sperm cells (Goldberg et al., 1993).

Identification of the gene for HD in 1993 (MacDonald et al., 1993), has meant that since then it has been possible to determine the presence or absence of the abnormal expansion from a blood test. Prior to this, and since 1986, linkage analysis had been possible. Diagnostic gene testing can be carried out to provide confirmation of cases where there is a Huntington family history and there are signs and symptoms of the disease. Where there is a family history of HD but as yet no noticeable signs or symptoms, a predictive genetic test can be conducted to find out whether or not the individual carries the expanded HD mutation. If the abnormal expansion is not inherited, then the risk of HD is effectively eradicated in future generations of that section of the family tree. If the abnormal expansion is indeed inherited, then this means that HD will almost certainly develop in the affected child's natural life time, as the gene is fully penetrant; and the next generation will also inherit the 50% risk of developing HD.

What is not known, however, is the specific phenotype and how this will evolve over the protracted course of the disease. Another unknown element is when the symptoms of HD will emerge for each individual. There are various formulae addressing the known relationship between CAG repeat size and age to estimate where people may be on the HD disease trajectory, and to estimate predicted age of motor onset in research, including the Disease Burden Score (Penney, Vonsattel, Macdonald, Gusella & Myers, 1997), Cag Age Product (Ying et al., 2011), and Prognostic Index (Long et al., 2016). However, at a clinical level it would be inappropriate to apply these to individual cases given the large degree of variability and factors not yet captured by these equations. Genetic modifiers from recent genome wide association studies can temper the age of disease onset (Lee et al., 2015). Furthermore, the role of environmental factors and epigenetic influences should not be underestimated, as monozygotic HD twins with the same CAG repeat size can differ markedly both in onset and presentation (Georgiou et al., 1999).

As there is no known cure or established disease-modifying treatment at present, the vast majority of people at risk of HD choose not to take the test. Predictive testing of individuals who have a close biological relative with HD, and are therefore at risk for the disease is still consistently the exception rather than the norm worldwide, with less than 20% of these individuals choosing to find out their genetic status (Baig et al., 2016). Those who do take the test usually do so when the costs of not knowing and being able to plan ahead outweigh any burden of knowing, and also when there is a specific reason such as starting a family. Therefore, whether or not to take a genetic test, and deciding when the time to do so is, is a highly personal decision. Genetic counselling is part of the standard genetic testing process in order to ensure that people fully understand what taking the test means and also the implications of the results obtained (MacLeod et al., 2013). When it comes to reproductive decision making, the choice to undertake preimplantation genetic diagnosis and in vitro fertilisation because of a positive status for HD is an option. Nonetheless, it is also very uncommon, just like the low uptake of predictive genetic testing (Nance, 2017).

Juvenile-onset Huntington's disease

Juvenile HD, or more accurately, juvenile-onset HD, refers to a variant that emerges before the age of 21 years, typically in adolescence and less commonly in childhood and infancy. Juvenile-onset HD is associated with higher CAG repeats, often in the 60s or much higher. Very high repeat values typically occur in the very young, and this usually occurs through a process of 'anticipation' whereby paternal transmission results in a large increase in the number of CAG repeats transmitted.

With a younger age of onset of symptoms comes the ethical issue of predictive testing for minors. While the testing of minors is not recommended in HD, it does occur in exceptional circumstances, usually when the individual concerned is just below the age of 18, and where a case can be made that proceeding with testing would be more helpful to the individual than waiting (Quarrell et al., 2018).

The course of juvenile-onset HD, also sometimes referred to as the Westphal variant, is typically more accelerated than adult-onset disease. Younger onset age is associated with poorer prognosis, increased likelihood of seizure disorder and shorter course of illness. Juvenile HD is characterised by rigidity and akinesia (with chorea being less prominent) resulting in awkward gait, clumsiness and falls, deterioration in handwriting and speech that is hesitant and dysarthric. Behavioural and emotional issues commonly include mood changes, anxiety and depression, impulsiveness and aggression. Challenging behaviour and cognitive changes, particularly in executive function, also present early, and together can be very disruptive in educational settings and can interact negatively with developmental issues (Nance & Myers, 2001). These issues collectively pose an extremely high burden of care on parents and the wider family, particularly on the non HD-affected spouse (who may also be caring for their HD-affected partner), as the juvenile patient becomes progressively incapacitated into adulthood (Brewer et al., 2008).

Neuropathology, neurophysiology and potential biomarkers

While the whole brain is affected by the downstream effects of the over expanded CAG repeat size and over production of the protein huntingtin, the brunt of the neuropathological consequences of HD is borne by a small group of structures located deep within the brain, the basal ganglia. The GABA (gamma-aminobutyric acid)-ergic medium spiny neurons here are particularly vulnerable and reductions in putamen and caudate nuclei of 50% and 30% respectively, have been found in early to moderate HD (Harris et al., 1992). These neuropathological changes can be found a decade or more before clinical manifestation of HD and become increasingly pronounced with closer proximity to motor onset (Aylward et al., 2004).

The basal ganglia are intimately connected to many key cortical regions, and are therefore critically involved in the control and regulation of movement, thinking and emotional responses through cortico-striato-pallido-thalamo-cortical loops (Alexander & Crutcher, 1990; Lehéricy et al., 2004; Mehrabi, Singh-Bains,

Waldvogel & Faull, 2016). These basal ganglia-thalamocortical circuits are functionally and structurally segregated and organised in parallel, each with functionally and structurally distinct components. The sensorimotor circuit features excitatory glutamatergic projections from the motor, premotor, supplementary motor area and sensory cortical areas to the posterior part of the putamen. The cognitive associative loop involves medial, ventral and dorsal prefrontal cortex projections to the head of the caudate nucleus and anterior part of the putamen. The limbic circuit is characterised by the medial orbitofrontal cortex, the amygdala and anterior cingulate cortex projecting to the ventral striatum. Together, these loops account for the motor, cognitive and emotional-behavioural changes seen in HD as their neuromodulatory influence is disrupted.

Malfunctioning along any point within these circuits can impact on the synergistic roles of the direct pathway (through D1 cells), the indirect (D2) pathway of these basal ganglia-thalamocortical loops, and also the hyperdirect cortico-subthalamo-pallidal pathway (Nambu, Tokuno & Takada, 2002). Activation of the direct ('go') pathway facilitates motor, cognitive and behavioural function. This occurs through putaminal inhibition of the globus pallidus interna, which then reduces its inhibitory influence over the thalamus, thus allowing thalamo-cortical excitation to facilitate behaviour. On the other hand, activation of the indirect ('stop') pathway exerts inhibitory control over these functions. This occurs through putaminal inhibition of the globus pallidus externa, which then reduces its inhibitory influence over the subthalamic nucleus. This in turn elicits the subthalamic nucleus to send an excitatory projection to the globus pallidus interna, which then inhibits the thalamus and reduces thalamocortical excitatory activity. This inhibitory process is critical for suppressing inappropriate movement, cognitions and behaviour. Disruption along this indirect pathway causes striatal dysregulation which perturbs the normal equilibrium of the direct and indirect pathways, giving rise to insufficient inhibitory control. This is reflected in the hyperkinetic motor manifestation of HD via the impaired sensorimotor circuit where unwanted involuntary movements are not suppressed. Hypokinesia, or slowed voluntary movement, can also coexist with ongoing striatal dysfunction affecting the direct pathway (Thompson et al., 1988). Likewise, dysfunction of the cognitive associative circuit gives rise to changes in executive function and working memory (Lawrence et al., 1996), and dysfunction in the limbic circuit is associated with changes in mood (Unschuld et al., 2012) and disinhibition (Duff et al., 2010b).

While damage in the basal ganglia and their circuits is pathognomonic of HD, neuropathological and neurophysiological changes are not confined here. Even early on in the course of disease cortical thickness is reduced throughout the brain, particularly in posterior regions (Rosas et al., 2002), and cerebellar neurons including deep nuclei are also affected (Rüb et al., 2013). Although these studies show substantial changes, the high variability across individuals has been found to correspond well to the clinical presentation in patients (Mehrabi, Waldvogel et al., 2016). Widespread cortical changes are also found in preclinical HD including the posterior cerebral cortex and associative visual cortical areas underlying visuospatial performance (Coppen, van der Grond, Hart, Lakke & Roos, 2018). White matter atrophy can be seen up to 15 years prior to estimated disease onset (Paulsen et al., 2010) and there is increasing evidence that white matter is structurally disorganised in premanifest individuals (Reading et al., 2005). The integrity of structural and functional connectivity in the motor corpus callosum and striatum are also found to be compromised early on, with a demonstrable link to motor control (Garcia-Gorro et al., 2018). Longitudinal diffusion MRI changes in the connectivity of structural networks that are associated with clinical measures may prove to be another useful biomarker with further research interrogation (Odish et al., 2015).

Changes in the pattern of task-dependent brain activation using functional magnetic resonance imaging (fMRI) and fluorodeoxyglucose (FDG) – positron emission tomography (PET) in premanifest and manifest individuals with HD have been reliably reported in the literature. However, interpretation of the findings is not entirely clear as over- or under-activation in cortical and striatal areas relative to controls could reflect varying degrees of impairment and/or compensation (Paulsen, 2009; Poudel et al., 2015). Resting state fMRI (which does not require individuals to perform a task in the scanner) more convincingly suggests reduced functional connectivity within the default mode and executive control networks in individuals with premanifest and manifest HD (Dumas et al., 2013). PET imaging, using specific tracers has shown evidence for striatal pathology (Russell et al., 2015), reduced D2 dopamine receptor binding (Pavese et al., 2003), and increased microglial activation (Pavese et al., 2006). Electrophysiological markers capturing changes in cortical activity are less invasive but require further development (Beste et al., 2013; Hart et al., 2015; Nguyen, Bradshaw, Stout, Croft & Georgiou-Karistianis, 2010).

Other recent potential biomarkers include proteins in cerebrospinal fluid such as mutant huntingtin (Wild et al., 2015), tau (Rodrigues et al., 2016) and neurofilament light protein (Byrne et al., 2017), as well as Magnetic Resonance Spectroscopy (MRS) to detect lowered N-acetyl aspartate in the putamen of premanifest and manifest individuals (Sturrock et al., 2015). While further work is needed to validate these, the most robust potential biomarkers to date are caudate volume and white matter volume (Georgiou-Karistianis, Scahill, Tabrizi, Squitieri & Aylward, 2013; Tabrizi et al., 2012), which are closely linked to changes in clinical disease severity.

Clinical symptoms

HD most typically emerges when people are in their thirties or forties and are in the prime of their life. The onset of disease is insidious, progression is very slow and survival time can span a period of up to two decades. The changes in motor, cognitive and neuropsychiatric/behavioural profiles are variable between patients, and gradually evolve over the long trajectory of disease; eventually the symptoms interfere with all aspects of function and behaviour. There is considerable variability as to which signs and symptoms present first and also on the course that the disease takes for each individual affected (Mehrabi, Waldvogel et al., 2016).

Motor symptoms

The hallmark of HD is chorea, characterised by writhing, jerky, or dance-like movements. These irrepressible, extraneous hyperkinetic movements are unintended, and often the most striking feature of the disease. Typically, the first motor symptoms noticed by patients, or others around them, are subtle twitches that may affect the hands, legs, face or trunk that over time increase in frequency and extent, heralding the emergence of chorea (Young et al., 1986). As the disease progresses, chorea can reduce in some patients, while in others it remains a prominent feature until late into the disease. Interestingly, patients may not be fully aware of the extent of their chorea even though it may be obvious to others around them (Snowden, Craufurd, Griffiths & Neary, 1998). This is particularly striking at the point of motor onset, where 50% of gene positive individuals naive to their gene status do not report any HD movement symptoms when explicitly asked (McCusker et al., 2013). Another dyskinetic motor feature that patients may not be aware of and can be difficult to differentiate from chorea is increased muscle tone and dystonia, which refers to slow writhing or twisting movements and prolonged abnormal posturing of the limbs, shoulder and trunk, that can often cause discomfort and even pain. While there is interindividual variability, dystonia tends to worsen over the course of disease (Louis, Lee, Quinn & Marder, 1999).

Although HD is essentially a hyperkinetic disorder with positive symptomatology, a more negative or debilitating aspect of motor impairment is reflected in how intentional voluntary movement is hesitant (akinetic), slowed (hypokinetic, bradykinetic), reduced in extent (hypometric) rigid, effortful, and uncoordinated (Bradshaw et al., 1992; Georgiou, Phillips, Bradshaw, Cunnington & Chiu, 1997). While bradykinesia may not be as striking as chorea, it correlates with poorer striatal D2 binding (Sanchez-Pernaute et al., 2000), and becomes increasingly problematic for patients as the disease progresses.

Changes in motor performance have been detected more than ten years before expected motor onset (Paulsen et al., 2007). Early on during the prodromal period, and progressively over the course of disease, the smooth execution of movements (Kirkwood et al., 2000) including eye movements is compromised (Leigh, Newman, Folstein, Lasker & Jensen, 1983), particularly along the vertical plane. Other sensitive motor measures are variability of tongue protrusion force (Reilmann et al., 2010), grip force variability and finger tapping (Antoniades, Xu, Mason, Carpenter & Barker, 2010), which become progressively more impaired in terms of extent, speed and smoothness of execution, as coordination progressively breaks down (Tabrizi et al., 2012). All motor systems are affected, with gradual impairment of function of the upper and lower limbs, affecting gait. Facial expression, postural and trunk control, speech (dysarthria) (Ludlow, Connor & Bassich, 1987), swallowing (dysphagia) (Kagel & Leopold, 1992) and respiration can also be affected by chorea and bradykinesia. This causes problems with the smooth execution of many everyday tasks relying on seamlessly coordinated motor sequences, such as handwriting, walking, dressing, eating and conversing clearly with others.

Swallowing difficulties often result in choking, so for safety, thickened fluids and pureed food are often recommended in moderate to severe disease (Hamilton et al., 2012). Clarity of speech is compromised as articulation becomes increasingly slurred and effortful. Due to hyperkinesia affecting the respiratory/speech motor system and poor coordination, unintended sub-vocal emissions can be part of the motor presentation in some patients. Speech eventually becomes hesitant, often leading to simple yes or no responses, towards the end stage of disease (Murray, 2000). By then, most patients require extensive support with mobility, feeding and also communication, and aids such as wheeled walkers/chairs, communication devices and a feeding tube may be employed.

Throughout the disease the most commonly used measure of motor function remains the total motor score of the Unified Huntington's Disease Rating Scale (UHDRS) (Huntington Study Group, 1996), where individuals are rated from 0 (no abnormalities) to 124 on the ability to perform a range of set tasks in a motor examination.

Cognition

Cognitive changes in HD are complex and multi-faceted, emerging and evolving only very gradually over the course of disease. Subtle changes early in the course of disease may be present ten or more years before anticipated clinical motor onset (Paulsen et al., 2007; Stout et al., 2011). In a subset of prodromal individuals, these early cognitive changes may occur even before any early motor changes (Paulsen & Long, 2014). However, what is more typically found is preservation of cognitive performance despite underlying neuropathological changes (Gray et al., 2013; Wolf, Vasic, Schönfeldt-Lecuona, Landwehrmeyer & Ecker, 2007). This has been attributed to neural compensation in terms of increased efficiency or versatility in the use of adapted brain networks that buffer against any decrement in performance (Papoutsi, Labuschagne, Tabrizi & Stout, 2014). The role of cognitive reserve has not yet been fully explored in HD but there are early indications of a possible neuroprotective effect (Soloveva, Jamadar, Poudel & Georgiou-Karistianis, 2018). Higher levels of cognitive reserve as defined by higher pre-morbid intelligence, as well as higher educational and occupational attainment, have been found to be associated with a neuroprotective effect on executive function and a slower rate of striatal atrophy over a 6-year period (Bonner-Jackson et al., 2013).

Due to subtle motor changes early on, it is perhaps somewhat unsurprising that the most susceptible cognitive change during the preclinical phase lies within a hybrid psychomotor domain. Tasks that illustrate this rely primarily on visuomotor processing speed, and involve fairly low-level cognitive processing and rapid execution of relevant motor responses. These include naming aloud patches of colour (Stroop Colour Naming), reading aloud words (Stroop Word Reading) (Stroop, 1935), and using a printed coding key to write down the corresponding codes on a page (Symbol Digit Modalities Task, SDMT) (Smith, 1968), which are all part of the UHDRS (Huntington Study Group, 1996) Cognitive Assessment. Further psychomotor tasks include connecting jumbled letters of the alphabet successively (Trail Making Test A) (Reitan, 1958) and various permutations of timed finger/button tapping. More recently, the Huntington's Disease Cognitive Assessment Battery (HD-CAB) has been assembled as a cognitive test battery (Stout et al., 2014), and features SDMT and paced tapping. Speed in both cognitive and motor elements, often in parallel, contribute to performance and are therefore particularly sensitive to preclinical and early HD. Although differences are small during the preclinical and early phases of HD, slowed performance of these speeded tasks tend to differentiate preclinical individuals from controls (Duff et al., 2010a; Snowden, Craufurd, Thompson & Neary, 2002; Stout et al., 2011), and further slowing can be found when performance is monitored longitudinally over successive years (Kirkwood et al., 1999; Rowe et al., 2010; Tabrizi et al., 2013). After clinical motor onset, impairment in psychomotor speed becomes clear (Snowden et al., 2002) and steadily increases over time (Bachoud-Levi et al., 2001; Ho et al., 2003).

Another area of cognition that becomes markedly compromised in HD is higher order executive function. Higher order executive function skills are crucial to effectively manage and control mental processes and resources to achieve a goal. They are involved in focusing attention to allow for appropriate encoding, working memory, accessing from memory relevant information, co-ordinating multiple mental tasks, mental flexibility, abstract thinking, problem solving, decision making and forward planning. Some of the more commonly used executive function tests in the HD literature include verbal (letter/phonemic) fluency (Benton, 1968) which is part of the UHDRS (Huntington Study Group, 1996) Cognitive Assessment, semantic (category) fluency (Butters, Granholm, Salmon, Grant & Wolfe, 1987), suppressing prepotent responses on the Stroop colour-word interference condition (Stroop, 1935), and alternating between numbers and letters of the alphabet successively (Trail Making Test B) (Reitan, 1958). Poor performance on these executive function tests in particular is found cross-sectionally and longitudinally in clinically symptomatic (Bachoud-Levi et al., 2001; Ho et al., 2003; Ho et al., 2002) and non-symptomatic HD (Stout et al., 2011; Tabrizi et al., 2013).

As brief screens, the Mini Mental State Examination (MMSE) (Folstein, Folstein & McHugh, 1975), Repeatable Battery for the Assessment of Neuropsychological Status (RBANS) (Randolph, Tierney, Mohr & Chase, 1998) and Montreal Cognitive Assessment (MoCA) (Nasreddine et al., 2005) have also been used in HD with the latter being a good alternative to the MMSE, which has a ceiling effect in preclinical or early disease (Mickes et al., 2010). However, within the MMSE, recall is sensitive to longitudinal decline largely due to changes in attention and working memory; progressive impairment in working memory was also shown in poorer retention and execution of multi-step instructions on the Token Test (Ho et al., 2003). The Frontal Assessment Battery (FAB) (Dubois, Slachevsky, Litvan & Pillon, 2000) has also demonstrated dysexecutive decline in symptomatic patients (Rodrigues et al., 2009). The HD-CAB (Stout et al., 2014) includes two executive function tasks such as the Trail Making Test B (Reitan, 1958) and the Stocking of Cambridge task (Robbins et al., 1994).

Executive function impairment is subtle and variable with some studies report-ing early deviation from matched control performance (Kirkwood et al., 2000; Lawrence et al., 1998; Snowden et al., 2002), particularly for individuals closer to estimated onset (Stout et al., 2011; Tabrizi et al., 2013). This could in part be due to variability in performance or in neural compensation mentioned earlier. Social cognition (Eddy & Rickards, 2015) and theory of mind have been found to be affected relatively early on (Brune, Blank, Witthaus & Saft, 2011), and executive function impairment is common in the manifest stage (Lawrence et al., 1996), becoming increasingly prominent as the disease takes hold (Bachoud-Levi et al., 2001; Ho et al., 2003). Another 'frontal' impairment that can be striking is lack of insight or self-awareness (Craufurd, Thompson & Snowden, 2001; Ho, Robbins & Barker, 2006; Hoth et al., 2007). Gradual and collective dysexecutive changes can manifest in complex work environments early in HD and at the prodromal stage with individuals feeling increased stress in maintaining performance in pressured and demanding situations (Goh et al., 2018).

Although less commonly examined, visuospatial function including visual scan-ning and visuospatial processing has been found to be compromised early in the course of disease (Coppen et al., 2018; Lawrence, Watkins, Sahakian, Hodges & Robbins, 2000). Also affected is odour identification (Moberg et al., 1987; Stout et al., 2011) and taste perception (Hayes, Stevenson & Coltheart, 2007; Mitchell, Heims, Neville & Rickards, 2005). Negative emotion recognition has been found to be affected relatively early on (Hayes et al., 2007; Sprengelmeyer et al., 1996; Tabrizi et al., 2013), and is represented in the HD-CAB (Stout et al., 2014).

Episodic memory can also be vulnerable early in the course of HD and even preclinically. As HD progresses neuropathologically, more cortical elements of cognition are at risk, with the variability in the literature reflecting heterogeneity in individual performance and assessments employed. Any decrements that occur unfold at a slow pace, and immediate memory impairment is affected in both visual and verbal domains becoming more pronounced over time (Beglinger et al., 2010; Ho et al., 2003; Stout et al., 2011; Tabrizi et al., 2013). Common meas-ures include list learning tasks such as the Hopkins Verbal Learning Test (HVLT) (Brandt, 1991), which features in the HD-CAB (Stout et al., 2014).

Despite the impact of considerable brain pathology at the early to mid-stage of HD, where motor symptomatology has been a long-standing feature, perfor-mance on language and semantic memory is relatively well-preserved. However, as the burden of brain pathology increases, impairment in more global cogni-tive functioning ensues. Only at these later stages of disease does a more cortical dementia set in and overall MMSE scores fall (Rodrigues et al., 2009), having been relatively stable up to this point (Bachoud-Levi et al., 2001; Ho et al., 2003). However, the level of clinical impairment seen is variable between patients and can be easily underestimated by those not familiar with them, particularly when patients' attentional resources are low and verbal output is commonly scant. At this late stage, lexico-semantic memory and language function tends to be compro-mised and spontaneous speech is short, simple and minimal (Chenery, Copland &

Murdoch, 2002; Podoll, Caspary, Lange & Noth, 1988). Nevertheless, even towards end stage, when patients are chair or bed bound, many patients can still recognise close family members and familiar key figures, even if speech and communication is markedly reduced.

In summary, the hallmark sub-cortical cognitive changes in HD centre on psychomotor and processing speed, attention and executive function, verbal memory, visuospatial, emotion and odour processing; a more global dementia is usually only evident towards end stage of the disease.

Behavioural, emotional and neuropsychiatric aspects

The neuropsychiatric or behavioural aspects of HD are common and often the most distressing to patients and their families. These changes are not specific to HD, and may primarily be behavioural consequences of underlying pathophysiology affecting the pathways governing emotional and motivational control. However, they may also be a secondary reaction to other changes brought on by HD, or possibly by a complex combination of both factors. Psychological distress may also interact with the patient's circumstances and may indeed be exacerbated by dealing with the stress of genetic testing, diagnosis and symptom onset, symptom progression and loss of function, as well as dealing with uncertainty and the future. This could be particularly relevant for anxiety, and depressive mood, and may in part contribute to the variability in research findings. While the estimates of prevalence vary widely depending on different definitions, measures and patient samples (Paoli et al., 2017), the behavioural changes most commonly associated with HD are depressed mood, apathy, anxiety, irritability/aggression and obsessive compulsive tendencies, with psychosis being relatively rare (Orth et al., 2010; Paulsen, Ready, Hamilton, Mega & Cummings, 2001).

Depressed mood is a commonly reported behavioural change, particularly during the earlier to moderate stages of disease (Dale et al., 2016; van Duijn et al., 2008) including the preclinical phase (Epping et al., 2013), and tends to be less apparent towards the later stages (Kirkwood, Su, Conneally & Foroud, 2001; Paulsen, Nehl, et al., 2005). As this is likely to be treated pharmacologically, there is variability in studies with some reporting no change in depressive mood over time (Thompson et al., 2012). There is some evidence that those aware of the earliest motor symptoms at diagnosis also register lower mood (McCusker et al., 2013). Depression is the best predictor of suicide in HD, which is typically elevated early on prior to clinical diagnosis and in the mid stages when function and independence are reduced (Farrer, 1986; Paulsen, Hoth, Nehl & Stierman, 2005; van Duijn, Vrijmoeth, Giltay, Bernhard Landwehrmeyer & Network, 2018).

Anxiety in the form of a generalised anxiety disorder and panic disorder can occur in the preclinical stage (Julien et al., 2007; Marshall et al., 2007) as well as symptomatic stages. While anxiety has not been found to correspond with disease progression in some studies (Dale et al., 2016), it has been linked to depressive mood (Craufurd et al., 2001) and key disease milestones such as diagnostic testing (Decruyenaere et al.,

2003), the emergence of symptoms close to disease onset (Julien et al., 2007) and progression of symptoms affecting everyday functioning (Paulsen, Nehl, et al., 2005). While the emotional impact of genetic testing for HD is generally found to be minimal in the literature, some studies have indicated that there may be a higher risk for behavioural issues further down the line (Timman, Roos, Maat-Kievit & Tibben, 2004), regardless of test outcome (Decruyenaere et al., 2003).

Apathy, on the other hand, is conceptually different, and independent from depressive mood (Mason & Barker, 2015; Naarding, Janzing, Eling, van der Werf & Kremer, 2009), in that it centres on the lack of drive and engagement. Apathy may be more characteristic of HD, being tightly linked to neural changes progressing in tandem with duration of disease and overall motor disease progression (Craufurd et al., 2001; Tabrizi et al., 2013; Thompson et al., 2012).

Irritability is another key feature of HD and has been found to be increased during the early stages (Thompson et al., 2012). This feature has been associated with aggression and impulsivity, involving the orbitofrontal cortex and amygdala in the limbic circuit (Klöppel et al., 2010). This affects families as they often describe themselves as 'walking on eggshells' around patients who are prone to emotional outbursts and mood swings. Irritability has also been linked with disinhibition (Paulsen et al., 2001). This altered emotional control parallels affected cognitive control, which can manifest in disinhibited and inappropriate behaviour, as well as perseverative behaviour, with patients 'getting stuck' on specific thoughts or actions, and being unusually preoccupied or rigid in their thinking, lacking the ability to let go and move on (Craufurd et al., 2001). Over time, some patients may develop a preference for keeping to set routines and a low tolerance for disruption, where dealing with new or unplanned events can be problematic.

Obsessive compulsive tendencies in HD can occur prior to or after motor onset, and have been reported to occur later on in the illness accompanied by depression and other neuropsychiatric changes (Anderson et al., 2010). Psychotic symptoms comprising delusions and hallucinations are relatively rare in HD and tend to occur towards the latter stages (van Duijn et al., 2014), and may also be related to medication.

Common measures used to monitor neuropsychiatric disturbance in HD include the Beck Depression Inventory (BDI) (Beck, Steer & Brown, 1996; Beck, Ward, Mendelson, Mock & Erbaugh, 1961), Hospital Anxiety and Depressions Scale (HADS) (Zigmond & Snaith, 1983), Apathy Evaluation Scale (AES) (Marin, 1990), Snaith Irritability Scale (SIS) (Snaith, Constantopoulos, Jardine & McGuffin, 1978), Schedule of Compulsions, Obsessions and Pathological Impulses (SCOPI) (Watson & Wu, 2005) as well as several multi-domain HD-specific measures such as the UHDRS behavioural scale (Huntington Study Group, 1996), and Problem Behaviours Assessment (PBA) (Craufurd et al., 2001).

Everyday functioning, care and health-related quality of life

A range of other symptoms can also occur in HD, most notably unintended weight loss which is common and thought to be related to hypermetabolism (Aziz et al.,

2008; Robbins, Ho & Barker, 2006). Autonomic system changes like excessive sweating may be less well-known but again, are not uncommon as there is research showing that presymptomatic and symptomatic individuals report more issues than non-HD controls in gastrointestinal, urinary, cardiovascular and (for men) sexual domains (Aziz, Anguelova, Marinus, Van Dijk & Roos, 2010). Sleep disruption and disintegration of the usual sleep-wake cycle (Morton, 2013) are also common-place and can have a major impact on everyday functioning.

Indeed, the myriad changes associated with HD span the full spectrum of human behaviour and they slowly but inexorably progress over the long course of the dis-ease. Deterioration may not be linear, uniform nor constant (Marder et al., 2000), and there is considerable variability both within and between individuals. The collective impact of these HD related changes on an individual's functional abil-ity is profound. Progressive loss of independence can be felt even early on in the disease as work and lifestyle can be affected, as well as driving (Devos et al., 2014). Over time further changes evolve, firstly in instrumental activities of daily living such as the ability to handle finances and household chores; eventually activities of daily living are compromised as patients need help with personal care. The most commonly used measures of functional ability are from the UHDRS (Huntington Study Group, 1996), specifically the Total Functional Capacity (TFC) score, where individuals are rated from 13 (normal function) to 0 (needing full-time care).

Functional ability and mood are key determinants of health-related quality of life in HD patients (Ho, Gilbert, Mason, Goodman & Barker, 2009). This latter is a patient-reported outcome that provides the overall perspective of the individual with respect to the impact of disease. Due to the heritability, complexity, and multifaceted repercussions of HD, generic health-related quality of life scales are unlikely to capture the full impact of Huntington's (Ho et al., 2004). In a recent review by Mestre et al. (2018), commissioned by the International Movement Disorders Society's Committee on Rating Scale Development, the Huntington's Disease Health-Related Quality of Life (HDQoL) questionnaire (Ho, Horton, Landwehrmeyer, Burgunder & Tennant, in press; Hocaoglu, Gaffan & Ho, 2012) was the key HD specific questionnaire suggested. The HDQoL comes with a parallel version for carers and partners to provide their perspective on the patient (Hocaoglu, Gaffan & Ho, 2012).

The clinical experience of people living with HD as they navigate the health sys-tem is important in terms of how this affects everyday quality of life. Management and care can play an important part in mitigating disease impact as the symptoms of HD can be treated and managed by exploring the full arsenal of existing phar-macological options for individual complaints (Anderson et al., 2018; Schiefer, Werner & Reetz, 2015). While there remains a paucity of non-pharmacological interventions, particularly in the cognitive (Andrews, Domínguez, Mercieca, Georgiou-Karistianis & Stout, 2015) and psychological (Berardelli et al., 2015) domains, early work on multidisciplinary rehabilitation programmes (Zinzi et al., 2007), and particularly on exercise (Fritz et al., 2017) are promising. Further work is needed in non-pharmacological interventions to explore the concept of neuroplasticity in the context of HD and to understand how behavioural and environmental influences might impact symptoms, underlying processes and pathology. Both behavioural and pharmacological approaches have a role to play and can be used in combination to enhance functioning and health-related quality of life.

While there has been limited success in identifying an effective disease modifying therapy for HD thus far, there is growing optimism with an increasing number of laboratory studies and clinical trials. In addition to pharmacological research, there is promise in Huntingtin protein lowering approaches such as gene editing, which aims to provide neuroprotection by intervening upstream to prevent the activation of pathology in the first place (Kieburtz, Reilmann & Olanow, 2018). As the momentum of HD-relevant research continues to increase, there is good reason to hope that this will transform the future of care, treatment, and the lives of countless individuals living with the presence or risk of HD, as well as their families.

Concluding remarks

Returning to the vignette of Marielle, a few years on from her father's funeral, she soldiers on, dealing with her daily life while keeping up with scientific developments in HD as she watches and waits for what could be a clear indication of chorea – there are days when she wonders if this has already occurred, with her increasingly erratic movements. In addition to keeping a watchful eye on the latest scientific developments, she has also told her family and close friends, and has decided to take steps to get connected with the HD community. She now proactively seeks to take part in research studies and clinical trials as she tries to carve out a life on her own terms while waiting and hoping for a 'cure', if not for her then perhaps for her son, should this eventually be needed for him. She prioritises exercising regularly in order to do what she can to try to delay the effects of her increasingly compromised neurophysiology, and tries not to dwell too much on how badly affected her uncles are now. We leave her feeling just a little more accepting of life at present, even though she does not want to look too far into the future, and instead keeps herself busy living one day at a time, trying not to see HD every time she gazes at her young son.

HD is a life-changing disease on many different levels. In fact, the mere presence of HD in the family, rendering an individual at risk of this disease is in itself life-changing, not to mention the repercussions of having a parent, and possibly other family members affected by the disease. The consequences of a long-term multi-system brain disorder on a single individual cannot in reality be neatly parcelled into the motor, cognitive and behavioural categories, which are useful in clinical care and research. These seemingly discrete manifestations of disease will impact and influence related aspects of disease, and interact with the backdrop of personal history as they are played out on the real-world stage of a person's evolving everyday life. We see in the vignette, a glimpse of the multi-generational burden shouldered by patients and their families, as they live with the shadow of HD, and so it behoves us to progress both scientific research and clinical care innovations, as the emergence of new behavioural interventions and disease modifying treatments cannot come soon enough.

Abbreviations

AES	Apathy Evaluation Scale
BDI	Beck Depression Inventory
BG	basal ganglia
CAG	cytosine-adenine-guanine
FAB	frontal assessment battery
FDG-PET	fluorodeoxyglucose-positron emission tomography
fMRI	functional magnetic resonance imaging
GABA	gamma-aminobutyric acid
HADS	Hospital Anxiety and Depressions Scale
HD	Huntington's disease
HD-CAB	Huntington's Disease Cognitive Assessment Battery
HDQoL	Huntington's Disease Health-Related Quality of Life questionnaire
HTT	huntingtin gene
MMSE	Mini Mental State Examination
MoCA	Montreal Cognitive Assessment
MRS	magnetic resonance spectroscopy
PBA	Problem Behaviours Assessment
RBANS	Repeatable Battery for the Assessment of Neuropsychological Status
SCOPI	Schedule of Compulsions, Obsessions and Pathological Impulses
SDMT	Symbol Digit Modalities Task
SIS	Snaith Irritability Scale
TFC	total functional capacity
UHDRS	Unified Huntington's Disease Rating Scale

Further reading

Dumas, E. M., van den Bogaard, S. J. A., Middelkoop, H. A. M. & Roos, R. A. C. (2013). A review of cognition in Huntington's disease. *Frontiers in Bioscience (Scholar edition)*, *5*, 1–18. Retrieved from http://europepmc.org/abstract/MED/23277034. doi:10.2741/S355

McColgan, P. & Tabrizi, S. J. (2018). Huntington's disease: A clinical review. *European Journal of Neurology*, *25*(1), 24–34. doi:10.1111/ene.13413

Nance, M. A. (2017). Genetic counseling and testing for Huntington's disease: A historical review. *American Journal of Medical Genetics Part B: Neuropsychiatric Genetics*, *174*(1), 75–92. doi:10.1002/ajmg.b.32453

Nance, M. A. & Myers, R. H. (2001). Juvenile-onset Huntington's disease – clinical and research perspectives. *Mental Retardation and Developmental Disabilities Research Reviews*, *7*(3), 153–157. doi:10.1002/mrdd.1022

Paoli, R. A., Botturi, A., Ciammola, A., Silani, V., Prunas, C., Lucchiari, C., . . . Caletti, E. (2017). Neuropsychiatric burden in Huntington's disease. *Brain Sciences*, 7(6). pii: E67. doi: 10.3390/brainsci7060067

Papp, K. V., Kaplan, R. F. & Snyder, P. J. (2011). Biological markers of cognition in prodromal Huntington's disease: A review. *Brain Cognition*, 77(2), 280–291. doi:S0278-2626(11)00126-6

References

Alexander, G. E. & Crutcher, M. D. (1990). Preparation for movement: Neural representations of intended direction in three motor areas of the monkey. *Journal of Neurophysiology*, 64(1), 133–150.

Anderson, K. E., Gehl, C. R., Marder, K. S., Beglinger, L. J., Paulsen, J. S. & Huntington's Study Group (2010). Comorbidities of obsessive and compulsive symptoms in Huntington's disease. *The Journal of Nervous and Mental Disease*, 198(5), 334–338. doi:10.1097/NMD.0b013e3181da852a

Anderson, K. E., van Duijn, E., Craufurd, D., Drazinic, C., Edmondson, M., Goodman, N., . . . Goodman, L. V. (2018). Clinical management of neuropsychiatric symptoms of Huntington disease: Expert-based consensus guidelines on agitation, anxiety, apathy, psychosis and sleep disorders. *Journal of Huntington's Disease*, 7(3), 239–250. doi:10.3233/jhd-180293

Andrews, S. C., Domínguez, J. F., Mercieca, E.-C., Georgiou-Karistianis, N. & Stout, J. C. (2015). Cognitive interventions to enhance neural compensation in Huntington's disease. *Neurodegenerative Disease Management*, 5(2), 155–164. doi:10.2217/nmt.14.58

Antoniades, C. A., Xu, Z., Mason, S. L., Carpenter, R. H. S. & Barker, R. A. (2010). Huntington's disease: Changes in saccades and hand-tapping over 3 years. *Journal of Neurology*, 257(11), 1890–1898. doi:10.1007/s00415-010-5632-2

Aylward, E. H., Sparks, B. F., Field, K. M., Yallapragada, V., Shpritz, B. D., Rosenblatt, A., . . . Ross, C. A. (2004). Onset and rate of striatal atrophy in preclinical Huntington disease. *Neurology*, 63(1), 66–72. doi:10.1212/01.wnl.0000132965.14653.d1

Aziz, N. A., Anguelova, G. V., Marinus, J., Van Dijk, J. G. & Roos, R. A. C. (2010). Autonomic symptoms in patients and pre-manifest mutation carriers of Huntington's disease. *European Journal of Neurology*, 17(8), 1068–1074. doi:10.1111/j.1468-1331. 2010.02973.x

Aziz, N. A., van der Burg, J. M., Landwehrmeyer, G. B., Brundin, P., Stijnen, T. & Roos, R. A. (2008). Weight loss in Huntington disease increases with higher CAG repeat number. *Neurology*, 71(19), 1506–1513.

Bachoud-Levi, A. C., Maison, P., Bartolomeo, P., Boisse, M. F., Dalla Barba, G., Ergis, A. M., . . . Peschanski, M. (2001). Retest effects and cognitive decline in longitudinal follow-up of patients with early HD. *Neurology*, 56(8), 1052–1058.

Baig, S. S., Strong, M., Rosser, E., Taverner, N. V., Glew, R., Miedzybrodzka, Z., . . . Quarrell, O. W. (2016). 22 years of predictive testing for Huntington's disease: The experience of the UK Huntington's Prediction Consortium. *European Journal of Human Genetics*, 24(10), 1396–1402. doi:10.1038/ejhg.2016.36

Beck, A. T., Steer, R. & Brown, G. (1996). *BDI-11 Manual*. San Antonio, TX: The Psychological Corporation.

Beck, A. T., Ward, C. H., Mendelson, M., Mock, J. & Erbaugh, J. (1961). An inventory for measuring depression. *Archives of General Psychiatry*, 4, 561–571.

Beglinger, L. J., Duff, K., Allison, J., Theriault, D., O'Rourke, J. J., Leserman, A. & Paulsen, J. S. (2010). Cognitive change in patients with Huntington disease on the

Repeatable Battery for the Assessment of Neuropsychological Status. *Journal of Clinical and Experimental Neuropsychology, 32*(6), 573–578. doi:10.1080/13803390903313564

Benton, A. (1968). Differential behavioural effects in frontal lobe disease. *Neuropsychologia, 6*, 53–60.

Berardelli, I., Pasquini, M., Roselli, V., Biondi, M., Berardelli, A. & Fabbrini, G. (2015). Cognitive behavioral therapy in movement disorders: A review. *Movement Disorders Clinical Practice, 2*(2), 107–115.

Beste, C., Stock, A.-K., Ness, V., Hoffmann, R., Lukas, C. & Saft, C. (2013). A novel cognitive-neurophysiological state biomarker in premanifest Huntington's disease validated on longitudinal data. *Scientific Reports, 3*, 1797. doi:10.1038/srep01797

Bonner-Jackson, A., Long, J. D., Westervelt, H., Tremont, G., Aylward, E., Paulsen, J. S., . . . Coordinators of the Huntington Study Group (2013). Cognitive reserve and brain reserve in prodromal Huntington's disease. *Journal of the International Neuropsychological Society: JINS, 19*(7), 739–750. doi:10.1017/S1355617713000507

Bradshaw, J. L., Phillips, J. G., Dennis, C., Mattingley, J. B., Andrewes, D., Chiu, E., . . . Bradshaw, J. A. (1992). Initiation and execution of movement sequences in those suffering from and at-risk of developing Huntington's disease. *Journal of Clinical and Experimental Neuropsychology, 14*(2), 179–192. doi:10.1080/01688639208402822

Brandt, J. (1991). The Hopkins Verbal Learning Test: Development of a new memory test with six equivalent forms. *Clinical Neuropsychology, 5*, 125–142.

Brewer, H. M., Eatough, V., Smith, J. A., Stanley, C. A., Glendinning, N. W. & Quarrell, O. W. (2008). The impact of juvenile Huntington's disease on the family: The case of a rare childhood condition. *Journal of Health Psychology, 13*(1), 5–16.

Brune, M., Blank, K., Witthaus, H. & Saft, C. (2011). 'Theory of mind' is impaired in Huntington's disease. *Movement Disorders, 26*(4), 671–678. doi:10.1002/mds.23494

Butters, N., Granholm, E., Salmon, D. P., Grant, I. & Wolfe, J. (1987). Episodic and semantic memory: A comparison of amnesic and demented patients. *Journal of Clinical and Experimental Neuropsychology, 9*(5), 479–497.

Byrne, L. M., Rodrigues, F. B., Blennow, K., Durr, A., Leavitt, B. R., Roos, R. A. C., . . . Wild, E. J. (2017). Neurofilament light protein in blood as a potential biomarker of neurodegeneration in Huntington's disease: A retrospective cohort analysis. *The Lancet Neurology, 16*(8), 601–609. doi:10.1016/S1474-4422(17)30124-2

Chenery, H. J., Copland, D. A. & Murdoch, B. E. (2002). Complex language functions and subcortical mechanisms: Evidence from Huntington's disease and patients with non-thalamic subcortical lesions. *International Journal of Language and Communication Disorders, 37*(4), 459–474.

Coppen, E. M., van der Grond, J., Hart, E. P., Lakke, E. A. J. F. & Roos, R. A. C. (2018). The visual cortex and visual cognition in Huntington's disease: An overview of current literature. *Behavioural Brain Research, 351*, 63–74. doi:10.1016/j.bbr.2018.05.019

Craufurd, D., Thompson, J. C. & Snowden, J. S. (2001). Behavioural changes in Huntington disease. *Neuropsychiatry Neuropsychology and Behavioral Neurology, 14*(4), 219–226.

Dale, M., Maltby, J., Shimozaki, S., Cramp, R., Rickards, H. & REGISTRY investigators of the European Huntington's Disease Network (2016). Disease stage, but not sex, predicts depression and psychological distress in Huntington's disease: A European population study. *Journal of Psychosomatic Research, 80*, 17–22. doi:10.1016/j.jpsychores.2015.11.003

Decruyenaere, M., Evers-Kiebooms, G., Cloostermans, T., Boogaerts, A., Demyttenaere, K., Dom, R. & Fryns, J. P. (2003). Psychological distress in the 5-year period after predictive testing for Huntington's disease. *European Journal of Human Genetics, 11*(1), 30–38.

Devos, H., Nieuwboer, A., Vandenberghe, W., Tant, M., De Weerdt, W. & Uc, E. Y. (2014). On-road driving impairments in Huntington disease. *Neurology, 82*(11), 956–962. doi:10.1212/wnl.0000000000000220

Dubois, B., Slachevsky, A., Litvan, I. & Pillon, B. (2000). The FAB: A Frontal Assessment Battery at bedside. *Neurology, 55*(11), 1621–1626.

Duff, K., Paulsen, J., Mills, J., Beglinger, L. J., Moser, D. J., Smith, M. M., . . . Harrington, D. L. (2010a). Mild cognitive impairment in prediagnosed Huntington disease. *Neurology, 75*(6), 500–507.

Duff, K., Paulsen, J. S., Beglinger, L. J., Langbehn, D. R., Wang, C., Stout, J. C., . . . Predict-HD Investigators of the Huntington Study Group (2010b). 'Frontal' behaviors before the diagnosis of Huntington's disease and their relationship to markers of disease progression: Evidence of early lack of awareness. *The Journal of Neuropsychiatry and Clinical Neurosciences, 22*(2), 196–207. doi:10.1176/jnp.2010.22.2.196

Dumas, E. M., van den Bogaard, S. J. A., Hart, E. P., Soeter, R. P., van Buchem, M. A., van der Grond, J., . . . Roos, R. A. C. (2013). Reduced functional brain connectivity prior to and after disease onset in Huntington's disease. *NeuroImage: Clinical, 2*, 377–384. doi:10.1016/j.nicl.2013.03.001

Eddy, C. M. & Rickards, H. E. (2015). Interaction without intent: The shape of the social world in Huntington's disease. *Social Cognitive and Affective Neuroscience, 10*(9), 1228–1235. doi:10.1093/scan/nsv012

Epping, E. A., Mills, J. A., Beglinger, L. J., Fiedorowicz, J. G., Craufurd, D., Smith, M. M., . . . Paulsen, J. S. (2013). Characterization of depression in prodromal Huntington disease in the neurobiological predictors of HD (PREDICT-HD) study. *Journal of Psychiatric Research, 47*(10), 1423–1431. doi:10.1016/j.jpsychires.2013.05.026

Farrer, L. A. (1986). Suicide and attempted suicide in Huntington disease: Implications for preclinical testing of persons at risk. *American Journal of Medical Genetics, 24*(2), 305–311. doi:10.1002/ajmg.1320240211

Fisher, E. R. & Hayden, M. R. (2014). Multisource ascertainment of Huntington disease in Canada: Prevalence and population at risk. *Movement Disorders, 29*(1), 105–114. doi:10.1002/mds.25717

Folstein, M. F., Folstein, S. E. & McHugh, P. R. (1975). 'Mini-mental state': A practical method for grading the cognitive state of patients for the clinician. *Journal of Psychiatric Research, 12*(3), 189–198.

Fritz, N. E., Rao, A. K., Kegelmeyer, D., Kloos, A., Busse, M., Hartel, L., . . . Quinn, L. (2017). Physical therapy and exercise interventions in Huntington's disease: A mixed methods systematic review. *Journal of Huntington's Disease, 6*(3), 217–235.

Garcia-Gorro, C., de Diego-Balaguer, R., Martínez-Horta, S., Pérez-Pérez, J., Kulisevsky, J., Rodríguez-Dechicha, N., . . . Camara, E. (2018). Reduced striato-cortical and inhibitory transcallosal connectivity in the motor circuit of Huntington's disease patients. *Human Brain Mapping, 39*(1), 54–71. doi:10.1002/hbm.23813

Georgiou, N., Bradshaw, J. L., Chiu, E., Tudor, A., O'Gorman, L. & Phillips, J. G. (1999). Differential clinical and motor control function in a pair of monozygotic twins with Huntington's disease. *Movement Disorders, 14*(2), 320–325. doi:10.1002/1531-8257(199903)14:2<320::aid-mds1018>3.0.co;2-z

Georgiou, N., Phillips, J. G., Bradshaw, J. L., Cunnington, R. & Chiu, E. (1997). Impairments of movement kinematics in patients with Huntington's disease: A comparison with and without a concurrent task. *Movement Disorders, 12*(3), 386–396.

Georgiou-Karistianis, N., Scahill, R., Tabrizi, S. J., Squitieri, F. & Aylward, E. (2013). Structural MRI in Huntington's disease and recommendations for its potential use in clinical trials. *Neuroscience & Biobehavioral Reviews, 37*(3), 480–490. doi:10.1016/j. neubiorev.2013.01.022

Goh, A. M. Y., You, E., Perin, S., Clay, F. J., Loi, S., Ellis, K., . . . Lautenschlager, N. (2018). Predictors of workplace disability in a premanifest Huntington's disease cohort. *The Journal of Neuropsychiatry and Clinical Neurosciences, 30*(2), 115–121. doi:10.1176/ appi.neuropsych.17040086

Goldberg, Y. P., Kremer, B., Andrew, S. E., Theilmann, J., Graham, R. K., Squitieri, F., . . . Hayden, M. R. (1993). Molecular analysis of new mutations for Huntington's disease: Intermediate alleles and sex of origin effects. *Nature Genetics, 5,* 174. doi:10.1038/ ng1093-174

Gray, M. A., Egan, G. F., Ando, A., Churchyard, A., Chua, P., Stout, J. C. & Georgiou-Karistianis, N. (2013). Prefrontal activity in Huntington's disease reflects cognitive and neuropsychiatric disturbances: The IMAGE-HD study. *Experimental Neurology, 239,* 218–228. doi:10.1016/j.expneurol.2012.10.020

Gusella, J. F. & MacDonald, M. E. (2006). Huntington's disease: Seeing the pathogenic process through a genetic lens. *Trends in Biochemical Sciences, 31*(9), 533–540. doi:10.1016/j. tibs.2006.06.009

Hamilton, A., Heemskerk, A.-W., Loucas, M., Twiston-Davies, R., Matheson, K. Y., Simpson, S. A. & Rae, D. (2012). Oral feeding in Huntington's disease: A guideline document for speech and language therapists. *Neurodegenerative Disease Management, 2*(1), 45–53. doi:10.2217/nmt.11.77

Harper, P. S. (1992). The epidemiology of Huntington's disease. *Human Genetics, 89*(4), 365–376. doi:10.1007/bf00194305

Harris, G. J., Pearlson, G. D., Peyser, C. E., Aylward, E. H., Roberts, J., Barta, P. E., . . . Folstein, S. E. (1992). Putamen volume reduction on magnetic resonance imaging exceeds caudate changes in mild Huntington's disease. *Annals of Neurology, 31*(1), 69–75.

Hart, E. P., Dumas, E. M., Zwet, E. W., Hiele, K., Jurgens, C. K., Middelkoop, H. A. M., . . . Roos, R. A. C. (2015). Longitudinal pilot-study of Sustained Attention to Response Task and P300 in manifest and pre-manifest Huntington's disease. *Journal of Neuropsychology, 9*(1), 10–20. doi:10.1111/jnp.12031

Hayes, C. J., Stevenson, R. J. & Coltheart, M. (2007). Disgust and Huntington's disease. *Neuropsychologia, 45*(6), 1135–1151. doi:10.1016/j.neuropsychologia.2006.10.015

Ho, A. K., Gilbert, A. S., Mason, S. L., Goodman, A. O. & Barker, R. A. (2009). Health-related quality of life in Huntington's disease: Which factors matter most? *Movement Disorders, 24*(4), 574–578. doi:10.1002/mds.22412

Ho, A. K., Horton, M. C., Landwehrmeyer, G. B., Burgunder, J. M. & Tennant, A. (in press). Meaningful and measurable health domains in Huntington's: Large-scale validation of the Huntington's Disease health-related Quality of Life questionnaire (HDQoL) across severity stages. *Value in Health.*

Ho, A. K., Robbins, A. O. & Barker, R. A. (2006). Huntington's disease patients have selective problems with insight. *Movement Disorders, 21*(3), 385–389.

Ho, A. K., Robbins, A. O., Walters, S. J., Kaptoge, S., Sahakian, B. J. & Barker, R. A. (2004). Health-related quality of life in Huntington's disease: A comparison of two generic instruments, SF-36 and SIP. *Movement Disorders, 19*(11), 1341–1348.

Ho, A. K., Sahakian, B. J., Brown, R. G., Barker, R. A., Hodges, J. R., Ane, M. N., . . . Bodner, T. (2003). Profile of cognitive progression in early Huntington's disease. *Neurology, 61*(12), 1702–1706.

Ho, A. K., Sahakian, B. J., Robbins, T. W., Barker, R. A., Rosser, A. E. & Hodges, J. R. (2002). Verbal fluency in Huntington's disease: A longitudinal analysis of phonemic and semantic clustering and switching. *Neuropsychologia, 40*(8), 1277–1284.

Hocaoglu, M., Gaffan, E. & Ho, A. (2012). Health-related quality of life in Huntington's disease patients: A comparison of proxy assessment and patient self-rating using the disease-specific Huntington's disease health-related quality of life questionnaire (HDQoL). *Journal of Neurology, 259*(9), 1793–1800. doi:10.1007/s00415-011-6405-2

Hocaoglu, M. B., Gaffan, E. A. & Ho, A. K. (2012). The Huntington's Disease health-related Quality of Life questionnaire (HDQoL): A disease-specific measure of health-related quality of life. *Clinical Genetics, 81*(2), 117–122. doi:10.1111/j.1399-0004.2011.01823.x

Hoth, K. F., Paulsen, J. S., Moser, D. J., Tranel, D., Clark, L. A. & Bechara, A. (2007). Patients with Huntington's disease have impaired awareness of cognitive, emotional, and functional abilities. *Journal of Clinical and Experimental Neuropsychology, 29*(4), 365–376.

Huntington Study Group. (1996). Unified Huntington's disease rating scale: Reliability and consistency. *Movement Disorders, 11*(2), 136–142.

Julien, C. L., Thompson, J. C., Wild, S., Yardumian, P., Snowden, J. S., Turner, G. & Craufurd, D. (2007). Psychiatric disorders in preclinical Huntington's disease. *Journal of Neurology Neurosurgery and Psychiatry, 78*(9), 939–943. doi:10.1136/jnnp.2006.103309

Kagel, M. C. & Leopold, N. A. (1992). Dysphagia in Huntington's disease: A 16-year retrospective. *Dysphagia, 7*(2), 106–114.

Kieburtz, K., Reilmann, R. & Olanow, C. W. (2018). Huntington's disease: Current and future therapeutic prospects. *Movement Disorders, 33*(7), 1033–1041. doi:10.1002/mds.27363

Kirkwood, S. C., Siemers, E., Bond, C., Conneally, P. M., Christian, J. C. & Foroud, T. (2000). Confirmation of subtle motor changes among presymptomatic carriers of the Huntington disease gene. *Archives of Neurology, 57*(7), 1040–1044.

Kirkwood, S. C., Siemers, E., Stout, J. C., Hodes, M. E., Conneally, P. M., Christian, J. C. & Foroud, T. (1999). Longitudinal cognitive and motor changes among presymptomatic Huntington disease gene carriers. *Archives of Neurology, 56*(5), 563–568. doi:10.1001/archneur.56.5.563

Kirkwood, S. C., Su, J. L., Conneally, P. & Foroud, T. (2001). Progression of symptoms in the early and middle stages of Huntington disease. *Archives of Neurology, 58*(2), 273–278. doi:10.1001/archneur.58.2.273

Klöppel, S., Stonnington, C. M., Petrovic, P., Mobbs, D., Tüscher, O., Craufurd, D., . . . Frackowiak, R. S. J. (2010). Irritability in pre-clinical Huntington's disease. *Neuropsychologia, 48*(2), 549–557. doi:10.1016/j.neuropsychologia.2009.10.016

Lawrence, A. D., Hodges, J. R., Rosser, A. E., Kershaw, A., Ffrench-Constant, C., Rubinsztein, D. C., . . . Sahakian, B. J. (1998). Evidence for specific cognitive deficits in preclinical Huntington's disease. *Brain, 121*(Pt 7), 1329–1341.

Lawrence, A. D., Sahakian, B. J., Hodges, J. R., Rosser, A. E., Lange, K. W. & Robbins, T. W. (1996). Executive and mnemonic functions in early Huntington's disease. *Brain, 119* (Pt 5), 1633–1645.

Lawrence, A. D., Watkins, L. H., Sahakian, B. J., Hodges, J. R. & Robbins, T. W. (2000). Visual object and visuospatial cognition in Huntington's disease: Implications for information processing in corticostriatal circuits. *Brain, 123*(Pt 7), 1349–1364. doi:10.1093/brain/123.7.1349

Lee, J.-M., Wheeler, Vanessa C., Chao, Michael J., Vonsattel, Jean Paul G., Pinto, Ricardo M., Lucente, D., . . . Myers, Richard H. (2015). Identification of genetic factors that modify clinical onset of Huntington's disease. *Cell, 162*(3), 516–526. doi:10.1016/j.cell.2015.07.003

Lehéricy, S., Ducros, M., Van De Moortele, P. F., Francois, C., Thivard, L., Poupon, C., ... Kim, D. S. (2004). Diffusion tensor fiber tracking shows distinct corticostriatal circuits in humans. *Annals of Neurology, 55*(4), 522–529. doi:10.1002/ana.20030

Leigh, R. J., Newman, S. A., Folstein, S. E., Lasker, A. G. & Jensen, B. A. (1983). Abnormal ocular motor control in Huntington's disease. *Neurology, 33*(10), 1268–1268.

Long, J. D., Langbehn, D. R., Tabrizi, S. J., Landwehrmeyer, B. G., Paulsen, J. S., Warner, J. & Sampaio, C. (2016). Validation of a prognostic index for Huntington's disease. *Movement Disorders, 32*(2), 256–263. doi:10.1002/mds.26838

Louis, E. D., Lee, P., Quinn, L. & Marder, K. (1999). Dystonia in Huntington's disease: Prevalence and clinical characteristics. *Movement Disorders, 14*(1), 95–101. doi:10.1002/1531-8257(199901)14:1<95::AID-MDS1016>3.0.CO;2-8

Ludlow, C. L., Connor, N. P. & Bassich, C. J. (1987). Speech timing in Parkinson's and Huntington's disease. *Brain and Language, 32*(2), 195–214.

MacDonald, M. E., Ambrose, C. M., Duyao, M. P., Myers, R. H., Lin, C., Srinidhi, L., ... Harper, P. S. (1993). A novel gene containing a trinucleotide repeat that is expanded and unstable on Huntington's disease chromosomes. *Cell, 72*(6), 971–983. doi:10.1016/0092-8674(93)90585-E

MacLeod, R., Tibben, A., Frontali, M., Evers-Kiebooms, G., Jones, A., Martinez-Descales, A. & Roos, R. (2013). Recommendations for the predictive genetic test in Huntington's disease. *Clinical Genetics, 83*(3), 221–231.

Marder, K., Zhao, H., Myers, R. H., Cudkowicz, M., Kayson, E., Kieburtz, K., ... Shoulson, I. (2000). Rate of functional decline in Huntington's disease. Huntington Study Group. *Neurology, 54*(2), 452–458.

Marin, R. S. (1990). Differential diagnosis and classification of apathy. *The American Journal of Psychiatry, 147*(1), 22–30. doi:10.1176/ajp.147.1.22

Marshall, J., White, K., Weaver, M., Flury Wetherill, L., Hui, S., Stout, J. C., ... Foroud, T. (2007). Specific psychiatric manifestations among preclinical Huntington disease mutation carriers. *Archives of Neurology, 64*(1), 116–121. doi:10.1001/archneur.64.1.116

Mason, S. & Barker, R. A. (2015). Rating apathy in Huntington's disease: Patients and companions agree. *Journal of Huntington's Disease, 4*(1), 49–59.

McCusker, E. A., Gunn, D. G., Epping, E. A., Loy, C. T., Radford, K., Griffith, J., ... Paulsen, J. S. (2013). Unawareness of motor phenoconversion in Huntington disease. *Neurology, 81*(13), 1141–1147. doi:10.1212/WNL.0b013e3182a55f05

McCusker, E. A. & Loy, C. T. (2017). Huntington disease: The complexities of making and disclosing a clinical diagnosis after premanifest genetic testing. *Tremor and Other Hyperkinetic Movements (New York, NY), 7*, 467. Retrieved from http://europepmc.org/abstract/MED/28975045 doi:10.7916/D8PK0TDD

Mehrabi, N., Singh-Bains, M., Waldvogel, H. & Faull, R. (2016). Cortico-basal ganglia interactions in Huntington's disease. *Annals of Neurodegenerative Disorders, 1*(2), 1007.

Mehrabi, N. F., Waldvogel, H. J., Tippett, L. J., Hogg, V. M., Synek, B. J. & Faull, R. L. M. (2016). Symptom heterogeneity in Huntington's disease correlates with neuronal degeneration in the cerebral cortex. *Neurobiology of Disease, 96*, 67–74. doi:10.1016/j.nbd.2016.08.015

Mestre, T. A., Carlozzi, N. E., Ho, A. K., Burgunder, J. M., Walker, F., Davis, A. M., ... Sampaio, C. (2018). Quality of life in Huntington's disease: Critique and recommendations for measures assessing patient health-related quality of life and caregiver quality of life. *Movement Disorders, 33*(5), 742–749.

Mickes, L., Jacobson, M., Peavy, G., Wixted, J. T., Lessig, S., Goldstein, J. L. & Corey-Bloom, J. (2010). A comparison of two brief screening measures of cognitive impairment in Huntington's disease. *Movement Disorders, 25*(13), 2229–2233. doi:10.1002/mds.23181

Mitchell, I. J., Heims, H., Neville, E. A. & Rickards, H. (2005). Huntington's disease patients show impaired perception of disgust in the gustatory and olfactory modalities. *The Journal of Neuropsychiatry and Clinical Neurosciences, 17*(1), 119–121. doi:10.1176/appi.neuropsych.17.1.119

Moberg, P. J., Pearlson, G. D., Speedie, L. J., Lipsey, J. R., Strauss, M. E. & Folstein, S. E. (1987). Olfactory recognition: Differential impairments in early and late Huntington's and Alzheimer's diseases. *Journal of Clinical and Experimental Neuropsychology, 9*(6), 650–664. doi:10.1080/01688638708405208

Morton, A. J. (2013). Circadian and sleep disorder in Huntington's disease. *Experimental Neurology, 243*, 34–44. doi:10.1016/j.expneurol.2012.10.014

Murray, L. L. (2000). Spoken language production in Huntington's and Parkinson's diseases. *Journal of Speech Language and Hearing Research, 43*(6), 1350–1366.

Naarding, P., Janzing, J. G. E., Eling, P., van der Werf, S. & Kremer, B. (2009). Apathy is not depression in Huntington's disease. *The Journal of Neuropsychiatry and Clinical Neurosciences, 21*(3), 266–270. doi:10.1176/jnp.2009.21.3.266

Nambu, A., Tokuno, H. & Takada, M. (2002). Functional significance of the cortico-subthalamo-pallidal 'hyperdirect' pathway. *Neuroscience Research, 43*(2), 111–117. doi:10.1016/S0168-0102(02)00027-5

Nance, M. A. (2017). Genetic counseling and testing for Huntington's disease: A historical review. *American Journal of Medical Genetics Part B: Neuropsychiatric Genetics, 174*(1), 75–92. doi:10.1002/ajmg.b.32453

Nance, M. A. & Myers, R. H. (2001). Juvenile-onset Huntington's disease – clinical and research perspectives. *Mental Retardation and Developmental Disabilities Research Reviews, 7*(3), 153–157. doi:10.1002/mrdd.1022

Nasreddine, Z. S., Phillips, N. A., Bédirian, V., Charbonneau, S., Whitehead, V., Collin, I., . . . Chertkow, H. (2005). The Montreal Cognitive Assessment, MoCA: A brief screening tool for mild cognitive impairment. *Journal of the American Geriatrics Society, 53*(4), 695–699.

Nguyen, L., Bradshaw, J. L., Stout, J. C., Croft, R. J. & Georgiou-Karistianis, N. (2010). Electrophysiological measures as potential biomarkers in Huntington's disease: Review and future directions. *Brain Research Reviews, 64*(1), 177–194. doi:10.1016/j.brainresrev.2010.03.004

Odish, O. F. F., Caeyenberghs, K., Hosseini, H., van den Bogaard, S. J. A., Roos, R. A. C. & Leemans, A. (2015). Dynamics of the connectome in Huntington's disease: A longitudinal diffusion MRI study. *NeuroImage: Clinical, 9*, 32–43. doi:10.1016/j.nicl.2015.07.003

Orth, M., Handley, O. J., Schwenke, C., Dunnett, S. B., Craufurd, D., Ho, A. K., . . . Landwehrmeyer, G. B. (2010). Observing Huntington's disease: The European Huntington's Disease Network's registry. *PLoS Curr, 2*. doi:10.1371/currents.RRN1184

Paoli, R. A., Botturi, A., Ciammola, A., Silani, V., Prunas, C., Lucchiari, C., . . . Caletti, E. (2017). Neuropsychiatric burden in Huntington's disease. *Brain Sciences, 7*(6). pii: E67. doi: 10.3390/brainsci7060067.

Papoutsi, M., Labuschagne, I., Tabrizi, S. J. & Stout, J. C. (2014). The cognitive burden in Huntington's disease: Pathology, phenotype, and mechanisms of compensation. *Movement Disorders, 29*(5), 673–683. doi:10.1002/mds.25864

Patrick, D. L., Curtis, J. R., Engelberg, R. A., Nielsen, E. & McCown, E. (2003). Measuring and improving the quality of dying and death. *Ann Intern Med, 139*(5 Pt 2), 410–415.

Paulsen, J. S. (2009). Functional imaging in Huntington's disease. *Experimental Neurology, 216*(2), 272–277.

Paulsen, J. S., Hoth, K. F., Nehl, C. & Stierman, L. (2005). Critical periods of suicide risk in Huntington's disease. *American Journal of Psychiatry, 162*(4), 725–731.

Paulsen, J. S., Langbehn, D. R., Stout, J. C., Aylward, E., Ross, C. A., Nance, M., . . . Hayden, M. (2007). Detection of Huntington's disease decades before diagnosis: The Predict HD study. *Journal of Neurology Neurosurgery and Psychiatry*, *79*(8), 874–880.

Paulsen, J. S. & Long, J. D. (2014). Onset of Huntington's disease: Can it be purely cognitive? *Movement Disorders*, *29*(11), 1342–1350. doi:10.1002/mds.25997

Paulsen, J. S., Nehl, C., Hoth, K. F., Kanz, J. E., Benjamin, M., Conybeare, R., . . . Turner, B. (2005). Depression and stages of Huntington's disease. *Journal of Neuropsychiatry and Clinical Neuroscience*, *17*(4), 496–502.

Paulsen, J. S., Nopoulos, P. C., Aylward, E., Ross, C. A., Johnson, H., Magnotta, V. A., . . . Nance, M. (2010). Striatal and white matter predictors of estimated diagnosis for Huntington disease. *Brain Research Bulletin*, *82*(3), 201–207. doi:10.1016/j.brainresbull. 2010.04.003

Paulsen, J. S., Ready, R. E., Hamilton, J. M., Mega, M. S. & Cummings, J. L. (2001). Neuropsychiatric aspects of Huntington's disease. *Journal of Neurology Neurosurgery and Psychiatry*, *71*(3), 310–314.

Pavese, N., Andrews, T. C., Brooks, D. J., Ho, A. K., Rosser, A. E., Barker, R. A., . . . Piccini, P. (2003). Progressive striatal and cortical dopamine receptor dysfunction in Huntington's disease: A PET study. *Brain*, *126*(Pt 5), 1127–1135.

Pavese, N., Gerhard, A., Tai, Y. F., Ho, A. K., Turkheimer, F., Barker, R. A., . . . Piccini, P. (2006). Microglial activation correlates with severity in Huntington disease: A clinical and PET study. *Neurology*, *66*(11), 1638–1643.

Penney, J. B., Vonsattel, J.-P., Macdonald, M. E., Gusella, J. F. & Myers, R. H. (1997). CAG repeat number governs the development rate of pathology in Huntington's disease. *Annals of Neurology*, *41*(5), 689–692. doi:10.1002/ana.410410521

Podoll, K., Caspary, P., Lange, H. W. & Noth, J. (1988). Language functions in Huntington's disease. *Brain*, *111*(Pt 6), 1475–1503.

Poudel, G. R., Stout, J. C., Domínguez D. J. F., Gray, M. A., Salmon, L., Churchyard, A., . . . Georgiou-Karistianis, N. (2015). Functional changes during working memory in Huntington's disease: 30-month longitudinal data from the IMAGE-HD study. *Brain Structure and Function*, *220*(1), 501–512. doi:10.1007/s00429-013-0670-z

Quarrell, O. W., Clarke, A. J., Compton, C., de Die-Smulders Christine, E. M., Fryer, A., Jenkins, S., . . . Bijlsma, E. K. (2018). Predictive testing of minors for Huntington's disease: The UK and Netherlands experiences. *American Journal of Medical Genetics Part B: Neuropsychiatric Genetics*, *177*(1), 35–39. doi:10.1002/ajmg.b.32582

Quarrell, O. W. J., Rigby, A. S., Barron, L., Crow, Y., Dalton, A., Dennis, N., . . . Warner, J. (2007). Reduced penetrance alleles for Huntington's disease: A multi-centre direct observational study. *Journal of Medical Genetics*, *44*(3), e68–e68. doi:10.1136/jmg.2006.045120

Randolph, C., Tierney, M. C., Mohr, E. & Chase, T. N. (1998). The Repeatable Battery for the Assessment of Neuropsychological Status (RBANS): Preliminary clinical validity. *Journal of Clinical and Experimental Neuropsychology*, *20*(3), 310–319. doi:10.1076/jcen.20.3.310.823

Reading, S. A. J., Yassa, M. A., Bakker, A., Dziorny, A. C., Gourley, L. M., Yallapragada, V., . . . Ross, C. A. (2005). Regional white matter change in pre-symptomatic Huntington's disease: A diffusion tensor imaging study. *Psychiatry Research: Neuroimaging*, *140*(1), 55–62. doi:10.1016/j.pscychresns.2005.05.011

Reilmann, R., Bohlen, S., Klopstock, T., Bender, A., Weindl, A., Saemann, P., . . . Lange, H. W. (2010). Tongue force analysis assesses motor phenotype in premanifest and symptomatic Huntington's disease. *Movement Disorders*, *25*(13), 2195–2202. doi:10.1002/mds.23243

Reilmann, R., Leavitt, B. R. & Ross, C. A. (2014). Diagnostic criteria for Huntington's disease based on natural history. *Movement Disorders, 29*(11), 1335–1341. doi:10.1002/mds.26011

Reitan, R. M. (1958). Validity of the Trail Making Test as an indicator of organic brain damage. *Perceptual and Motor Skills, 8,* 271–276.

Robbins, A. O., Ho, A. K. & Barker, R. A. (2006). Weight changes in Huntington's disease. *European Journal of Neurology, 13*(8), e7.

Robbins, T. W., James, M., Owen, A. M., Sahakian, B. J., McInnes, L. & Rabbitt, P. (1994). Cambridge Neuropsychological Test Automated Battery (CANTAB): A factor analytic study of a large sample of normal elderly volunteers. *Dementia, 5*(5), 266–281.

Rodrigues, F. B., Byrne, L., McColgan, P., Robertson, N., Tabrizi, S. J., Leavitt, B. R., . . . Wild, E. J. (2016). Cerebrospinal fluid total tau concentration predicts clinical phenotype in Huntington's disease. *Journal of Neurochemistry, 139*(1), 22–25. doi:10.1111/jnc.13719

Rodrigues, G. R., Souza, C. P., Cetlin, R. S., de Oliveira, D. S., Pena-Pereira, M., Ujikawa, L. T., . . . Tumas, V. (2009). Use of the frontal assessment battery in evaluating executive dysfunction in patients with Huntington's disease. *Journal of Neurology, 256*(11), 1809–1815. doi:10.1007/s00415-009-5197-0

Rosas, H., Liu, A., Hersch, S., Glessner, M., Ferrante, R., Salat, D., . . . Fischl, B. (2002). Regional and progressive thinning of the cortical ribbon in Huntington's disease. *Neurology, 58*(5), 695–701.

Rowe, K. C., Paulsen, J. S., Langbehn, D. R., Duff, K., Beglinger, L. J., Wang, C., . . . Moser, D. J. (2010). Self-paced timing detects and tracks change in prodromal Huntington disease. *Neuropsychology, 24*(4), 435–442. doi:10.1037/a0018905

Rüb, U., Hoche, F., Brunt, E. R., Heinsen, H., Seidel, K., Del Turco, D., . . . Dunnen, W. F. (2013). Degeneration of the cerebellum in Huntington's disease (HD): Possible relevance for the clinical picture and potential gateway to pathological mechanisms of the disease process. *Brain Pathology, 23*(2), 165–177. doi:10.1111/j.1750-3639.2012.00629.x

Russell, D., Jennings, D., Barret, O., Tamagnan, G., Carroll, V., Alagille, D., . . . Marek, K. (2015). Monitoring loss of striatal phosphodiesterase 10A (PDE10A) with [^{18}F]MNI-659 and PET: A biomarker of early Huntington disease (HD) progression. (I11-4A). *Neurology, 84*(14 Supplement).

Sanchez-Pernaute, R., Kunig, G., del Barrio Alba, A., de Yebenes, J. G., Vontobel, P. & Leenders, K. L. (2000). Bradykinesia in early Huntington's disease. *Neurology, 54*(1), 119–125.

Schiefer, J., Werner, C. J. & Reetz, K. (2015). Clinical diagnosis and management in early Huntington's disease: A review. *Degenerative Neurological and Neuromuscular Disease, 5,* 37–50.

Smith, A. (1968). The Symbol Digit Modalities Test: A neuropsychologic test for economic screening of learning and other cerebral disorders. *Learning Disorders, 3,* 83–91.

Snaith, R. P., Constantopoulos, A. A., Jardine, M. Y. & McGuffin, P. (1978). A clinical scale for the self-assessment of irritability. *The British Journal of Psychiatry, 132,* 164–171. doi:10.1192/bjp.132.2.164

Snowden, J. S., Craufurd, D., Griffiths, H. L. & Neary, D. (1998). Awareness of involuntary movements in Huntington disease. *Archives of Neurology, 55*(6), 801–805. doi:10.1001/archneur.55.6.801

Snowden, J. S., Craufurd, D., Thompson, J. & Neary, D. (2002). Psychomotor, executive, and memory function in preclinical Huntington's disease. *Journal of Clinical and Experimental Neuropsychology, 24*(2), 133–145. doi:10.1076/jcen.24.2.133.998

Soloveva, M. V., Jamadar, S. D., Poudel, G. & Georgiou-Karistianis, N. (2018). A critical review of brain and cognitive reserve in Huntington's disease. *Neuroscience & Biobehavioral Reviews, 88,* 155–169. doi:10.1016/j.neubiorev.2018.03.003

Sprengelmeyer, R., Young, A. W., Calder, A. J., Karnat, A., Lange, H., Homberg, V., . . . Rowland, D. (1996). Loss of disgust: Perception of faces and emotions in Huntington's disease. *Brain, 119*(Pt 5), 1647–1665.

Stout, J. C., Paulsen, J. S., Queller, S., Solomon, A. C., Whitlock, K. B., Campbell, J. C., . . . Aylward, E. H. (2011). Neurocognitive signs in prodromal Huntington disease. *Neuropsychology, 25*(1), 1–14. doi:10.1037/a0020937

Stout, J. C., Queller, S., Baker, K. N., Cowlishaw, S., Sampaio, C., Fitzer-Attas, C., . . . Investigators, H.-C. (2014). HD-CAB: A cognitive assessment battery for clinical trials in Huntington's disease. *Movement Disorders, 29*(10), 1281–1288. doi:10.1002/mds.25964

Stroop, J. (1935). Studies of interference in serial verbal interactions. *Journal of Experimental Psychology, 18,* 643–662.

Sturrock, A., Laule, C., Wyper, K., Milner, R. A., Decolongon, J., Santos, R. D., . . . Leavitt, B. R. (2015). A longitudinal study of magnetic resonance spectroscopy Huntington's disease biomarkers. *Movement Disorders, 30*(3), 393–401. doi:10.1002/mds.26118

Tabrizi, S. J., Reilmann, R., Roos, R. A. C., Durr, A., Leavitt, B., Owen, G., . . . Langbehn, D. R. (2012). Potential endpoints for clinical trials in premanifest and early Huntington's disease in the TRACK-HD study: Analysis of 24 month observational data. *The Lancet Neurology, 11*(1), 42–53. doi:10.1016/s1474-4422(11)70263-0

Tabrizi, S. J., Scahill, R. I., Owen, G., Durr, A., Leavitt, B. R., Roos, R. A., . . . Johnson, H. (2013). Predictors of phenotypic progression and disease onset in premanifest and early-stage Huntington's disease in the TRACK-HD study: Analysis of 36-month observational data. *Lancet Neurology, 12.* doi:10.1016/s1474-4422(13)70088-7

Thompson, J. C., Harris, J., Sollom, A. C., Stopford, C. L., Howard, E., Snowden, J. S. & Craufurd, D. (2012). Longitudinal evaluation of neuropsychiatric symptoms in Huntington's disease. *Journal of Neuropsychiatry and Clinical Neuroscience, 24*(1), 53–60. doi:10.1176/appi.neuropsych.11030057

Thompson, P. D., Berardelli, A., Rothwell, J., Day, B., Dick, J., Benecke, R. & Marsden, C. (1988). The coexistence of bradykinesia and chorea in Huntington's disease and its implications for theories of basal ganglia control of movement. *Brain, 111*(2), 223–244.

Timman, R., Roos, R., Maat-Kievit, A. & Tibben, A. (2004). Adverse effects of predictive testing for Huntington disease underestimated: Long-term effects 7–10 years after the test. *Health Psychology, 23*(2), 189–197.

Unschuld, P. G., Joel, S. E., Pekar, J. J., Reading, S. A., Oishi, K., McEntee, J., . . . Redgrave, G. W. (2012). Depressive symptoms in prodromal Huntington's Disease correlate with Stroop-interference related functional connectivity in the ventromedial prefrontal cortex. *Psychiatry Research: Neuroimaging, 203*(2), 166–174. doi:10.1016/j.pscychresns.2012.01.002

Van Duijn, E., Craufurd, D., Hubers, A. A. M., Giltay, E. J., Bonelli, R., Rickards, H., . . . Landwehrmeyer, G. B. (2014). Neuropsychiatric symptoms in a European Huntington's disease cohort (REGISTRY). *Journal of Neurology Neurosurgery and Psychiatry, 85*(12), 1411–1418. doi:10.1136/jnnp-2013-307343

Van Duijn, E., Kingma, E. M., Timman, R., Zitman, F. G., Tibben, A., Roos, R. A. & van der Mast, R. C. (2008). Cross-sectional study on prevalences of psychiatric disorders in mutation carriers of Huntington's disease compared with mutation-negative first-degree relatives. *The Journal of Clinical Psychiatry, 69*(11), 1804–1810.

Van Duijn, E., Vrijmoeth, E. M., Giltay, E. J., Bernhard Landwehrmeyer, G. & REGISTRY investigators of the European Huntington's Disease Network (2018). Suicidal ideation and suicidal behavior according to the C-SSRS in a European cohort of Huntington's disease gene expansion carriers. *Journal of Affective Disorders, 228*, 194–204. doi:10.1016/j.jad.2017.11.074

Watson, D. & Wu, K. D. (2005). Development and validation of the Schedule of Compulsions, Obsessions, and Pathological Impulses (SCOPI). *Assessment, 12*(1), 50–65. doi:10.1177/1073191104271483

Wild, E. J., Boggio, R., Langbehn, D., Robertson, N., Haider, S., Miller, J. R. C., . . . Weiss, A. (2015). Quantification of mutant huntingtin protein in cerebrospinal fluid from Huntington's disease patients. *The Journal of Clinical Investigation, 125*(5), 1979–1986. doi:10.1172/JCI80743

Wolf, R. C., Vasic, N., Schönfeldt-Lecuona, C., Landwehrmeyer, G. B. & Ecker, D. (2007). Dorsolateral prefrontal cortex dysfunction in presymptomatic Huntington's disease: evidence from event-related fMRI. *Brain, 130*(11), 2845–2857. doi:10.1093/brain/awm210

Ying, Z., Long, J. D., Mills, J. A., Warner, J. H., Lu, W., Paulsen, J. S. & the PREDICT-HD Investigators and Coordinators of the Huntington Study Group. (2011). Indexing disease progression at study entry with individuals at-risk for Huntington disease. *American Journal of Medical Genetics Part B: Neuropsychiatric Genetics, 156*(7), 751–763. doi:10.1002/ajmg.b.31232

Young, A. B., Shoulson, I., Penney, J. B., Starosta-Rubinstein, S., Gomez, F., Travers, H., . . . Moreno, H. (1986). Huntington's disease in Venezuela neurologic features and functional decline. *Neurology, 36*(2), 244–249.

Zigmond, A. S. & Snaith, R. P. (1983). The Hospital Anxiety and Depression Scale. *Acta Psychiatrica Scandinavica, 67*(6), 361–370.

Zinzi, P., Salmaso, D., De Grandis, R., Graziani, G., Maceroni, S., Bentivoglio, A., . . . Jacopini, G. (2007). Effects of an intensive rehabilitation programme on patients with Huntington's disease: A pilot study. *Clinical Rehabilitation, 21*(7), 603–613.

5

EXPERIENCE-DEPENDENT MODULATION OF NEURODEGENERATIVE DISORDERS

Huntington's disease as an exemplar

Isaline Mees, Harvey Tran, Thibault Renoir and Anthony J. Hannan

Introduction

As described in Chapter 4, Huntington's disease (HD) is an autosomal dominant neurodegenerative disorder caused by an unstable expansion of a trinucleotide CAG repeat in the *huntingtin* (*HTT*) gene, leading to a mutant form of the huntingtin protein. Individuals with 40 CAG repeats or more in the *HTT* gene will develop HD whereas less than 36 glutamine-encoding CAG repeats are considered to be within the normal range. Individuals with CAG repeat lengths between 36 and 39 show incomplete penetrance. Those who inherit the mutated gene will gradually develop neuropathology but only show clinical manifestation (classically diagnosed via motor manifestations) when reaching a symptomatic threshold, which can be as early as 2 years of age (approximately 5% of cases are juvenile) (Myers, 2004). Indeed, the age at onset of motor symptoms has been negatively correlated with the number of CAG repeats (Trottier, Biancalana & Mandel, 1994). Diagnosis of HD via motor symptoms commonly occurs during the fourth or fifth decade of life. The disease is characterised by a triad of symptoms, including psychiatric, cognitive and motor impairments. The psychiatric and cognitive symptoms appear before the onset of motor degeneration (Pla, Orvoen, Saudou, David & Humbert, 2014; Van Duijn et al., 2014) and their intensity is less clearly correlated with the CAG repeat length.

The gene mutation causing this fatal neurodegenerative disorder was discovered over 25 years ago. Yet there is still no disease-modifying treatment available to delay onset or slow the progression of the disease. Most therapeutic studies have focused on the development of drug treatments, although cell therapies and other therapeutic approaches are also being pursued. Despite the monogenic origin of this neurodegenerative disorder, pre-clinical studies have shown that environmental factors impact the age of onset and progression of the disease. Although experience-dependent environmental factors have a great impact in other neurodegenerative diseases (e.g. Alzheimer's disease and Parkinson's disease), the focus of this chapter will be on HD. Environmental modulation has shown promising results in pre-clinical studies of HD (as reviewed below) and could be a possible lead to the development of interventions to delay and slow the progression of the disease, particularly in a pre-symptomatic population, as genetic testing can identify people at risk decades before the symptoms manifest.

Experience-dependent modulation of neurodegenerative diseases may occur via a wide range of lifestyle factors and environmental exposures. In this chapter, we will discuss the pre-clinical models of environmental modulation leading to clinical trials and to the potential findings of new therapeutic targets.

Preclinical models of Huntington's disease

Since the discovery of the causative gene mutation in 1993, many animal models of HD have been genetically engineered with the purpose of understanding the pathogenesis and evaluating new leads for the development of novel treatments. Rodents are the most studied animal models of HD, as they are for most human diseases. Genetic models can be divided into three types depending on how they were engineered: (1) transgenic animals expressing only the N-terminal region (containing the CAG repeat encoding a polyglutamine tract) of the human *HTT* gene; (2) full-length transgenic models incorporating the total length of the human *HTT* gene; and (3) knock-in models in which the CAG repeat is engineered to produce a CAG repeat expansion in the *HTT* gene homologue (*Htt*). All these models differentiate by the length of CAG repeats, the origin of the huntingtin protein (mouse or human), the promoter driving the expression of the protein, and the background strains. Interestingly, these models also appear to differ in their sensitivity to environmental factors compared to their wild-type[1] control littermates.

The first animal models of HD to be generated with genetic construct validity were the R6 transgenic mouse lines (Mangiarini et al., 1996). These mice only express exon 1 of the human *huntingtin* gene containing the expanded CAG repeats, under control of the human promoter. Different lines were created, depending on the number of CAG repeats. R6/1 and R6/2 are the most commonly used in preclinical studies, with 116 and 144 repeats at origin respectively. These mice show strong face validity, reflecting closely the human pathology at the molecular, cellular and behavioural level, presenting psychiatric motor and cognitive impairments. Studies on these mice have led to the discovery of the aggregates due to the polyglutamine expansion in the huntingtin protein (Davies et al., 1997), which were then shown on post-mortem brain samples from HD patients (DiFiglia et al., 1997).

The N171-82Q mouse model is another transgenic mouse model commonly used, containing 82 CAG repeats and whose transgene expression is controlled by the mouse prion protein promoter. However, the use of this prion promoter means that the spatiotemporal expression pattern of transgene expression is very different from *HTT* expression, which represents a major confound in this N171-82Q model. YAC128 and BACHD are two full-length gene models expressing the full mutated human huntingtin protein in either yeast artificial chromosome (YAC) or bacterial artificial chromosome (BAC) transgenes. These models present a better genetic construct validity compared to the fragmented (N-terminal) huntingtin models, however their face validity appears no better than the R6/1 HD mouse model, for example. The last models are the knock-in models, which present a slower progression of the phenotype. Mouse models of HD have been recently reviewed elsewhere (Hersch & Ferrante, 2004; Menalled & Brunner, 2014).

Experience-dependent modulators of Huntington's disease

Environmental enrichment

The paradigm of environmental enrichment (EE) in laboratories consists of housing conditions in which the animals experience enhanced cognitive, physical and sensory stimulation. Environmental enrichment is a relative term, as the enrichment involves an increased complexity and novelty compared to the standard housing conditions.

The neurobiological research in this field was born in the 1940s, when Donald Hebb found that rats free to roam in his home were more efficient at solving problems than laboratory rats. Since then, many studies have investigated the molecular, cellular and behavioural effects of environmental enrichment on animal models, in physiological and pathological conditions. The underlying molecular mechanisms are still not fully understood.

Enriched laboratory animals are generally housed in larger cages compared to standard housing and these cages contain a set of enrichment objects with different shapes, sizes and textures, changed regularly to enhance novelty and complexity. To enhance physical activity, ladders, tunnels and running wheels are often used. In some enrichment protocols, the cages are directly enriched, while in other protocols the animals are moved into enriched cages for a certain amount of time before returning to their home cages.

It is known that the duration of enrichment as well as the age of the animals when starting the enrichment directly impacts the intensity and persistence of its effects (Amaral, Vargas, Hansel, Izquierdo & Souza, 2008; Leger et al., 2015). There are different protocols of EE, depending on the dimensions of the cages used, the number of animals per cages, the objects used (i.e. the presence or absence of a running wheel), the duration of the enrichment and the frequency at which the objects are substituted. Some protocols also use a social enrichment paradigm by putting more animals in the enriched cages, which will not be reviewed in this chapter. The variability of the protocols used among different laboratories is high and contributes to inconsistencies between results from different studies (Van de

Weerd et al., 2002). Therefore, standardising the procedure for enrichment for rodent laboratories has become crucial for preclinical studies looking at environmental and genetics interactions (Sztainberg & Chen, 2010).

While environmental enrichment has been shown to have a beneficial impact on a wide variety of preclinical models of brain disorders, including neurodegenerative (e.g. Alzheimer's disease, Parkinson's disease and multiple sclerosis) and psychiatric disorders (e.g. schizophrenia, depression and autism spectrum disorders), this review will focus on its effects on HD. As a matter of fact, the first study highlighting the benefits of enrichment in a genetic model of disease was performed in a transgenic mouse model of HD (Van Dellen, Blakemore, Deacon, York & Hannan, 2000).

Until the year 2000, HD was considered primarily a genetic disorder, whose age of onset and progression was entirely determined by one single gene mutation. However, Van Dellen et al. (2000) showed that environmentally enriched HD transgenic mice had a delayed onset of motor symptoms and cerebral volume loss when compared to their standard-housed littermates (ibid.). In contrast, environmental enrichment did not induce any improvement in the body weight decline and protein aggregate formation. This study opened the way to investigate the mechanisms underlying the beneficial effects of environmental enrichment. The effects of EE on HD animal models have been reviewed multiple times (Nithianantharajah & Hannan, 2006, 2011). The results on the R6/1 mouse model of HD have been replicated (Spires et al., 2004) and also applied to other animal models of Huntington's disease, including the R6/2 and N171-82Q transgenic mouse models (Hockly et al., 2002; Schilling et al., 2004).

Taken together, several studies have shown that environmental enrichment delays the onset of motor symptoms and improves motor performance in mouse models of HD (Hockly et al., 2002; Kreilaus, Spiro, Hannan, Garner & Jenner, 2016; Spires et al., 2004; Van Dellen et al., 2000). Furthermore, novel and complex environments induce improvements on the cognitive decline and spatial memory deficits seen in HD mouse models (Nithianantharajah, Barkus, Murphy & Hannan, 2008; Pang, Stam, Nithianantharajah, Howard & Hannan, 2006).

Housing HD mouse models in an enriched environment has shown a wide range of beneficial effects on dysregulated molecular and cellular pathomechanisms (Table 5.1). Among these, HD mice housed in an enriched environment show amelioration in neurogenesis deficits (Lazic et al., 2006), delayed loss of cerebral volume, delayed deficit in hippocampal synaptic protein PSD-95, rescued BDNF and DARPP-32 expression (Spires et al., 2004), partially rescued CB1 expression (Glass, Van Dellen, Blakemore, Hannan & Faull, 2004) and reduced aggregate size (Benn et al., 2010). The R6/1 mouse model shows BDNF deficits in the striatum and hippocampus, which can be rescued by environmental enrichment (Spires et al., 2004). These results indicate a possible molecular mechanism leading to the therapeutic effects of EE. An increase in BDNF levels was also observed in striatal grafts of a rat model of HD (where rats received a neural cell suspension in the striatum), along with greater spine densities and larger cell volumes within the

TABLE 5.1 A summary of environmental enrichment exercise interventions in mouse models of Huntington's disease.

Environmental factor	Mouse model	Molecular/cellular outcome	Behaviour outcome
EE	R6/1	Delayed degenerative loss of cerebral volume (Van Dellen et al., 2000)	Delayed onset of motor symptoms (Van Dellen et al., 2000)
		Rescued striatal and hippocampal BDNF deficits (Spires et al., 2004)	Improved motor performance (Spires et al., 2004)
		Rescued cortical DARPP-32 deficits (Spires et al., 2004)	Improved motor performance in males only (Kreilaus et al., 2016)
		Amelioration of hippocampal type 1 (hrt1A+htr1B) 5-HT receptor expression in females (Pang et al., 2009)	Amelioration in spatial learning and long term spatial memory (Nithianantharajah et al., 2008)
		Corrected adrenal pathophysiology (Du et al., 2012)	Decreased anxiety (Nithianantharajah et al., 2008; Renoir et al., 2013) and corrected altered stress response (Renoir et al., 2013)
		Rescued expression of the glucocorticoid receptor in the adrenal glands (Du et al., 2012)	Rescued the depressive phenotype in females (Pang et al., 2009)
		Ameliorated deficit in neurogenesis, longer neurites and increased migration of DCX+ cells (Lazic et al., 2006)	
		Partially rescued CB1 receptor expression in the entopeduncular nucleus and substantia nigra (Glass et al., 2004)	
		Reduced aggregate size (Benn et al., 2010)	
	R6/2	Increased peristriatal volume (Hockly et al., 2002)	Slower decline in motor performance (Hockly et al., 2002)
			Improved long-term spatial memory in females (combined with handling) (Wood et al., 2010)
			Better survival (Wood et al., 2010)
			Increased body weight of males (combined with handling) (Wood et al., 2010)
	N171-82Q		Improved motor skills (Schilling et al., 2004)

	Model		
Physical exercise	R6/1	Normalised mitochondrial respiratory capacity (Herbst & Holloway, 2015) Enhanced level of monoamines (Renoir, Chevarin, Lanfumey & Hannan, 2011) Increased BDNF expression (Zajac et al., 2010) Rescued striatal deficit by wheel running (Pang et al., 2006)	Delayed on set of motor co-ordination and rescue deficit in open-field test (Van Dellen, Cordery, Spires, Blakemore & Hannan, 2008) Improved motor coordination, reduced striatal neuronal loss (Harrison et al., 2013)
	R6/2	Rescued reduction of striatal neuron (Cepeda et al., 2010) Physical exercise fail to rescue neurogenesis deficit in HD mice (Kohl et al., 2007)	Corrected deficit in spatial learning, improved survival rate (Wood et al., 2010) Delayed onset of general health deterioration (limited effect) (Skillings, Wood & Morton, 2014) Delayed circadian disruption (Cuesta, Aungier & Morton, 2014)
	N171-82Q	Exercise is not able to rescue reduced neurogenesis and intracellular inclusion (Potter, Yuan, Ottenritter, Mughal & van Praag, 2010)	Physical exercise is not able to rescue motor dysfunction (Potter et al., 2010)
	CAG140 knock-in	Restored D2 dopamine receptors and dopamine release, and reduced intracellular inclusions (Stefanko, Shah, Yamasaki, Petzinger & Jakowec, 2017)	Delayed onset of non-motor behaviours and striatal pathology (Stefanko et al., 2017)

graft (Döbrössy & Dunnett, 2006), suggesting that EE combined with striatal grafts might enhance cellular plasticity.

EE was also able to rescue DARPP-32 deficits in the cortex but not in the striatum of HD mice (Spires et al., 2004). DARPP-32 (dopamine and cAMP-regulated phosphoprotein) is a pivotal intracellular protein involved in dopaminergic, serotonergic and glutamatergic signalling (Svenningsson et al., 2004). These neurotransmitters are involved in mood regulation, emotion, cognition and reward. Consequently, deficits in this protein could potentially contribute to the psychiatric and cognitive symptoms seen in HD, and the enhancement of DARPP-32 levels might be a molecular component contributing to the cognitively positive and antidepressant effects of EE.

Indeed, studies have highlighted the effect of EE on depression and anxiety. The first symptoms of HD are, at the very early stages, psychiatric symptoms such as anxiety and depression, before the onset of motor symptoms. Antidepressants are efficient in patients suffering from HD and also in preclinical models of the disease. A study from our laboratory has shown that EE rescued the depressive-like phenotype observed in female HD mice only (Pang, Du, Zajac, Howard & Hannan, 2009). This change in behaviour was accompanied by an increase in the expression of 5-HT1A and 5-HT1B serotonin receptors (ibid.). In contrast, a study from Renoir and colleagues, also in our laboratory, showed that EE reduced anxiety-like behaviours but not depression-like behaviours in HD female mice (Renoir et al., 2013). These two studies from the same research group used exactly the same environmental enrichment protocol, with an exposure of 4 weeks, but aimed to study its effect on depression-like behaviour at different ages (12 and 8 weeks respectively), which might explain the inconsistency in the outcome of EE. Indeed, enrichment-induced improvements also depend on the age of the mice (Harburger, Lambert & Frick, 2007), and this may be particularly relevant when considering changes in hippocampal neuroplasticity (Frick & Fernandez, 2003).

When investigating the sex differences in depressive-like phenotypes seen in HD mice, Du and colleagues (2012) found evidence of female-specific dysregulated hypothalamic–pituitary–adrenal (HPA) axis, which might be a cause of depression (Palazidou, 2012). Interestingly, female mice housed in an enriched environment did not show any adrenal pathophysiology compared to their standard-housed littermates. This study is the first demonstration that EE also has beneficial effects on peripheral organs such as the adrenal gland, and this may be independent of any changes occurring in the brain (Du et al., 2012).

Beneficial effects of EE are also seen on wild-type rodents, including the wild-type littermates of the transgenic HD mice. Consequently, it is likely that many of the beneficial effects of EE seen on HD phenotype are due to compensative effects, including those involving neuroprotection. Although environmental enrichment shows many beneficial effects, at behavioural, cellular and molecular levels, it is not a cure. Enriched animals still eventually present with HD pathology and neurodegeneration, even if the onset is delayed and progression of the disease is slowed down. The therapeutic effects of this paradigm need further investigation and the mechanistic insights thus obtained could facilitate the development of new treatments.

One important caveat of such experimental interventions is that environmental enrichment is relative to a standard housing. Standard housing for laboratory rodents is generally very simple and does not allow much cognitive, sensory and motor enhancement. Therefore, these forms of laboratory rodent standard housing may have limitations in their 'environmental construct validity' when it comes to translating to the clinic. 'Standard housing', as used for most preclinical rodent studies, could represent a deprivation state, rather than an ethologically normal environmental condition. Moreover, while enrichment and standard housing are easy to distinguish in the laboratory, the situation is substantially more complex in humans, who generally lead more stimulating lives, although at widely variable levels across the population. We could then wonder if enrichment would have positive effects on clinical HD, as seen in the animal models. However, 'super-enrichment' (additional EE in external chambers, on top of home-cage EE) induced further therapeutic benefits in HD mice, which indicates that the level (or dose) of enrichment is important as well (Mazarakis et al., 2014), which may bode well for translation of these preclinical studies to clinical HD.

There are a limited number of clinical papers describing the effects of environmental factors such as cognitive and physical stimulation. Furthermore, some of these studies have been constrained by limitations of research design, sample sizes and suboptimal analyses of cognitive and functional capacity in patients, and in some cases, the lack of validated measurement tools to assess the therapy outcomes. The largest genetically related HD cohort in Venezuela was part of a study in 2004 (which was the first attempt to translate the preclinical HD study by Van Dellen and colleagues, 2000) which provided substantial new insights into the role of environmental modifiers in disease pathogenesis (US–Venezuela Collaborative Research Project & Wexler, 2004). Firstly, in studying this population Wexler and colleagues (US–Venezuela Collaborative Research Project & Wexler, 2004) were able to confirm the inverse correlation between age of onset and number of CAG repeats. More importantly, they were the first to highlight the contribution of environmental factors to the age of onset in a well-powered cohort of HD families. Indeed, they found that the fluctuation in age of onset cannot be entirely explained by the number of CAG repeats, and would be explained partly by environmental modifiers (60%) and genetic modifiers (40%) (ibid.).

Lifestyle factors seem to impact on HD patients, as reported in a retrospective study from Trembath and colleagues in 2010 (Trembath et al., 2010), which was also designed to translate the preclinical studies in HD mice. The authors found that the more passive in their activities the patients were, the earlier the onset of disease appeared. This difference is substantial, as patients with a more active lifestyle had a delay of 4.6 years in their age of onset compared with the most passive ones, taking into account the CAG repeats. This implies that environmental factors also play a role in age of onset in HD and the disease course can be modified by behavioural changes.

A rehabilitation therapy on HD patients, consisting of physical and occupational therapy and cognitive exercises, showed improvements in motor and functional ability in patients (Zinzi et al., 2007). This was confirmed in a recent clinical study by Cruickshank and colleagues, in which patients who received multidisciplinary therapy (physical and cognitive exercises) showed better dexterity and increased muscle strength (Cruickshank et al., 2018).

The same research group had previously shown that a long-term multidisciplinary therapy (9 months) increases the volume in grey matter and induces improvements in learning and memory tasks (Cruickshank et al., 2015). These preliminary findings suggest that, although it is not a cure, a multidisciplinary program including physical and cognitive activity can ameliorate some aspects of motor and cognitive deficits in patients and even have favourable effects on brain structures. However, these promising results need to be confirmed with larger randomised controlled trials.

Exercise

The environmental enrichment paradigms can be dissected into different components such as physical activity, and sensory and cognitive enhancement. However, it is difficult to separate these components in a natural environment. Nevertheless, understanding the effects of each on neuroplasticity, cognition, affective function and behaviour would help us comprehend the mechanisms mediating the beneficial effects of an enriched environment. Also, being aware of their molecular and cellular mediators could lead to potential new treatments.

Environmental enrichment cages for laboratory rodents often, but not always, include at least one running wheel per cage. As EE cages are larger and contain platforms and objects to explore, mice housed in enriched cages even without running wheels also show increased physical activity, considered as exploratory movements. Treadmill running and voluntary wheel running are two common paradigms used in laboratory rodents. Treadmill running is advantageous to quantify and unify the exercise for each individual, although forced running may increase stress levels. In contrast, the level of exercise with running wheels is highly inconsistent between different animals in a cage. When having access to a running wheel, mice run on average 4–10 km a day. However, motor impairment caused by certain neurodegenerative diseases such as HD reduces considerably the amount of exercise, which needs to be taken into account (Ransome & Hannan, 2013). Exercise can be studied alone, using one of these two paradigms, or with the enrichment paradigm when the cages contain a running wheel. However, EE interventions without running wheels may still enhance exercise to some extent, via enhanced exploratory physical activity.

Physical activity has shown beneficial effects on a number of neurological disorders such as Parkinson's disease and Alzheimer's disease (Paillard, Rolland & de Souto Barreto, 2015) and is the most translatable environmental modulator. In wild-type laboratory animals, exercise has been shown to stimulate hippocampal neurogenesis (van Praag, Kempermann & Gage, 1999) and induce angiogenesis in the neocortex, cerebellum and hippocampus (Ekstrand, Hellsten & Tingström, 2008). At the molecular and cellular levels, physical activity increases the release of BDNF (Lafenetre, Leske, Wahle & Heumann, 2011) and IGF-1 (van Praag, 2009) and induces changes in neurotransmitters (Lin & Kuo, 2013).

Adding running wheels to the cages of adult transgenic HD mice delays the onset of motor deficits (Pang et al., 2006; Van Dellen et al., 2008) and hippocampal-dependent cognitive impairments (Harrison et al., 2013; Pang et al., 2006). However, the effects of voluntary running wheels on the HD phenotype were less striking than those seen after EE, suggesting that the cognitive enhancement and physical activity (other than wheel running) induced by EE also contribute to the therapeutic effect. Increased voluntary physical activity also ameliorates the depressive-like behaviour seen in animal models of HD (females only) (Renoir et al., 2012) and normalises the altered sleep-wake patterns seen in HD mice (Cuesta et al., 2014).

At the cellular level, although physical activity enhances neurogenesis in WT mice, it did not compensate for the neurogenesis deficit seen in HD mice (Kohl et al., 2007; Renoir et al., 2012). This could be explained by the reduced amount of exercise due to the phenotype (Ransome & Hannan, 2013). Brain-derived neurotrophic factor (BDNF) is an important growth factor involved in the exercise-induced hippocampal neurogenesis (Liu & Nusslock, 2018) and accordingly, running did not induce significant changes of BDNF at the protein level in the hippocampus and striatum of HD mice (Cepeda et al., 2010; Harrison et al., 2013; Pang et al., 2006). Running corrected the deficit in hippocampal BDNF mRNA levels in female HD mice (Zajac et al., 2010). Chronic exercise training did not reduce the formation of aggregates in transgenic mice for HD (Van Dellen et al., 2008) but could prevent the loss of mitochondrial protein and normalise mitochondrial respiration in the striatum of R6/1 mice (Herbst & Holloway, 2015). Physical activity also reduced striatal neuron loss in the R6/1 mouse model of HD (Harrison et al., 2013) possibly by rescuing some membrane biophysical parameters in medium-sized spiny neurons such as cell capacitance, as seen in the R6/2 mouse model (Cepeda et al., 2010).

Despite the fact that exercise did not rescue BDNF protein levels and neurogenesis in HD mice, these running mice still showed beneficial cognitive outcome, including improvements in hippocampal-dependent memory tasks (Harrison et al., 2013; Pang et al., 2006). These results suggest that exercise-dependent hippocampal synaptic plasticity does not only rely on BDNF. In fact, a study has shown that mice with impaired hippocampal BDNF expression showed intact performance in spatial learning, working memory and fear conditioning (Sakata et al., 2013), implying that BDNF is not required for all forms of experience-dependent synaptic plasticity (Aarse, Herlitze & Manahan-Vaughan, 2016).

Increased voluntary physical activity also ameliorated the depressive-like behaviour seen in animal models of HD (females only) (Renoir et al., 2012) and normalised the altered sleep-wake patterns seen in HD mice (Cuesta et al., 2014).

Although most antidepressants, despite different pharmacological mechanisms, increase hippocampal neurogenesis (Yan, Cao, Gao & Zhu, 2011), the requirement of induced neurogenesis related to their efficacy has already been questioned. Indeed, hippocampal-neurogenesis ablated mice do not show any depressive-like phenotype (Santarelli et al., 2003), supporting the neurogenesis-independent antidepressive effect of exercise seen in HD mice.

Finally, adding running wheels in the cages of adult transgenic HD mice delayed the onset of motor deficits (Pang et al., 2006; Van Dellen et al., 2008). However, the effects of voluntary running wheels on the HD phenotype were less striking than the ones seen after EE, suggesting that the cognitive enhancement and physical activity (other than wheel running) induced by EE also contribute to the therapeutic effect.

A few clinical studies have investigated the impact of exercise on HD patients (reviewed in Busse, Khalil, Brooks, Quinn & Rosser, 2012), during early but also advanced stages of the disease. The first controlled feasibility study of a defined exercise intervention in HD patients found that a home-based exercise intervention was safe and feasible. Moreover, they found improvements in gait variability, walking speed, balance and physical functioning (Khalil et al., 2013). The safety of physical activity in HD patients has been questioned, as an HD patient training as a marathon runner developed myopathy well before any HD symptoms and developed HD around 20 years before median age of onset for the same CAG repeat number (Kosinski et al., 2007). Although it is a single case (and such case studies need to be interpreted cautiously), it is possible that this patient developed HD-associated myopathy due to the well reported mitochondria impairments seen in HD patient's brain and muscles and also seen in transgenic mice (Quintanilla & Johnson, 2009). It is also possible that light/moderate exercise is more beneficial than strenuous exercise, where the metabolic challenge becomes excessive for HD patients.

In summary, the underlying mechanisms of the behavioural benefits from exercise in HD are yet to be explored. Indeed, the positive outcomes of physical activity seen on psychiatric and cognitive symptoms do not seem to rely on BDNF or neurogenesis enhancement and could be due to more peripheral effects.

Cognitive stimulation

Cognitive stimulation is considered as another aspect of environmental enrichment. This paradigm is harder to assess on its own on laboratory rodents. Exercise and food rewards are often confounding factors in cognitive tasks. Studying the effect of cognitive stimulation would help to understand the mechanisms underlying the cognitive reserve paradigm. The concept of cognitive reserve is based on the fact that people with greater levels of education, intelligence and a mentally stimulating occupation will be less susceptible to functional deficits as a result of brain damage (Stern, 2002). Indeed, people with the same level of brain pathology may present completely different clinical signs (ibid.). The degree of cognitive stimulation an individual receives in early life, or even at later stages, is likely to have impacts on cognitive ability (Ball et al., 2002).

One study on the R6/2 mouse model of HD focused on the effects of cognitive stimulation by training the mice through an OX maze. As HD mice present with motor impairments, it is important to take into account these genotype differences when assessing the outcome of cognitive stimulation. Wood and colleagues in 2011 developed the OX maze[2] to cognitively stimulate the mice. The OX maze demands little movement and is presented with proximal visual cues, designed specifically to avoid any confounding factor due to genotype differences. During this training, mice received food rewards. When assessing the development of cognitive reserve after training in a cognitive task, only R6/2 males performed better at the Lashley III maze (a water escape task), had increased body weight and better survival compared to the control group (Wood, Glynn & Morton, 2011). However, the Lashley III maze, chosen to assess cognitive function after a cognitive stimulation, requires good physical condition and motor coordination as the mice have to swim to an escape platform, which could be a confounding factor for 12-week-old R6/2 mice. Moreover, the high sugar and lipid diet provided from the food rewards during the training could have influenced these results. Even though cognitive training in HD mouse models needs to be more extensively investigated, these positive results on male R6/2 mice would suggest that developing a cognitive reserve in HD patients, and delaying onset with a cognitive stimulation intervention, may be possible.

The PREDICT-HD study investigated the relationship between cognitive reserve and longitudinal change in cognitive capacity and brain volumes in prodromal HD patients. The cognitive reserve was assessed by the number of years of education, the occupational status and the outcome of tasks estimating premorbid intellectual level (Word Association Test and National Adult Reading Test). Results show that a higher cognitive reserve is associated with a slower decline in one cognitive measure (the Trail Making Test Part B[3]) and slower volume loss in the caudate and putamen (Bonner-Jackson et al., 2013). These results were confirmed by a large epidemiological study showing that the prevalence for Alzheimer's disease is lower in people with higher education level (Sando et al., 2008). López-Sendon and colleagues assessed the impact of education on HD patients in a large population in Europe ($n = 891$) and found that higher education levels leads to better cognitive and motor outcome on the Unified Huntington's Disease Rating Scale (UHDRS) (López-Sendon et al., 2011). Surprisingly, patients with higher education also had earlier age of onset, but this could be explained by other variables associated with early diagnosis (such as being more likely to seek medical assessment at an early stage).

Only a few studies have looked at the benefits of cognitive intervention in HD (Andrews, Dominguez, Mercieca, Georgiou-Karistianis & Stout, 2015). In these studies, cognitive intervention was only a small component in a multidisciplinary program, which makes it impossible to disentangle the actual benefits of cognitive stimulation alone. When delivered in the context of a multidisciplinary rehabilitation, cognitive intervention had positive impacts on patients, such as the absence of a significant cognitive decline in the two years following the intervention (Zinzi et al., 2007), and amelioration in cognitive performance and mood (Cruickshank et al., 2015; Piira et al., 2013). Altogether, cognitive intervention seems beneficial even if it cannot be ruled out that the other components of the rehabilitation program (including physical activity, physiotherapy and respiratory treatment) may play a central role in the outcome of the study. However, we need to take into account that the patients enrolled in these studies were all fully symptomatic and this type of intervention may be more successful in a premanifest population, in which the neurodegeneration is less advanced. The subjects would then be more able to engage in enhanced cognitive and physical activities, and compensatory beneficial effects induced by cognitive stimulation might lead to delayed disease onset (Papoutsi, Labuschagne, Tabrizi & Stout, 2014).

Stress

When referring to stress, the text book definition of stress, firstly coined by Hans Selye, is 'the non-specific response of the body to any demand for change' (Selye, 1936). He described stress not simply as 'nervous tension' but in a context of physiological changes whereby glucocorticoid and glucocorticoid receptors play an important role in stress response. The term was later elaborated by many others, putting 'stress' in the scheme of interactions of the central nervous system (CNS), the peripheral nervous system and the rest of the body. Stress, therefore, should not be considered as a negative factor that only brings out detrimental effects, but as a continuum ranging from positive to negative impacts. An inverted U-shape curve of stress intensity and its effects on an individual's performance is a best representation of stress response. However, in the scope of this review, we are only focusing on the negative effects of stress on neurodegenerative diseases and especially in HD patients. Stress also has significant impacts on other neurodegenerative diseases such as Alzheimer's disease and Parkinson's disease, which has been discussed widely in the literature. In Alzheimer's disease preclinical models, stressed animals show increased amyloid beta plaque aggregation (Kang, Cirrito, Dong, Csernansky & Holtzman, 2007; Rosa et al., 2005) and hyperphosphorylation of tau protein (Ikeda, Ishiguro & Fujita, 2007; Rissman, 2009). In Parkinson's disease animal models, exposure to either chronic restraint stress or social isolation exacerbates motor dysfunction in an MPTP-induced Parkinson's disease model (MPTP is a strong neurotoxin affecting dopaminergic neurons, which causes symptoms in mice similar to Parkinson's disease patients) (Lauretti, Di Meco, Merali & Praticò, 2016).

In HD, the effect of stress has been recently investigated. Our research group has shown that while acute stress led to an increase of depressive like behaviour (Pang et al., 2009), affecting short-term memory acquisition (Mo, Renoir, Pang & Hannan, 2013), prolonged stress (either by repeatedly injecting corticosterone (Mo et al., 2014) or using restraint paradigm (a way of inflicting stress whereby mice were being physically constrained in a Plexiglas tube) (Mo, Renoir &

Hannan, 2014) led to an accelerated onset of specific symptoms in R6/1 mice. Specifically, mice subjected to one episode of 10 minutes forced swimming display depressive-like behaviour and elevation of corticosterone – a stress hormone (Du et al., 2012; Pang et al., 2009). Chronic stress of confinement, where mice are kept in a ventilated tube for a period (2 hours a day for 7 days or 6 hours a day for 21 days), also aggravated motor deficit and stress response (Mo, Renoir, & Hannan, 2014; Yan et al., 2018).

Interestingly, when exercise is overloaded, it could do more harm than good. Potter et al. reported that running exercise did not improve motor dysfunction, rescue striatum volume loss or delay the age of onset in the N171-82Q mice model of HD (keeping in mind that this is not an ideal HD model, which uses a prion gene promotor, and the mice were socially isolated). Even though there is not a clear explanation for the negative impact of exercise on multiple symptoms of HD, the authors suggest that applying high levels of exercise on a vulnerable system such as mouse model of HD is in fact, inflicting stress (presumably exacerbated by social isolation) rather than promoting benefits (Sorrells, Caso, Munhoz & Sapolsky, 2009). This is in agreement with recent finding by Yan and colleagues (2018), using a pig knock-in model of HD. In this large animal model of HD, pigs subjected to treadmill exercise died after two days, indicating a susceptibility to excess exercise (or stress). It should be kept in mind that this new HD pig model amounts to a juvenile form of HD, since the pigs died early, between the ages of 5 to 10 months. Given the severity of HD, people with HD are likely to be suffering from the burdens of stress and stress-related disorder. In fact, one of the most prevalent clinical symptoms in HD patients is depression (Epping & Paulsen, 2011). Developing effective coping strategies that help patients to take off the heavy load of stress and build up resilience could therefore be of therapeutic benefit. While a cure for HD is still yet to be developed, the improvements made by understanding effects of environmental enrichment, exercise, cognitive stimulation and stress, in relation to boosting brain and cognitive reserve and building resilience, will have impacts not only in HD itself, but also in other neurodegenerative diseases.

Enviromimetics as a therapeutic lead for Huntington's disease

Beneficial environmental modulation, such as EE, has been shown to improve cognitive and motor functions in a wide range of neurological disorders, including HD, Alzheimer's disease, Parkinson's disease (Nithianantharajah & Hannan, 2006), schizophrenia (Burrows & Hannan, 2016) and autism spectrum disorder (Aronoff, Hillyer & Leon, 2016). Although all these disorders have distinct etiologies, enrichment and exercise have shown behavioural positive effects through different molecular mechanisms, as reviewed elsewhere (Nithianantharajah & Hannan, 2006).

While most studies focus on finding new treatments based on pathological molecular/cellular mechanisms, another interesting approach is to enhance the effect of positive environmental modulation by mimicking the molecular mechanisms of experience-dependent plasticity (McOmish & Hannan, 2007). Those drugs would therefore induce the beneficial effects seen after exposure to a stimulating environment, with less individual variability and more control over administration (ibid.).

As EE has been shown to rescue BDNF protein levels in striatum and hippocampus of preclinical models of HD, the development of treatments increasing BDNF signalling, either through enhancement of its expression or stimulation of its receptor, has gained interest. The fact that a deficiency in BDNF signalling is sufficient to cause neuronal loss and dendritic abnormalities in the striatum and cortex highlights its importance in the pathogenesis of HD (Baquet, 2004). Moreover, its role in neuronal survival and neurogenesis makes it an important therapeutic target for neurodegenerative disorders. However, targeting BDNF for the development of therapeutics is challenging due to treatment delivery challenges (low brain bioavailability) and the short half-life of the recombinant protein. Furthermore, levels of one of the BDNF receptors, TrkB (tropomyosin receptor kinase B), are reduced in HD patients and mouse models (Brito et al., 2013; Zuccato et al., 2008), implying that a TrkB ligand has to be administered as a therapy before severe TrkB loss to still have a therapeutic effect. Studies have tried different delivery methods that could potentially translate to the clinic. The use of an adeno-associated virus (AAV) to express BDNF in the striatum induced longer lifespan and increased neurogenesis in a rat model of HD (Benraiss et al., 2012), but using AAV for gene treatment in patients remains a challenge, mainly since these vectors can induce unwanted immune responses (Colella, Ronzitti & Mingozzi, 2018). Another approach was to use murine (Dey et al., 2010) and human (Pollock et al., 2016) mesenchymal stem cells engineered to produce BDNF. Implantation of these cells into the striatum of transgenic HD mice induced improvements in motor symptoms (Dey et al., 2010), increased neurogenesis and increased lifespan (Pollock et al., 2016). Stem cell-based therapy has shown safety when intracranially injected in patients for other diseases, but has various limitations, especially in the duration of the therapeutic effects. The use of this delivery system is awaiting FDA approval to start clinical trials on HD patients (Deng et al., 2016) and could potentially show efficacy in other neurodegenerative disorders such as Parkinson's disease, amyotrophic lateral sclerosis and Alzheimer's disease. Other researchers have focused on non-invasive administration methods for BDNF. For example, da Fonseca and colleagues looked at the efficacy of intra-nasal BDNF treatment on the YAC128 mouse model. Intranasal BDNF treatment could prevent the anhedonic and depressive-like phenotype in YAC128 mice although it did not induce changes in BDNF levels in the striatum and hippocampus and had no effect on hippocampal neurogenesis. While further studies are needed, it is possible that the effects observed are due to an alteration in BDNF signalling (i.e. activation of TrkB receptors) (da Fonsêca et al., 2018).

Indeed, another way to enhance BDNF signalling is to target its TrkB (Simmons, 2017) and p75[NTR] receptors (ibid.). Small molecules acting as TrkB ligands, that are able to cross the blood brain barrier, have been identified through screening methods. However, these molecules only act as partial agonists, initiating different signalling pathways than those induced by the endogenous neurotrophins. Among these, 7,8-dihydroxyflavone (7,8-DHF) has shown therapeutic efficacy in various models of neurodegenerative diseases related to deficient BDNF signalling (amyotrophic lateral sclerosis, Alzheimer's disease, Parkinson's disease and Rett syndrome) (Liu, Chan & Ye, 2016), including HD. Oral administration of 7,8-DHF ameliorated cerebral volume loss, increased neurogenesis and striatal DARPP-32 levels, and improved motor performance and survival in HD mouse models (N171-82Q and R6/1) (Barriga et al., 2017; Jiang et al., 2013). Another TrkB ligand tested on HD mouse models is the LM22A-4 molecule. This molecule improved motor functions, increased striatal neuron survival and decreased huntingtin aggregates in the R6/2 and BACHD mice (Simmons et al., 2013). Altogether, these results indicate that TrkB ligands are a potential new strategy to treat HD, although these molecules have not reached clinical trials yet.

The p75 neurotrophin receptor is also involved in disease progression, due to an imbalance in its deleterious and survival/trophic signalling. In contrast to the TrkB receptor, p75[NTR] expression and deleterious signalling are increased in HD mouse models and patients (Brito et al., 2013). A molecule targeting p75[NTR] and capable of enhancing its trophic signalling, LM11A-31, has shown beneficial effects on the R6/2 and BACHD mice. LM11A-31 reduced huntingtin aggregates, ameliorated cognitive and motor functions and improved survival. More interestingly, this molecule is currently in phase IIa clinical trials for Alzheimer's disease and has shown safety in phase I, making it a potential candidate molecule for HD (Simmons et al., 2016).

Other drugs have been shown to increase BDNF signalling in HD mice such as antidepressants (sertraline; Peng et al., 2008) and glutamate receptor modulators (ampakines; Simmons et al., 2009). A new study also showed that a 23 amino-acid peptide of the huntingtin protein, P42, prevents aggregate formation and reduces motor symptoms and neurodegeneration in the R6/2 mouse model, through the enhancement of the BDNF-TrkB signalling (Couly et al., 2018). These molecules/peptides support the idea of a BDNF-TrkB-based therapy for HD, but do not target BDNF or TrkB and therefore may be at the core of undesirable effects.

Another enviromimetic target is the cannabinoid receptor, especially cannabinoid receptor 1 (CB1). The CB1 is a G protein-coupled cannabinoid receptor, which is activated by cannabinoid agonist and can regulate aspects of mood, appetite, nociception, inflammation and memory (Aizpurua-Olaizola et al., 2017). As mentioned above, R6/1 mice under standard housing conditions show loss of cannabinoid CB1 receptor in comparison with their respective wild-type littermate controls. Being exposed to an enriched environment not only rescues the depletion of CB1 receptor but also improves the behavioural phenotype, suggesting that supplying cannabinoid pharmacologically can be beneficial (Glass et al., 2004). The effect of cannabinoid has been further investigated. A case report using nabilone, a CB1 agonist, has reported a therapeutic effect by mitigating chorea and irritability (Kluger, Triolo, Jones & Jankovic, 2015; Armstrong & Miyasaki, 2012). However, another line of evidence showed no effect of cannabinoid in a form of cannabidiol (Consroe et al., 1991), Sativex (López-Sendón Moreno et al., 2016), or even nabilone (Curtis, Mitchell, Patel, Ives & Rickards, 2009), on HD patients. Altogether, further research is required to elucidate the roles of cannabinoids and cannabinoid receptors, as well as a variety of other neurotransmitter systems, in HD. These approaches could identify molecular targets for enviromimetics, and thus facilitate development of effective treatments for HD, and possibly also related neurodegenerative diseases.

Concluding remarks

Since the discovery that environmental enrichment delays onset of disease, HD has provided an exemplar for gene–environment interactions in neurodegenerative diseases, as well as other brain disorders. If cognitive stimulation and physical activity can slow down a monogenic disorder such as HD (which until then was considered the epitome of genetic determinism) then the implication is that all such brain diseases are environmentally modifiable. These findings have proven robust across multiple preclinical models, and have been extended to specific investigations of cognitive stimulation and exercise interventions, as well as the role of stress as a disease modifier. While these preclinical studies in mouse models of HD have led to epidemiological and clinical trial studies, they also have implications for the development of enviromimetics, which can mimic or enhance the therapeutic effects of cognitive stimulation and physical activity. These enviromimetics will not only be effective for HD, but are predicted to exhibit therapeutic efficacy for other neurodegenerative diseases such as Alzheimer's disease, Parkinson's disease and amyotrophic lateral sclerosis.

Almost 150 years after George Huntington first described HD, and over 25 years since the gene mutation was discovered, we still have no disease modifying treatment for this devastating disease. While this thought is intensely sobering, it also provides inspiration to push forward with both preclinical and clinical studies, so as to deliver hope and eventual therapeutic efficacy for the many affected families around the word.

Abbreviations

5-HT1A	serotonin 1A receptor
5-HT1B	serotonin 1B receptor
AAV	adeno-associated virus
ALS	amyotrophic lateral sclerosis
BACHD	bacterial artificial chromosome
BDNF	brain-derived neurotrophic factor
CAG	cytosine-adenine-guanine
CB1	cannabinoid receptor 1

DARPP-32	dopamine and cAMP regulated neuronal phosphoprotein
EE	environmental enrichment
FDA	Food and Drug Administration
HD	Huntington's disease
HPA	hypothalamic-pituitary-adrenal
HTT	*huntingtin*
IGF-1	insulin-like growth factor 1
MPTP	1-methyl-4-phenyl-1,2,3,6-tetrahydropyridine
P75[NTR]	neurotrophin receptor p75
TrkB	tropomyosin receptor kinase B
WT	wild-type
YAC	yeast artificial chromosome

Notes

1 Wild-type refers to animals carrying the most prevalent or 'normal' allele, in contrast with mutants carrying the mutated allele.
2 The OX maze apparatus consists of a square box (60 cm × 60 cm × 30 cm) in which are positioned 6 holed blocks, each with a symbol (O, X, =, II). A reward (food pellet made of flour, sugar and sunflower oil) is located in one of the 4 symbols and the number of correct and incorrect nose pokes are recorded.
3 Test in which the participant has to connect dots with numbers and letters in order.

Further reading

Bates, G. P., Dorsey, R., Gusella, J. F., Hayden, M. R., Kay, C., Leavitt, B. R., . . . Tabrizi, S. J. (2015). Huntington disease. *Nature Reviews Disease Primers, 1.* doi:10.1038/nrdp.2015.5

Hannan, A. J. (2018). Tandem repeats mediating genetic plasticity in health and disease. *Nature Reviews Genetics, 19,* 286–298. doi:10.1038/nrg.2017.115

Mo, C., Hannan, A. J. & Renoir, T. (2015). Environmental factors as modulators of neurodegeneration: Insights from gene-environment interactions in Huntington's disease. *Neuroscience and Biobehavioral Reviews, 52,* 178–192. doi:10.1016/j.neubiorev.2015.03.003

Mo, C., Pang, T. Y., Ransome, M. I., Hill, R. A., Renoir, T. & Hannan, A. J. (2014). High stress hormone levels accelerate the onset of memory deficits in male Huntington's disease mice. *Neurobiology of Disease, 69,* 248–262. doi:10.1016/j.nbd.2014.05.004

Mo, C., Renoir, T. & Hannan, A. J. (2014). Effects of chronic stress on the onset and progression of Huntington's disease in transgenic mice. *Neurobiology of Disease, 71,* 81–94. doi:10.1016/j.nbd.2014.07.008

Mo, C., Renoir, T. & Hannan, A. J. (2016). What's wrong with my mouse cage? Methodological considerations for modeling lifestyle factors and gene-environment interactions in mice. *Journal of Neuroscience Methods, 265,* 99–108. doi:10.1016/j.jneumeth.2015.08.008

Nithianantharajah, J. & Hannan, A. J. (2006). Enriched environments, experience-dependent plasticity and disorders of the nervous system. *Nature Reviews Neuroscience, 7*(9), 697–709. doi:10.1038/nrn1970

Pang, T. Y. C., Stam, N. C., Nithianantharajah, J., Howard, M. L. & Hannan, A. J. (2006). Differential effects of voluntary physical exercise on behavioral and brain-derived neurotrophic factor expression deficits in Huntington's disease transgenic mice. *Neuroscience, 141*(2), 569–584. doi:10.1016/j.neuroscience.2006.04.013

Tyebji, S. & Hannan, A. J. (2017). Synaptopathic mechanisms of neurodegeneration and dementia: Insights from Huntington's disease. *Progress in Neurobiology, 153*, 18–45. doi:10.1016/j.pneurobio.2017.03.008

Van Dellen, A., Blakemore, C., Deacon, R., York, D. & Hannan, A. J. (2000). Delaying the onset of Huntington's in mice. *Nature, 404*(6779), 721–722. doi:10.1038/35008142

References

Aarse, J., Herlitze, S. & Manahan-Vaughan, D. (2016). The requirement of BDNF for hippocampal synaptic plasticity is experience-dependent. *Hippocampus, 26*(6), 739–751. doi:10.1002/hipo.22555

Aizpurua-Olaizola, O., Elezgarai, I., Rico-Barrio, I., Zarandona, I., Etxebarria, N. & Usobiaga, A. (2017). Targeting the endocannabinoid system: Future therapeutic strategies. *Drug Discovery Today*. doi:10.1016/j.drudis.2016.08.005

Amaral, O. B., Vargas, R. S., Hansel, G., Izquierdo, I. & Souza, D. O. (2008). Duration of environmental enrichment influences the magnitude and persistence of its behavioral effects on mice. *Physiology and Behavior, 93*(1–2), 388–394. doi:10.1016/j.physbeh.2007.09.009

Andrews, S. C., Dominguez, J. F., Mercieca, E. C., Georgiou-Karistianis, N. & Stout, J. C. (2015). Cognitive interventions to enhance neural compensation in Huntington's disease. *Neurodegenerative Disease Management, 5*(2), 155–164. doi:10.2217/nmt.14.58

Armstrong, M. J. & Miyasaki, J. M. (2012). Evidence-based guideline: Pharmacologic treatment of chorea in Huntington disease: Report of the Guideline Development Subcommittee of the American Academy of Neurology. *Neurology, 79*(6), 597–603. doi:10.1212/WNL.0b013e318263c443

Aronoff, E., Hillyer, R. & Leon, M. (2016). Environmental enrichment therapy for autism: Outcomes with increased access. *Neural Plasticity*. doi:10.1155/2016/2734915

Ball, K., Berch, D. B., Helmers, K. F., Jobe, J. B., Leveck, M. D., Marsiske, M., . . . Advanced Cognitive Training for Independent and Vital Elderly Study Group. (2002). Effects of cognitive training interventions with older adults: A randomized controlled trial. *JAMA, 288*(18), 2271–2281. doi:10.1001/jama.288.18.2271

Baquet, Z. C. (2004). Early striatal dendrite deficits followed by neuron loss with advanced age in the absence of anterograde cortical brain-derived neurotrophic factor. *Journal of Neuroscience, 24*(17), 4250–4258. doi:10.1523/JNEUROSCI.3920-03.2004

Barriga, G. G. D., Giralt, A., Anglada-Huguet, M., Gaja-Capdevila, N., Orlandi, J. G., Soriano, J., . . . Alberch, J. (2017). 7,8-dihydroxyflavone ameliorates cognitive and motor deficits in a Huntington's disease mouse model through specific activation of the PLCγ1 pathway. *Human Molecular Genetics, 26*(16), 3144–3160. doi:10.1093/hmg/ddx198

Benn, C. L., Luthi-Carter, R., Kuhn, A., Sadri-Vakili, G., Blankson, K. L., Dalai, S. C., . . . Cha, J. H. J. (2010). Environmental enrichment reduces neuronal intranuclear inclusion load but has no effect on messenger RNA expression in a mouse model of Huntington disease. *Journal of Neuropathology and Experimental Neurology, 69*(8), 817–827. doi:10.1097/NEN.0b013e3181ea167f

Benraiss, A., Bruel-Jungerman, E., Lu, G., Economides, A. N., Davidson, B. & Goldman, S. A. (2012). Sustained induction of neuronal addition to the adult rat neostriatum by AAV4-delivered noggin and BDNF. *Gene Therapy, 19*(5), 483–493. doi:10.1038/gt.2011.114

Bonner-Jackson, A., Long, J. D., Westervelt, H., Tremont, G., Aylward, E. & Paulsen, J. S. (2013). Cognitive reserve and brain reserve in prodromal Huntington's disease. *Journal*

of the International Neuropsychological Society, *19*(7), 739–750. doi:10.1017/S13556177
13000507

Brito, V., Puigdellívol, M., Giralt, A., Del Toro, D., Alberch, J. & Ginés, S. (2013). Imbalance
of p75^{NTR}/TrkB protein expression in Huntington's disease: Implication for neuroprotective therapies. *Cell Death and Disease*, *4*(4), e595. doi:10.1038/cddis.2013.116

Burrows, E. L. & Hannan, A. J. (2016). Cognitive endophenotypes, gene-environment
interactions and experience-dependent plasticity in animal models of schizophrenia.
Biological Psychology, *116*, 82–89. doi:10.1016/j.biopsycho.2015.11.015

Busse, M., Khalil, H., Brooks, S., Quinn, L. & Rosser, A. (2012). Practice, progress and
future directions for physical therapies in Huntington's disease. *Journal of Huntington's
Disease*, *1*(2), 175–185. doi:10.3233/JHD-120025

Cepeda, C., Cummings, D. M., Hickey, M. A., Kleiman-Weiner, M., Chen, J.,
Watson, J. B. & Levine, M. S. (2010). Rescuing the corticostriatal synaptic disconnection in the R6/2 mouse model of Huntington's disease: Exercise, adenosine receptors
and ampakines. *PLoS Currents*, (SEP). doi:10.1371/currents.RRN1182

Colella, P., Ronzitti, G. & Mingozzi, F. (2018). Emerging issues in AAV-mediated in
vivo gene therapy. *Molecular Therapy – Methods and Clinical Development*, *8*, 87–104.
doi:10.1016/j.omtm.2017.11.007

Consroe, P., Laguna, J., Allender, J., Snider, S., Stern, L., Sandyk, R., . . . Schram, K.
(1991). Controlled clinical trial of cannabidiol in Huntington's disease. *Pharmacology,
Biochemistry and Behavior*, *40*(3), 701–708. doi:10.1016/0091-3057(91)90386-G

Couly, S., Paucard, A., Bonneaud, N., Maurice, T., Benigno, L., Jourdan, C., . . . Maschat, F.
(2018). Improvement of BDNF signalling by P42 peptide in Huntington's disease.
Human Molecular Genetics, *27*(17), 3012–3028. doi:10.1093/hmg/ddy207

Cruickshank, T. M., Reyes, A. P., Penailillo, L. E., Pulverenti, T., Bartlett, D. M., Zaenker, P.,
. . . Ziman, M. R. (2018). Effects of multidisciplinary therapy on physical function
in Huntington's disease. *Acta Neurologica Scandinavica*, *138*(6), 500–507. doi:10.1111/
ane.13002

Cruickshank, T. M., Thompson, J. A., Domínguez D., J. F., Reyes, A. P., Bynevelt, M.,
Georgiou-Karistianis, N., . . . Ziman, M. R. (2015). The effect of multidisciplinary
rehabilitation on brain structure and cognition in Huntington's disease: An exploratory
study. *Brain and Behavior*, *5*(2), 1–10. doi:10.1002/brb3.312

Cuesta, M., Aungier, J. & Morton, A. J. (2014). Behavioral therapy reverses circadian deficits in a transgenic mouse model of Huntington's disease. *Neurobiology of Disease*, *63*,
85–91. doi:10.1016/j.nbd.2013.11.008

Curtis, A., Mitchell, I., Patel, S., Ives, N. & Rickards, H. (2009). A pilot study using
nabilone for symptomatic treatment in Huntington's disease. *Movement Disorders*, *24*(15),
2254–2259. doi:10.1002/mds.22809

Da Fonsêca, V. S., da Silva Colla, A. R., de Paula Nascimento-Castro, C., Plácido, E.,
Rosa, J. M., Farina, M., . . . Brocardo, P. S. (2018). Brain-derived neurotrophic factor
prevents depressive-like behaviors in early-symptomatic YAC128 Huntington's disease
mice. *Molecular Neurobiology*, *55*(9), 7201–7215. doi:10.1007/s12035-018-0890-6

Davies, S. W., Turmaine, M., Cozens, B. A., DiFiglia, M., Sharp, A. H., Ross, C. A., . . .
Bates, G. P. (1997). Formation of neuronal intranuclear inclusions underlies the neurological dysfunction in mice transgenic for the HD mutation. *Cell*, *90*(3), 537–548.
doi:10.1016/S0092-8674(00)80513-9

Deng, P., Torrest, A., Pollock, K., Dahlenburg, H., Annett, G., Nolta, J. A. & Fink, K. D.
(2016). Clinical trial perspective for adult and juvenile Huntington's disease using
genetically-engineered mesenchymal stem cells. *Neural Regeneration Research*, *11*(5),
702–705. doi:10.4103/1673-5374.182682

Dey, N. D., Bombard, M. C., Roland, B. P., Davidson, S., Lu, M., Rossignol, J., . . . Dunbar, G. L. (2010). Genetically engineered mesenchymal stem cells reduce behavioral deficits in the YAC 128 mouse model of Huntington's disease. *Behavioural Brain Research, 214*(2), 193–200. doi:10.1016/j.bbr.2010.05.023

DiFiglia, M., Sapp, E., Chase, K. O., Davies, S. W., Bates, G. P., Vonsattel, J. P. & Aronin, N. (1997). Aggregation of huntingtin in neuronal intranuclear inclusions and dystrophic neurites in brain. *Science, 277*(5334), 1990–1993. doi:10.1126/science.277.5334.1990

Döbrössy, M. D. & Dunnett, S. B. (2006). Morphological and cellular changes within embryonic striatal grafts associated with enriched environment and involuntary exercise. *European Journal of Neuroscience, 24*(11), 3223–3233. doi:10.1111/j.1460-9568.2006.05182.x

Du, X., Leang, L., Mustafa, T., Renoir, T., Pang, T. Y. & Hannan, A. J. (2012). Environmental enrichment rescues female-specific hyperactivity of the hypothalamic-pituitary-adrenal axis in a model of Huntington's disease. *Translational Psychiatry, 2.* doi:10.1038/tp.2012.58

Ekstrand, J., Hellsten, J. & Tingström, A. (2008). Environmental enrichment, exercise and corticosterone affect endothelial cell proliferation in adult rat hippocampus and prefrontal cortex. *Neuroscience Letters, 442*(3), 203–207. doi:10.1016/j.neulet.2008.06.085

Epping, E. A. & Paulsen, J. S. (2011). Depression in the early stages of Huntington disease. *Neurodegenerative Disease Management, 1*(5), 407–414. doi:10.2217/nmt.11.45

Frick, K. M. & Fernandez, S. M. (2003). Enrichment enhances spatial memory and increases synaptophysin levels in aged female mice. *Neurobiology of Aging, 24*(4), 615–626. doi:10.1016/S0197-4580(02)00138-0

Glass, M., Van Dellen, A., Blakemore, C., Hannan, A. J. & Faull, R. L. M. (2004). Delayed onset of Huntington's disease in mice in an enriched environment correlates with delayed loss of cannabinoid CB1 receptors. *Neuroscience, 123*(1), 207–212. doi:10.1016/S0306-4522(03)00595-5

Harburger, L. L., Lambert, T. J. & Frick, K. M. (2007). Age-dependent effects of environmental enrichment on spatial reference memory in male mice. *Behavioural Brain Research, 185*(1), 43–48. doi:10.1016/j.bbr.2007.07.009

Harrison, D. J., Busse, M., Openshaw, R., Rosser, A. E., Dunnett, S. B. & Brooks, S. P. (2013). Exercise attenuates neuropathology and has greater benefit on cognitive than motor deficits in the R6/1 Huntington's disease mouse model. *Experimental Neurology, 248*, 457–469. doi:10.1016/j.expneurol.2013.07.014

Herbst, E. A. F. & Holloway, G. P. (2015). Exercise training normalizes mitochondrial respiratory capacity within the striatum of the R6/1 model of Huntington's disease. *Neuroscience, 303*, 515–523. doi:10.1016/j.neuroscience.2015.07.025

Hersch, S. M. & Ferrante, R. J. (2004). Translating therapies for Huntington's disease from genetic animal models to clinical trials. *NeuroRx, 1*(3), 298–306.

Hockly, E., Cordery, P. M., Woodman, B., Mahal, A., Van Dellen, A., Blakemore, C., . . . Bates, G. P. (2002). Environmental enrichment slows disease progression in R6/2 Huntington's disease mice. *Annals of Neurology, 51*(2), 235–242. doi:10.1002/ana.10094

Ikeda, Y., Ishiguro, K. & Fujita, S. C. (2007). Ether stress-induced Alzheimer-like tau phosphorylation in the normal mouse brain. *FEBS Letters, 581*(5), 891–897. doi:10.1016/j.febslet.2007.01.064

Jiang, M., Peng, Q., Liu, X., Jin, J., Hou, Z., Zhang, J., . . . Duan, W. (2013). Small-molecule TrKB receptor agonists improve motor function and extend survival in a mouse model of Huntington's disease. *Human Molecular Genetics, 22*(12), 2462–2470. doi:10.1093/hmg/ddt098

Kang, J.-E., Cirrito, J. R., Dong, H., Csernansky, J. G. & Holtzman, D. M. (2007). Acute stress increases interstitial fluid amyloid-β via corticotropin-releasing factor and neuronal activity. *Proceedings of the National Academy of Sciences, 104*(25), 10673–10678. doi:10.1073/pnas.0700148104

Khalil, H., Quinn, L., van Deursen, R., Dawes, H., Playle, R., Rosser, A. & Busse, M. (2013). What effect does a structured home-based exercise programme have on people with Huntington's disease? A randomized, controlled pilot study. *Clinical Rehabilitation, 27*(7), 646–658. doi:10.1177/0269215512473762

Kluger, B., Triolo, P., Jones, W. & Jankovic, J. (2015). The therapeutic potential of cannabinoids for movement disorders. *Movement Disorders, 30*(3), 313–327. doi:10.1002/mds.26142

Kohl, Z., Kandasamy, M., Winner, B., Aigner, R., Gross, C., Couillard-Despres, S., . . . Winkler, J. (2007). Physical activity fails to rescue hippocampal neurogenesis deficits in the R6/2 mouse model of Huntington's disease. *Brain Research, 1155*(1), 24–33. doi:10.1016/j.brainres.2007.04.039

Kosinski, C. M., Schlangen, C., Gellerich, F. N., Gizatullina, Z., Deschauer, M., Schiefer, J., . . . Lindenberg, K. S. (2007). Myopathy as a first symptom of Huntington's disease in a marathon runner. *Movement Disorders, 22*(11), 1637–1640. doi:10.1002/mds.21550

Kreilaus, F., Spiro, A. S., Hannan, A. J., Garner, B. & Jenner, A. M. (2016). Therapeutic effects of anthocyanins and environmental enrichment in R6/1 Huntington's disease mice. *Journal of Huntington's Disease, 5*(3), 285–296. doi:10.3233/JHD-160204

Lafenetre, P., Leske, O., Wahle, P. & Heumann, R. (2011). The beneficial effects of physical activity on impaired adult neurogenesis and cognitive performance. *Frontiers in Neuroscience, 5*, 51. doi:10.3389/fnins.2011.00051

Lauretti, E., Di Meco, A., Merali, S. & Praticò, D. (2016). Chronic behavioral stress exaggerates motor deficit and neuroinflammation in the MPTP mouse model of Parkinson's disease. *Translational Psychiatry, 6*, e733. doi:10.1038/tp.2016.1

Lazic, S. E., Grote, H. E., Blakemore, C., Hannan, A. J., van Dellen, A., Phillips, W. & Barker, R. A. (2006). Neurogenesis in the R6/1 transgenic mouse model of Huntington's disease: Effects of environmental enrichment. *The European Journal of Neuroscience, 23*(7), 1829–1838. doi:10.1111/j.1460-9568.2006.04715.x

Leger, M., Paizanis, E., Dzahini, K., Quiedeville, A., Bouet, V., Cassel, J. C., . . . Boulouard, M. (2015). Environmental enrichment duration differentially affects behavior and neuroplasticity in adult mice. *Cerebral Cortex, 25*(11), 4048–4061. doi:10.1093/cercor/bhu119

Lin, T. W. & Kuo, Y. M. (2013). Exercise benefits brain function: The monoamine connection. *Brain Sciences, 3*(1), 39–53. doi:10.3390/brainsci3010039

Liu, C., Chan, C. B. & Ye, K. (2016). 7,8-dihydroxyflavone, a small molecular TrkB agonist, is useful for treating various BDNF-implicated human disorders. *Translational Neurodegeneration, 6*, 2. doi:10.1186/s40035-015-0048-7

Liu, P. Z. & Nusslock, R. (2018). Exercise-mediated neurogenesis in the hippocampus via BDNF. *Frontiers in Neuroscience, 12*, 52. doi:10.3389/fnins.2018.00052

López-Sendon, J. L., Royuela, A., Trigo, P., Orth, M., Lange, H., Reilmann, R., . . . European, H. D. N. (2011). What is the impact of education on Huntington's disease? *Movement Disorders, 26*(8), 1489–1495. doi:10.1002/mds.23385

López-Sendón Moreno, J. L., García Caldentey, J., Trigo Cubillo, P., Ruiz Romero, C., García Ribas, G., Alonso Arias, M. A. A., . . . García de Yébenes Prous, J. (2016). A double-blind, randomized, cross-over, placebo-controlled, pilot trial with Sativex in

Huntington's disease. *Journal of Neurology, 263*(7), 1390–1400. doi:10.1007/s00415-016-8145-9

Mangiarini, L., Sathasivam, K., Seller, M., Cozens, B., Harper, A., Hetherington, C., . . . Bates, G. P. (1996). Exon I of the HD gene with an expanded CAG repeat is sufficient to cause a progressive neurological phenotype in transgenic mice. *Cell, 87*(3), 493–506. doi:10.1016/S0092-8674(00)81369-0

Mazarakis, N. K., Mo, C., Renoir, T., Van Dellen, A., Deacon, R., Blakemore, C. & Hannan, A. J. (2014). 'Super-Enrichment' reveals dose-dependent therapeutic effects of environmental stimulation in a transgenic mouse model of Huntington's disease. *Journal of Huntington's Disease, 3*(3), 299–309. doi:10.3233/JHD-140118

McOmish, C. E. & Hannan, A. J. (2007). Enviromimetics: Exploring gene environment interactions to identify therapeutic targets for brain disorders. *Expert Opinion on Therapeutic Targets, 11*(7), 899–913. doi:10.1517/14728222.11.7.899

Menalled, L. & Brunner, D. (2014). Animal models of Huntington's disease for translation to the clinic: Best practices. *Movement Disorders, 29*(11), 1375–1390. doi:10.1002/mds.26006

Mo, C., Pang, T. Y., Ransome, M. I., Hill, R. A., Renoir, T. & Hannan, A. J. (2014). High stress hormone levels accelerate the onset of memory deficits in male Huntington's disease mice. *Neurobiology of Disease, 69*, 248–262. doi:10.1016/j.nbd.2014.05.004

Mo, C., Renoir, T., & Hannan, A. J. (2014). Effects of chronic stress on the onset and progression of Huntington's disease in transgenic mice. *Neurobiology of Disease, 71*, 81–94. doi:10.1016/j.nbd.2014.07.008

Mo, C., Renoir, T., Pang, T. Y. & Hannan, A. J. (2013). Short-term memory acquisition in female Huntington's disease mice is vulnerable to acute stress. *Behavioural Brain Research, 253*, 318–322. doi:10.1016/j.bbr.2013.07.041

Myers, R. H. (2004). Huntington's disease genetics. *NeuroRx, 1*(2), 255–262. doi:10.1602/neurorx.1.2.255

Nithianantharajah, J., Barkus, C., Murphy, M. & Hannan, A. J. (2008). Gene-environment interactions modulating cognitive function and molecular correlates of synaptic plasticity in Huntington's disease transgenic mice. *Neurobiology of Disease, 29*(3), 490–504. doi:10.1016/j.nbd.2007.11.006

Nithianantharajah, J. & Hannan, A. J. (2006). Enriched environments, experience-dependent plasticity and disorders of the nervous system. *Nature Reviews Neuroscience, 7*(9), 697–709. doi:10.1038/nrn1970

Nithianantharajah, J. & Hannan, A. J. (2011). Mechanisms mediating brain and cognitive reserve: Experience-dependent neuroprotection and functional compensation in animal models of neurodegenerative diseases. *Progress in Neuro-Psychopharmacology and Biological Psychiatry, 35*(2), 331–339. doi:10.1016/j.pnpbp.2010.10.026

Paillard, T., Rolland, Y. & de Souto Barreto, P. (2015). Protective effects of physical exercise in Alzheimer's disease and Parkinson's disease: A narrative review. *Journal of Clinical Neurology (Seoul, Korea), 11*(3), 212–219. doi:10.3988/jcn.2015.11.3.212

Palazidou, E. (2012). The neurobiology of depression. *British Medical Bulletin, 101*, 127–145. doi:10.1093/bmb/lds004

Pang, T. Y., Du, X., Zajac, M. S., Howard, M. L. & Hannan, A. J. (2009). Altered serotonin receptor expression is associated with depression-related behavior in the R6/1 transgenic mouse model of Huntington's disease. *Human Molecular Genetics, 18*(4), 753–766. doi:10.1093/hmg/ddn385

Pang, T. Y., Stam, N. C., Nithianantharajah, J., Howard, M. L. & Hannan, A. J. (2006). Differential effects of voluntary physical exercise on behavioral and brain-derived neurotrophic factor expression deficits in Huntington's disease transgenic mice. *Neuroscience, 141*(2), 569–584. doi:10.1016/j.neuroscience.2006.04.013

Papoutsi, M., Labuschagne, I., Tabrizi, S. J. & Stout, J. C. (2014). The cognitive burden in Huntington's disease: Pathology, phenotype, and mechanisms of compensation. *Movement Disorders, 29*(5), 673–683. doi:10.1002/mds.25864

Peng, Q., Masuda, N., Jiang, M., Li, Q., Zhao, M., Ross, C. A. & Duan, W. (2008). The antidepressant sertraline improves the phenotype, promotes neurogenesis and increases BDNF levels in the R6/2 Huntington's disease mouse model. *Experimental Neurology, 210*(1), 154–163. doi:10.1016/j.expneurol.2007.10.015

Piira, A., van Walsem, M. R., Mikalsen, G., Nilsen, K. H., Knutsen, S. & Frich, J. C. (2013). Effects of a one year intensive multidisciplinary rehabilitation program for patients with Huntington's disease: A prospective intervention study. *PLoS Currents, 20*, 5. doi:10.1371/currents.hd.9504af71e0d1f87830c25c394be47027

Pla, P., Orvoen, S., Saudou, F., David, D. J. & Humbert, S. (2014). Mood disorders in Huntington's disease: From behavior to cellular and molecular mechanisms. *Frontiers in Behavioral Neuroscience, 8*. doi:10.3389/fnbeh.2014.00135

Pollock, K., Dahlenburg, H., Nelson, H., Fink, K. D., Cary, W., Hendrix, K., . . . Nolta, J. A. (2016). Human mesenchymal stem cells genetically engineered to over-express brain-derived neurotrophic factor improve outcomes in Huntington's disease mouse models. *Molecular Therapy: The Journal of the American Society of Gene Therapy, 24*(5), 965–977. doi:10.1038/mt.2016.12

Potter, M. C., Yuan, C., Ottenritter, C., Mughal, M. & van Praag, H. (2010). Exercise is not beneficial and may accelerate symptom onset in a mouse model of Huntington's disease. *PLoS Currents, 7*, 2. doi:10.1371/currents.RRN1201

Quintanilla, R. A. & Johnson, G. V. (2009). Role of mitochondrial dysfunction in the pathogenesis of Huntington's disease. *Brain Research Bulletin, 80*(4–5), 242–247. doi:10.1016/j.brainresbull.2009.07.010

Ransome, M. I. & Hannan, A. J. (2013). Impaired basal and running-induced hippocampal neurogenesis coincides with reduced Akt signaling in adult R6/1 HD mice. *Molecular and Cellular Neuroscience, 54*, 93–107. doi:10.1016/j.mcn.2013.01.005

Renoir, T., Chevarin, C., Lanfumey, L. & Hannan, A. J. (2011). Effect of enhanced voluntary physical exercise on brain levels of monoamines in Huntington disease mice. *PLoS Currents, 8*(3), RRN1281. doi:10.1371/currents.RRN1281

Renoir, T., Pang, T. Y., Mo, C., Chan, G., Chevarin, C., Lanfumey, L. & Hannan, A. J. (2013). Differential effects of early environmental enrichment on emotionality related behaviours in Huntington's disease transgenic mice. *The Journal of Physiology, 591*(1), 41–55. doi:10.1113/jphysiol.2012.239798

Renoir, T., Pang, T. Y., Zajac, M. S., Chan, G., Du, X., Leang, L., . . . Hannan, A. J. (2012). Treatment of depressive-like behaviour in Huntington's disease mice by chronic sertraline and exercise. *British Journal of Pharmacology, 165*(5), 1375–1389. doi:10.1111/j.1476-5381.2011.01567.x

Rissman, R. A. (2009). Stress-induced tau phosphorylation: Functional neuroplasticity or neuronal vulnerability? *Journal of Alzheimer's Disease, 18*(2), 453–457. doi:10.3233/JAD-2009-1153

Rosa, M. L., Guimarães, F. S., de Oliveira R. M., Padovan, C. M., Pearson, R. C. & Del Bel, E. A. (2005). Restraint stress induces β-amyloid precursor protein mRNA expression in the rat basolateral amygdala. *Brain Research Bulletin, 65*(1), 69–75. doi:10.1016/j.brainresbull.2004.11.011

Sakata, K., Martinowich, K., Woo, N. H., Schloesser, R. J., Jimenez, D. V., Ji, Y., . . . Lu, B. (2013). Role of activity-dependent BDNF expression in hippocampal-prefrontal cortical regulation of behavioral perseverance. *Proceedings of the National Academy of Sciences, 110*(37), 15103–15108. doi:10.1073/pnas.1222872110

Sando, S. B., Melquist, S., Cannon, A., Hutton, M., Sletvold, O., Saltvedt, I., . . . Aasly, J. (2008). Risk-reducing effect of education in Alzheimer's disease. *International Journal of Geriatric Psychiatry, 23*(11), 1156–1162. doi:10.1002/gps.2043

Santarelli, L., Saxe, M., Gross, C., Surget, A., Battaglia, F., Dulawa, S., . . . Hen, R. (2003). Requirement of hippocampal neurogenesis for the behavioral effects of antidepressants. *Science, 301*(5634), 805–809. doi:10.1126/science.1083328

Schilling, G., Savonenko, A. V., Coonfield, M. L., Morton, J. L., Vorovich, E., Gale, A., . . . Borchelt, D. R. (2004). Environmental, pharmacological, and genetic modulation of the HD phenotype in transgenic mice. *Experimental Neurology, 187*(1), 137–149. doi:10.1016/j.expneurol.2004.01.003

Selye, H. (1936). A syndrome produced by Diverse Nocuous Agents. *Nature, 138,* 32. doi:10.1038/138032a0

Simmons, D. A. (2017). Modulating neurotrophin receptor signaling as a therapeutic strategy for Huntington's disease. *Journal of Huntington's Disease, 6,* 303–325. doi:10.2174/1 871527315666161107 0930

Simmons, D. A., Belichenko, N. P., Ford, E. C., Semaan, S., Monbureau, M., Aiyaswamy, S., . . . Longo, F. M. (2016). A small molecule p75[NTR] ligand normalizes signalling and reduces Huntington's disease phenotypes in R6/2 and BACHD mice. *Human Molecular Genetics, 25*(22), 4920–4938. doi:10.1093/hmg/ddw316

Simmons, D. A., Belichenko, N. P., Yang, T., Condon, C., Monbureau, M., Shamloo, M., . . . Longo, F. M. (2013). A small molecule TrkB ligand reduces motor impairment and neuropathology in R6/2 and BACHD mouse models of Huntington's disease. *Journal of Neuroscience, 33*(48), 18712–18727. doi:10.1523/JNEUROSCI.1310-13.2013

Simmons, D. A., Rex, C. S., Palmer, L., Pandyarajan, V., Fedulov, V., Gall, C. M. & Lynch, G. (2009). Up-regulating BDNF with an ampakine rescues synaptic plasticity and memory in Huntington's disease knockin mice. *Proceedings of the National Academy of Sciences, 106*(12), 4906–4911. doi:10.1073/pnas.0811228106

Skillings, E. A., Wood, N. I. & Morton, A. J. (2014). Beneficial effects of environmental enrichment and food entrainment in the R6/2 mouse model of Huntington's disease. *Brain and Behavior, 4*(5), 675–686. doi:10.1002/brb3.235

Sorrells, S. F., Caso, J. R., Munhoz, C. D. & Sapolsky, R. M. (2009). The stressed CNS: When glucocorticoids aggravate inflammation. *Neuron, 64*(1), 33–39. doi:10.1016/j. neuron.2009.09.032

Spires, T. L., Grote, H. E., Varshney, N. K., Cordery, P. M., van Dellen, A., Blakemore, C. & Hannan, A. J. (2004). Environmental enrichment rescues protein deficits in a mouse model of Huntington's disease, indicating a possible disease mechanism. *Journal of Neuroscience, 24*(9), 2270–2276. doi:10.1523/JNEUROSCI.1658-03.2004

Stefanko, D. P., Shah, V. D., Yamasaki, W. K., Petzinger, G. M. & Jakowec, M. W. (2017). Treadmill exercise delays the onset of non-motor behaviors and striatal pathology in the CAG140 knock-in mouse model of Huntington's disease. *Neurobiology of Disease, 105,* 15–32. doi:10.1016/j.nbd.2017.05.004

Stern, Y. (2002). What is cognitive reserve? Theory and research application of the reserve concept. *Journal of the International Neuropsychological Society, 8*(3), 448–460. doi:10.1017/ S1355617702813248

Svenningsson, P., Nishi, A., Fisone, G., Girault, J.-A., Nairn, A. C. & Greengard, P. (2004). DARPP-32: An integrator of neurotransmission. *Annual Review of Pharmacology and Toxicology, 44*(1), 269–296. doi:10.1146/annurev.pharmtox.44.101802.121415

Sztainberg, Y. & Chen, A. (2010). An environmental enrichment model for mice. *Nature Protocols, 5*(9), 1535–1539. doi:10.1038/nprot.2010.114

Trembath, M. K., Horton, Z. A., Tippett, L., Hogg, V., Collins, V. R., Churchyard, A., . . . Delatycki, M. B. (2010). A retrospective study of the impact of lifestyle on age at onset of Huntington disease. *Movement Disorders, 25*(10), 1444–1450. doi:10.1002/mds.23108

Trottier, Y., Biancalana, V. & Mandel, J. (1994). Instability of CAG repeats in Huntington's disease: Relation to parental transmission and age of onset. *Journal of Medical Genetics, 31*(5), 377–382.

US–Venezuela Collaborative Research Project & Wexler, N. S. (2004). Venezuelan kindreds reveal that genetic and environmental factors modulate Huntington's. *Proceedings of the National Academy of Sciences of the United States of America, 101*(10), 3498–3503. doi:10.1073/pnas.0308679101

Van de Weerd, H. A., Aarsen, E. L., Mulder, A., Kruitwagen, C. L. J. J., Hendriksen, C. F. M. & Baumans, V. (2002). Effects of environmental enrichment for mice: Variation in experimental results. *Journal of Applied Animal Welfare Science, 5*(2), 87–109. doi:10.1207/S15327604JAWS0502_01

Van Dellen, A., Blakemore, C., Deacon, R., York, D. & Hannan, A. J. (2000). Delaying the onset of Huntington's in mice. *Nature, 404*(6779), 721–722. doi:10.1038/35008142

Van Dellen, A., Cordery, P. M., Spires, T. L., Blakemore, C. & Hannan, A. J. (2008). Wheel running from a juvenile age delays onset of specific motor deficits but does not alter protein aggregate density in a mouse model of Huntington's disease. *BMC Neuroscience, 9*. doi:10.1186/1471-2202-9-34

Van Duijn, E., Craufurd, D., Hubers, A. A. M., Giltay, E. J., Bonelli, R., Rickards, H., . . . Landwehrmeyer, G. B. (2014). Neuropsychiatric symptoms in a European Huntington's disease cohort (REGISTRY). *Journal of Neurology, Neurosurgery and Psychiatry, 85*(12), 1411–1418. doi:10.1136/jnnp-2013-307343

Van Praag, H. (2009). Exercise and the brain: Something to chew on. *Trends in Neurosciences, 32*(5), 283–290. doi:10.1016/j.tins.2008.12.007

Van Praag, H., Kempermann, G. & Gage, F. H. (1999). Running increases cell proliferation and neurogenesis in the adult mouse dentate gyrus. *Nature Neuroscience, 2*(3), 266–270. doi:10.1038/6368

Wood, N. I., Carta, V., Milde, S., Skillings, E. A., McAllister, C. J., Mabel Ang, Y. L., . . . Morton, J. (2010). Responses to environmental enrichment differ with sex and genotype in a transgenic mouse model of Huntington's disease. *PLoS ONE, 5*(2). doi:10.1371/journal.pone.0009077

Wood, N. I., Glynn, D. & Morton, A. J. (2011). 'Brain training' improves cognitive performance and survival in a transgenic mouse model of Huntington's disease. *Neurobiology of Disease, 42*(3), 427–437. doi:10.1016/j.nbd.2011.02.0051

Yan, H.-C., Cao, X., Gao, T.-M. & Zhu, X.-H. (2011). Promoting adult hippocampal neurogenesis: A novel strategy for antidepressant drug screening. *Current Medicinal Chemistry, 18*(28), 4359–4367. doi:10.2174/092986711797200471

Yan, S., Tu, Z., Liu, Z., Fan, N., Yang, H., Yang, S., . . . Li, X.-J. (2018). A Huntingtin knockin pig model recapitulates features of selective neurodegeneration in Huntington's disease. *Cell, 173*(4), 989–1002.e13. doi:10.1016/j.cell.2018.03.005

Zajac, M. S., Pang, T. Y. C., Wong, N., Weinrich, B., Leang, L. S. K., Craig, J. M., . . . Hannan, A. J. (2010). Wheel running and environmental enrichment differentially modify exon-specific BDNF expression in the hippocampus of wild-type and pre-motor symptomatic male and female Huntington's disease mice. *Hippocampus, 20*(5), 621–636. doi:10.1002/hipo.20658

Zinzi, P., Salmaso, D., De Grandis, R., Graziani, G., Maceroni, S., Bentivoglio, A., . . . Jacopini, G. (2007). Effects of an intensive rehabilitation programme on patients with Huntington's disease: A pilot study. *Clinical Rehabilitation, 21*, 603–613. doi:10.1177/0269215507075495

Zuccato, C., Marullo, M., Conforti, P., MacDonald, M. E., Tartari, M. & Cattaneo, E. (2008). Systematic assessment of BDNF and its receptor levels in human cortices affected by Huntington's disease. *Brain Pathology, 18*(2), 225–238. doi:10.1111/j.1750-3639.2007.00111.x

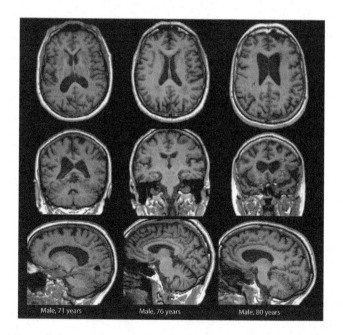

PLATE 1 Mismatch between chronological age and brain age. Structural T1 MR images of three cognitively healthy older men. Brain ageing is immediately apparent as cortical thinning and ventricular enlargement, as highlighted by the arrows. The youngest (left) and oldest (right) men show substantial ventricular enlargement and cortical thinning. The 76-year-old man shows relative sparing of the cortex, but may show some evidence of cerebellar thinning. Thus, signs of brain ageing are variable between individuals, and are not tightly linked to the individual's chronological age.

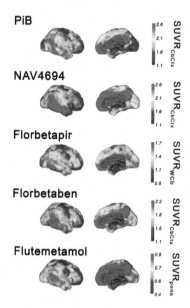

PLATE 2 Surface projection of PET images of patients with Alzheimer's disease obtained with different Aβ imaging radiotracers.

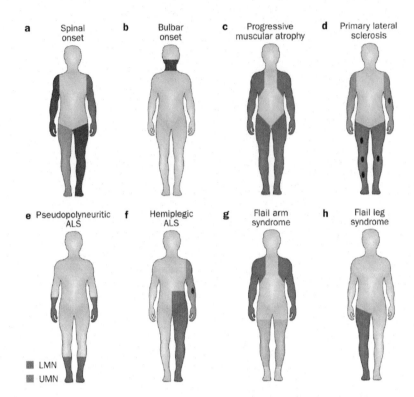

PLATE 3 Pattern of motor involvement in different ALS phenotypes. Red indicates LMN involvement, blue indicates UMN involvement. Darker shading indicates more-severe involvement. (a) In spinal-onset ALS, patchy UMN and LMN involvement is observed in all limbs. (b) In bulbar-onset ALS, UMN and LMN involvement is observed in the bulbar muscles. (c) In progressive muscular atrophy, LMNs in arms and legs are involved, often proximally. (d) In primary lateral sclerosis, UMNs of arms and legs are primarily involved, but later in the disease, discrete LMN involvement can be detected. (e) In pseudopolyneuritic ALS, only LMNs restricted to the distal limbs are involved. (f) In hemiplegic ALS, unilateral UMN involvement with sparing of the face, and sometimes discrete LMN involvement, can be observed. (g) In flail arm syndrome, LMN involvement is restricted to the upper limbs, but mild UMN signs can be detected in the legs. (h) In flail leg syndrome, LMN involvement is restricted to the lower limbs, and is often asymmetric. ALS, amyotrophic lateral sclerosis; LMN, lower motor neuron; UMN, upper motor neuron.

Source: Swinnen & Robberecht (2014); reproduced with permission (copyright licence 4342890349018)

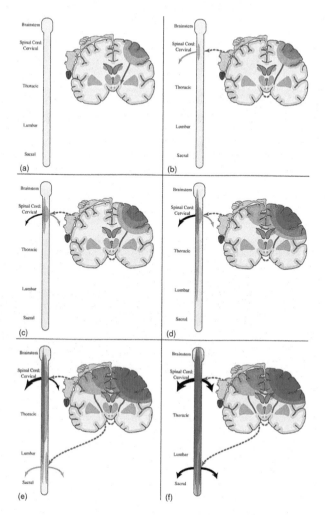

PLATE 4 Patterns of disease and the pathogenesis of motor neuron disease.
(a) Representation of the hypothesis of contiguous cortical and spinal
spread as an explanation of clinical patterns of disease, with the focus of
disease onset in the motor cortex representing the right upper limb.
(b) Pathology may then spread within the ipsilateral motor cortex and
involve the spinal cord through the corticospinal tract. (c) Independently,
pathology may spread within the spinal cord both through contiguous
anatomic spread from the initial focus in the right cervical spinal cord.
(d) Pathology may continue to spread within the motor cortex involving
the contralateral hemisphere by spreading across the corpus callosum, and
(e,f) through ongoing descending transmission through the corticospinal
tract. This mechanism of spread may help explain the complex patterns of
clinical involvement and spread seen in amyotrophic lateral sclerosis patients.

Source: Simon, Huynh, Vucic, Talbot & Kiernan (2015); reproduced with permission (copyright licence
4340750880994)

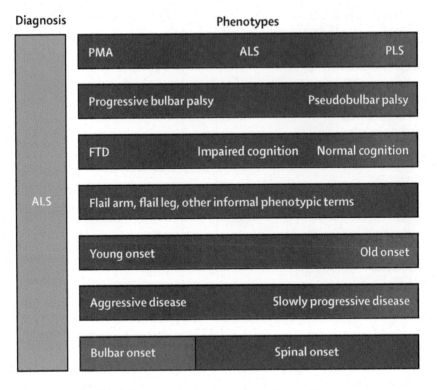

Diagnosis

Phenotypes

ALS

| PMA | ALS | PLS |

| Progressive bulbar palsy | Pseudobulbar palsy |

| FTD | Impaired cognition | Normal cognition |

| Flail arm, flail leg, other informal phenotypic terms |

| Young onset | Old onset |

| Aggressive disease | Slowly progressive disease |

| Bulbar onset | Spinal onset |

PLATE 5 Diagnosis and phenotypes of motor neuron disease. The term amyotrophic lateral sclerosis (ALS) is an overarching diagnosis, and is used interchangeably with motor neuron disease in the UK and some other countries. The term ALS is also used to distinguish the ALS phenotype from progressive muscular atrophy (PMA), primary lateral sclerosis (PLS), and other clinical manifestations. Whether PLS and PMA should be regarded as phenotypes of ALS or as diseases in their own right is not clear. The terms bulbar palsy and pseudobulbar palsy are sometimes used as diagnoses, but they are actually phenotypes of ALS. Cognitive impairment presents as a continuum but criteria define a cut-off for the diagnosis of frontotemporal dementia (FTD). Whether ALS–FTD should be regarded as a phenotype of ALS or as a diagnosis is also not clear. Flail arm, flail leg, and other terms are used to describe specific patterns of symmetrical limb weakness that are seen fairly frequently. Cut-offs for other continuous variables, such as age of onset and disease progression, are not defined by existing criteria. Bulbar onset accounts for about 25% of cases of ALS; bulbar onset and spinal onset can occur simultaneously, and other sites of onset, such as respiratory muscles, are sometimes seen.

Source: Al-Chalabi, Hardiman, Kiernan, Chio, Rix-Brooks & van den Berg (2016); reproduced with permission (copyright licence 4353570431941)

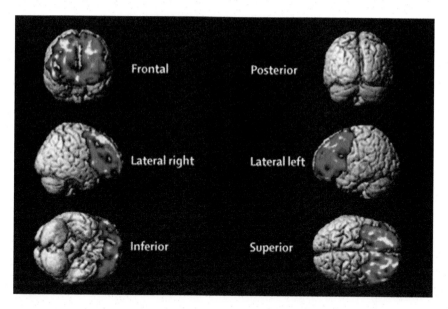

PLATE 6 18F-fluorodeoxyglucose PET analysis in MND patients demonstrating hypometabolism. The images show three-dimensional rendering of the brain cortical surface of the clusters of voxels in which patients with MND show hypometabolism compared with healthy controls. Uptake is substantially impaired mainly in the frontal and anterior cingulate cortex.

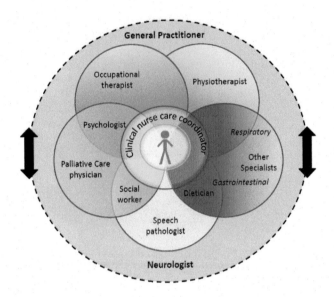

PLATE 7 MND multidisciplinary care model. The multidisciplinary care model centres around the MND patient. It involves dynamic integration of medical, nursing and allied health professionals for optimal patient management. Care is often coordinated by the clinical nurse, with the neurologist and general practitioner overseeing all aspects of care.

6

FRAGILE X-ASSOCIATED TREMOR ATAXIA SYNDROME

Rachael C. Cvejic, Julian N. Trollor and Darren R. Hocking

Introduction

Fragile X-associated disorders are a family of X-linked disorders caused by expansions of a CGG repetitive sequence in the Fragile X Mental Retardation 1 (*FMR1*) gene (Verkerk et al., 1991), which codes for the Fragile X Mental Retardation Protein (FMRP). The Fragile X Mental Retardation Protein (FMRP) has been found to have an important role in the regulation of a number of neuronal processes associated with healthy brain development, including synaptic development and neuroplasticity (Huber, Gallagher, Warren & Bear, 2002; Zalfa & Bagni, 2004). Perhaps the most widely known abnormal phenotype associated with the *FMR1* gene is fragile X syndrome (FXS), the most common form of inherited intellectual disability. However, less marked expansions within this same gene produce other clinical phenotypes distinct from FXS. These include the neurodegenerative phenotype of fragile X-associated tremor ataxia syndrome (FXTAS), and clinical signs of ovarian dysfunction (fragile X-associated primary ovarian insufficiency; FXPOI).

The *FMR1* gene and it expansions can be classified according to CGG repeat sizes. These can be within the normal (6–44 CGG repeats), grey zone (45–54 CGG repeats), premutation (PM; 55–200 CGG repeats), or full mutation range (>200 CGG repeats) (Human Genetics Society of Australasia, 2012). Normal repeats are typically stable when transmitted from parent to offspring, with 29–30 repeats being the most commonly found alleles (as reviewed in Peprah, 2012). Grey zone alleles are also common in the general population, found in approximately 1 in 66 females and 1 in 112 males (Tassone et al., 2012). The phenotypic impact of grey zone alleles is unclear; while a number of studies have reported no difference in the number of grey zone alleles identified in target populations compared to control population rates (Reis et al., 2008; Kurz et al., 2007; Biancalana et al., 2005), some studies have indicated that grey zone *FMR1* repeat expansions may be over-represented in people with idiopathic Parkinson's disease and other causes of Parkinsonism (Hall et al., 2011; Loesch et al., 2009; Zhang et al., 2012). Approximately 1 in 209 females and 1 in 430 males (Tassone et al., 2012) carry PM expansions of the *FMR1* gene; unstable alleles that during maternal transmission may expand into the full mutation range in subsequent generations (Nolin et al., 2003). Although it was previously thought that PM alleles were not associated with any specific clinical phenotype, PM alleles are now known to be associated with both FXTAS and FXPOI. Unlike the full mutation, PM expansions are associated with increased transcription and elevated levels of *FMR1* messenger ribonucleic acid (mRNA), and normal or slightly reduced levels of FMRP (Tassone et al., 2000). Full mutation of the *FMR1* gene results in aberrant methylation and transcriptional silencing of the gene (Verkerk et al., 1991), disrupting the production of FMRP, and causing FXS.

Preliminary considerations

The *FMR1* PM confers health risks that are distinct from FXS. Approximately 10–30% of women who carry the PM develop FXPOI (Cronister et al., 1991; Rodriguez-Revenga et al., 2009; Schwartz et al., 1994). This term encompasses a range of clinical signs of ovarian dysfunction, including irregular menses, increased follicle stimulating hormone, fertility problems, and cessation of menstruation prior to 40 years of age (Schwartz et al., 1994; Allingham-Hawkins et al., 1999). While this phenotype has been known to be associated with the PM in women since the early 1990s, early investigations failed to identify a distinct clinical phenotype in men. However, in 2001, Hagerman et al. (2001) described a case series of five elderly PM males all of whom showed a distinct profile of motor and cognitive features. These individuals presented with cerebellar and parkinsonian features including intention and resting tremor, bradykinesia, wide based gait and inability to tandem walk. Neuropsychological evaluation indicated impairments on the Wisconsin Card Sorting Task, a measure of executive function tapping abstract reasoning and set-shifting ability. Cognitive deficits were described as progressive and two cases met diagnostic criteria for dementia. It was proposed that this progressive neurological syndrome, termed FXTAS, represented a previously unrecognised phenotype associated with the PM caused by elevated production of *FMR1* mRNA (Hagerman et al., 2001).

Clinical vignette

A 66-year-old man presented with a history of tremor and balance problems. He reported that he first noticed the tremor beginning in his dominant hand at the age of 56 and that this progressed bilaterally, followed by the onset of a postural head tremor and mild balance problems by 63 years of age. He also described sensory loss in both lower limbs developing over the last 12 months. His medical history included diagnoses of major depressive disorder, generalised anxiety disorder, high blood pressure, and high cholesterol. There was no history of other significant health conditions such as diabetes, epilepsy, thyroid disorder, transient ischemic attack, stroke, or heart attack. He was an ex-smoker with a 9-year pack-a-day history and reported consuming three to six alcoholic beverages per week. There was no history of illicit substance use.

Genetic testing for an *FMR1* premutation was undertaken at the age of 60 years when his grandson was diagnosed with fragile X syndrome. Prior to her death, his mother was diagnosed with an unspecified type of dementia. There was no other remarkable family history in terms of risk for neurological or psychiatric disorder.

A neurological examination revealed multiple cerebellar and parkinsonian signs. He walked with a normal posture, stride, and speed, but showed a loss of arm swing. His handwriting was moderately abnormal with considerable tremor (Figure 6.1). He exhibited moderate intention tremor bilaterally in the upper extremities; bilateral action tremor in the lower extremities; intermittent bilateral resting tremor in the upper extremities; and infrequent resting tremor in the right leg. Difficulties with tandem walking (>3 deviations) were also observed.

Cognitive testing revealed deficits in executive function, speed of information processing, and visuospatial processing. His wife denied noticing any cognitive

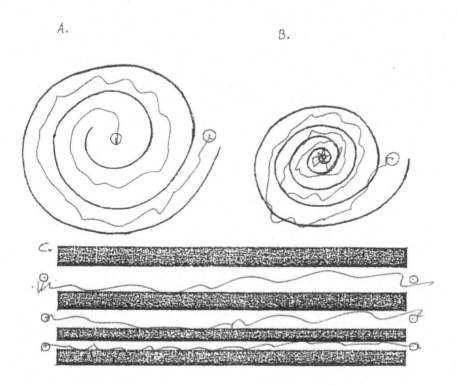

FIGURE 6.1 Abnormal handwriting demonstrated on a drawing task.

changes but reported psychiatric symptoms including moderate depression, moderate anxiety, and mild irritability and agitation. Diagnoses of current and lifetime history of major depression and generalised anxiety disorder were confirmed during a formal psychiatric interview.

On the brain MRI, T1-weighted and T2 FLAIR sequences showed moderate diffuse cerebral hemispheric and cerebellar volume loss (Figure 6.2A); white matter hyperintensities in the middle cerebellar peduncles (Figure 6.2B).

Onset and prevalence

FXTAS affects approximately 45% of PM males over 50 years of age and 8–16% of PM females over 40 years of age (Rodriguez-Revenga et al., 2009). The penetrance increases with age, such that approximately 17% of PM males in their 50s will have FXTAS, but this number rises to 38% in their 60s, 47% in their 70s and 75% of PM males in their 80s (Jacquemont et al., 2004).

Clinical signs and symptoms

Motor signs of FXTAS include intention tremor (increasing in amplitude toward the end point of a movement), and cerebellar ataxia (wide-based, unsteady gait), with less pronounced signs of parkinsonism (rigidity, bradykinesia, hypomimia, resting tremor) (Jacquemont et al., 2003; Leehey et al., 2008). Although less common, dystonia, spasticity and muscle weakness may also be present (Jacquemont

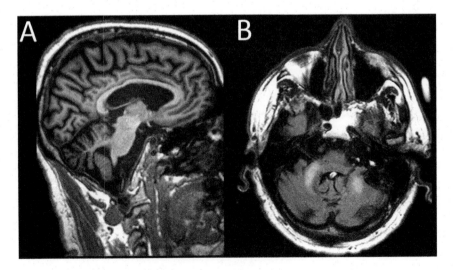

FIGURE 6.2 Slices from brain magnetic resonance imaging. (A) T-weighted image showing bilateral volume loss in the cerebral cortex and cerebellum. (B) T2-weighted fluid-attenuated inversion recovery image showing white matter hyperintensities in the middle cerebellar peduncles.

et al., 2003; Jacquemont et al., 2005; Zhang et al., 2014). Generally, neurological symptoms are more frequent and severe in males compared to females, possibly due to the random inactivation of the expanded X chromosome (Alvarez-Mora et al., 2016), a neuroprotective effect of oestrogen (Hagerman et al., 2004; Berry-Kravis, Potanos, Weinberg, Zhou & Goetz, 2005; Jacquemont et al., 2005; Horvath et al., 2007), or other, as yet unknown factors.

Cognitive features of FXTAS include poorer performance on measures of executive function, working memory, information processing speed, and fine motor function relative to matched controls (as reviewed in Birch, Cornish, Hocking & Trollor, 2014). Psychiatric features may include depression, anxiety and obsessive-compulsive symptoms (Bourgeois et al., 2009, 2011; Bacalman et al., 2006; Adams et al., 2010), as well as agitation, aggression, irritability and disinhibition (Bacalman et al., 2006; Grigsby et al., 2016). This neuropsychiatric profile is similar to other neurodegenerative disorders with primary cognitive and motor features including Parkinson's disease and dementia with Lewy bodies, and is suggestive of dysfunction to fronto–subcortical neural circuits modulating affect and behaviour (Bacalman et al., 2006).

Diagnostic instruments and clinical rating scales

Diagnostic criteria for FXTAS (Table 6.1) describing core clinical and radiological features were formulated in 2003 based on a study of 20 PM males presenting with at least one clinical sign (intention tremor, gait ataxia) and white matter lesions

TABLE 6.1 Diagnostic criteria for FXTAS. Inclusion criteria = FMR1 grey zone, premutation or full mutation. MRI: magnetic resonance imaging.

Examination	Degree	Observation
Radiological	Major	MRI white matter lesions in MCPs and or brain stem
	Major	MRI white matter lesions in the splenium of the corpus callosum
	Minor	MRI white matter lesions in cerebral white matter
	Minor	Moderate-to-severe generalised atrophy
Clinical	Major	Intention tremor
	Major	Gait ataxia
	Minor	Parkinsonism
	Minor	Neuropathy
	Minor	Moderate-to-severe short-term memory deficiency
	Minor	Executive function deficit

Diagnostic categories:

Definite:
a) One major clinical + one major radiological sign, or
b) One major clinical sign + presence of intranuclear neuronal and astrocytic inclusions on post-mortem examination of brain tissue

Probable:
a) One major radiological sign + one minor clinical symptom, or
b) Two major clinical symptoms

Possible:
a) One major clinical + one minor radiological sign

Sources: Jacquemont et al. (2003); Hall et al. (2014); Hagerman & Hagerman (2004)

in the middle cerebellar peduncles (MCP) (Jacquemont et al., 2003). Using these criteria, individuals were classified as having 'definite', 'probable', or 'possible' FXTAS according to clinical and radiological signs. Neuropathological features were subsequently included and may be used to make diagnoses of FXTAS where post-mortem brain tissue was available (Hagerman & Hagerman, 2004). Most recently, diagnostic criteria were updated to include white matter lesions in the splenium of the corpus callosum as a major radiological criterion, and neuropathy was added as a minor clinical criterion (Hall et al., 2014; Apartis et al., 2012). Criteria were also extended to include not only carriers of the premutation, but also the rare situations in which FXTAS develops in individuals with grey zone and full mutation expansions (Hall et al., 2014).

A seven-point clinical staging scale for FXTAS has also been developed whereby individuals are assigned a score according to the severity of motor symptoms (Bacalman et al., 2006). These clinical stages are defined as follows:

0   Normal.
1   Subtle or questionable signs (i.e. subtle tremor and/or mild balance problems) but no interference with activities of daily living (ADLs).
2   Minor, but clear tremor and/or balance problems producing minor interference with ADLs.
3   Moderate tremor and/or balance problems and at least occasional falls.
4   Severe tremor and/or balance problems requiring the use of cane or walker.
5   Uses wheelchair on a daily basis.
6   Bedridden.

Neuropsychology

As described above, cognitive features associated with FXTAS include poorer performance on measures of executive function (Grigsby et al., 2007, 2008; Brega et al., 2008; Cornish et al., 2008, 2009; Schneider et al., 2011; Yang et al., 2013a, 2013c), working memory (Grigsby et al., 2007, 2008; Brega et al., 2008; Cornish et al., 2008, 2009; Schneider et al., 2011; Yang et al., 2013a; Hashimoto, Javan, Tassone, Hagerman & Rivera., 2011b), information processing speed (Grigsby et al., 2007, 2008; Brega et al., 2008; Schneider et al., 2011; Yang et al., 2013a), and fine motor function (Grigsby et al., 2008; Schneider et al., 2011; Wang et al., 2013a) relative to matched controls. These features suggest difficulties with problem solving, behavioural regulation, psychomotor speed and manual dexterity. Deficits in verbal memory (Seritan et al., 2008) and visuospatial function (Grigsby et al., 2008) have also been described, although controlled studies exploring these domains are lacking (Birch et al., 2014). It has been proposed that changes in cognitive function represent an early and progressive feature of FXTAS, with one study reporting cognitive impairment in 31% and 67% of possible and definite FXTAS cases, respectively (Juncos et al., 2011). Estimates suggest that in 40% of PM males with FXTAS, cognitive changes may be sufficiently severe to impact on

ADLs, meeting diagnostic criteria for dementia under DSM-IV criteria (Seritan et al., 2008; American Psychiatric Association, 2000). Deficits in executive function in particular appear to contribute to functional disability (Brega et al., 2009).

Subtle deficits in cognitive function have also been described among adult PM males and females who do not meet diagnostic criteria for FXTAS. These include deficits in executive function (Cornish, Hocking, Moss & Kogan et al., 2011; Kraan et al., 2014a; Cornish et al., 2008), working memory (Kogan & Cornish, 2010; Cornish et al., 2009) and visuospatial processing (Hocking, Kogan & Cornish., 2012; Goodrich-Hunsaker et al., 2011; Wong et al., 2012) among both PM males and females, and decrements in verbal memory, motor sequence learning (Grigsby et al., 2008; Hippolyte et al., 2014), movement and reaction time (Shickman et al., 2018) among PM males. Although retrospective reports suggest that motor symptoms typically precede changes in cognitive function among PM males with FXTAS (Juncos et al., 2011; Leehey et al., 2005), findings of early cognitive changes in otherwise asymptomatic PM carriers suggest that subtle deficits in cognitive function may be observable prior to the onset of tremor and ataxia. Studies revealing worsening performance on measures of executive function (Cornish et al., 2011) and reaction time (Shickman et al., 2018) with advancing age and increasing CGG repeat length suggest that these measures may serve as important predictors of decline associated with FXTAS. Meanwhile low-level visual processing deficits reported among infant and toddler PM males and females that resemble those seen in the full mutation (Gallego, Burris & Rivera., 2014) suggest that the PM may also be associated with a neurodevelopmental cognitive phenotype. Further longitudinal studies are needed to distinguish neurodevelopmental versus neurodegenerative pathways associated with the PM as this will prove invaluable in informing the development of predictive models to ascertain risk for FXTAS.

Neuropathology/neurobiological mechanisms

Neuroimaging findings

Characteristic radiological changes observed among PM males with FXTAS include cerebral and cerebellar volume loss, hyperintensities in the MCP and splenium of the corpus callosum, and increased white matter hyperintensity volume in the whole brain (Juncos et al., 2011; Cohen et al., 2006; Jacquemont et al., 2003; Brunberg et al., 2002; Apartis et al., 2012; Renaud et al., 2015). White matter degeneration and disease appears to be prominent even in the early stages of disease (Battistella et al., 2013; Filley et al., 2015). Decreased grey matter density within specific regions implicated in fronto-subcortical and cortico-cerebellar pathways among PM males with FXTAS has also been described, including volume loss in the cingulate cortex, dorsomedial prefrontal cortex, orbito-frontal cortex, premotor cortex, thalamus, putamen, caudate, pallidum and multiple subregions of the cerebellum (Hashimoto et al., 2011b; Birch et al., 2017; Brunberg et al., 2002; Cohen et al., 2006; Moore et al., 2004; Wang et al., 2013b).

Neuropathology

Characteristic neuropathological changes associated with FXTAS include ubiquitin-positive intranuclear inclusions in neurons and astrocytes throughout the central and peripheral nervous systems (with the highest load found in the hippocampus), which may also extend to the reproductive and neuroendocrine systems (Greco et al., 2002, 2006, 2007; Gokden, Al-Hinti & Harik, 2009; Hunsaker et al., 2011; Louis, Moskowitz, Friez, Amaya & Vonsattel, 2006). Broadly distributed white matter disease may also be evident on post-mortem examination including loss of axons and myelin, mild to moderate cortical atrophy, perivascular widening, spongiosis of the MCP and white matter, and variable degrees of glial and purkinje cell loss (Greco et al., 2006).

The observation of significantly elevated levels of *FMR1* mRNA and normal or slightly reduced levels of FMRP described in the PM (Tassone et al., 2000; Kenneson, Zhang, Hagedorn & Warren, 2001) informed the development of the ribonucleic acid (RNA) toxicity pathogenic model for FXTAS (Hagerman et al., 2001). According to this model, RNA toxicity occurs as a result of expanded CGG repeats sequestering RNA binding proteins. Sequestration of these proteins interrupts their normal functions, and may lead to decreased cell viability or cell death (Galloway & Nelson, 2009; Jin et al., 2007; Sellier et al., 2010, 2013; Sofola et al., 2007). Exactly which proteins are affected, and the downstream effects of interruption to their processes on clinical phenotypes, has yet to be completely understood (Hagerman, 2012). Similarly, the mechanism underlying the formation of intranuclear inclusions, the neuropathological hallmark of FXTAS, remains unknown. Post-mortem studies suggest that the percentage of intranuclear inclusions in neurons and astrocytes in the central nervous system correlates with CGG repeat expansion size (Greco et al., 2002). Moreover, *FMR1* mRNA and RNA binding proteins have been detected in inclusions in human brain tissue (Iwahashi et al., 2006; Tassone, Iwahashi & Hagerman, 2004). More recent evidence from Drosophila and cell-based models suggest a role of CGG-repeat-associated toxicity and disruption of protein quality control pathways in the pathogenesis of FXTAS (Oh et al., 2015; Todd et al., 2013).

Neurobiological correlates

A number of studies suggest that structural and functional brain changes observed in carriers of the PM may be associated with *FMR1* molecular measures including greater CGG repeat length and elevated *FMR1* mRNA levels. Among PM carriers with and without FXTAS, greater CGG repeat length has been associated with decreased grey matter density in the dorsomedial prefrontal cortex (Hashimoto et al., 2011b) and cerebellum (Adams et al., 2007; Birch et al., 2015; Moore et al., 2004; Cohen et al., 2006) in addition to reduced structural connectivity in the MCP (Battistella et al., 2013) and global cortical network (Leow et al., 2014). Elevated *FMR1* mRNA levels have been linked to white matter integrity within the superior cerebellar peduncles (Wang et al., 2013a) and decreased right ventral inferior frontal cortex activity (Hashimoto et al., 2011a).

In line with findings of relationships between *FMR1* molecular measures and the structure and function of multiple brain regions involved in motor control (e.g. the cerebellum), there is also accumulating evidence that *FMR1* CGG repeat length and *FMR1* mRNA level may be associated with specific aspects of motor function. Larger CGG repeat lengths have been associated with younger age of onset of tremor and/or ataxia (Tassone et al., 2007) and greater severity of motor symptoms (Grigsby et al., 2006; Leehey et al., 2008; Apartis et al., 2012). Larger expansions have also been linked to various measures of postural control including body sway (Allen et al., 2008; O'Keefe et al., 2015) and step initiation time (Hocking et al., 2017) in PM males with and without FXTAS, and gait variability (Kraan et al., 2014b) and medial-lateral sway (Kraan et al., 2013) in asymptomatic PM females. Further, elevated *FMR1* mRNA levels have been associated with greater movement time variability during voluntary stepping among PM carriers with and without FXTAS (Hocking et al., 2015, 2017). The relationships between CGG expansion length and measures of postural control appear to be mediated by CGG-related reductions in cerebellar volume (Birch et al., 2015; Hocking et al., 2017). Collectively these findings point to possible dose-effects of larger PM expansions (CGG repeat length and *FMR1* mRNA levels) on neuromotor function among carriers both with and without FXTAS.

Several studies provide evidence of the biological determinants of cognitive and psychiatric features among PM carriers. Among PM males with and without FXTAS, larger CGG repeat expansions have been associated with increased risk for cognitive impairment (Sevin et al., 2009; Seritan, Kim, Benjamin, Seritan & Hagerman, 2016), and poorer performance on measures of general intelligence (Hessl et al., 2005; Cohen et al., 2006; Sevin et al., 2009), response inhibition (Cornish et al., 2011), working memory (Kogan & Cornish, 2010; Cornish et al., 2009), visuospatial function (Hocking et al., 2012), and verbal fluency (Grigsby et al., 2006). Both elevated levels of *FMR1* mRNA (Hessl et al., 2005, 2011; Koldewyn et al., 2008), and reductions in FMRP (Hessl et al., 2011) have been positively associated with psychiatric symptoms in the PM. Further, among PM females without FXTAS, studies have shown links between greater CGG repeats and poorer performance on measures of auditory information processing speed (Shelton et al., 2017), as well as epigenetic (specifically *FMR1* intron 1 methylation) effects on executive function and social anxiety (Cornish et al., 2015). Collectively these findings point to a role for CGG and RNA-associated toxicity, epigenetic effects, and reductions in levels of FMRP in the development of cognitive and psychiatric features in the PM.

In addition to relationships between *FMR1* molecular measures and clinical features, neural correlates of specific clinical features among PM carriers have also been described. For example, atrophy in the orbitofrontal cortex, cerebellar lobules VI/VII, vermis (Hashimoto et al., 2011b), thalamus, putamen and left caudate (Wang et al., 2013b) as well as white matter pathology in the MCP and fornix (Hashimoto, Srivastava, Tassone, Hagerman & Rivera, 2011c) have been associated with greater severity of FXTAS symptoms. As mentioned above, CGG-related reductions in cerebellar volume have been linked to poorer performance on measures of gait and postural control which provide an indication of increased risk for falls (Birch et al., 2015; Birch et al., 2017; Hocking et al., 2017). Volume loss in the anterior cingulate cortex and left inferior frontal cortex have been linked to lower working memory performance (Hashimoto et al., 2011b). Reduced event-related potential P300 amplitude and prolonged latency in the frontal lobes have also been reported among carriers with FXTAS, which correlate with performance on executive function tasks (Yang et al., 2013a, 2013c). Negative associations between white matter integrity of the dorsolateral prefrontal cortex and performance on a verbal memory encoding task (Hippolyte et al., 2014), and between white matter integrity of the genu and performance on measures of executive function and processing speed (Filley et al., 2015), support the view that white matter disease and degeneration has an important role in the pathogenesis of dementia associated with FXTAS (Filley, 2016; Filley et al., 2015). Psychiatric symptoms may be associated with subcortical pathology, particularly in the amygdalo-hippocampal complex. Greater psychiatric symptomatology has been described among PM males who show decreased hippocampal volume (Adams et al., 2010), and reduced activation of this region while performing a memory recall task (Koldewyn et al., 2008). Reduced amygdala activation and volume in PM males have also been associated with greater psychiatric symptomatology and autism spectrum symptoms (Hashimoto et al., 2011b; Hessl et al., 2007, 2011). Collectively, these findings suggest a complex interplay between molecular factors associated with the PM, structural and functional integrity of brain regions implicated in fronto-subcortical and cortico-cerebellar circuits, and impairments in associated processes among PM carriers with and without FXTAS.

Treatment including psychopharmacology

Currently there is no treatment targeting the pathophysiological mechanisms underlying FXTAS. Treatment is symptomatic, addressing specific motor, cognitive or psychiatric signs (Hall et al., 2006). A randomised controlled trial exploring treatment efficacy of Memantine, a glutamate receptor antagonist approved for use in the management of Alzheimer's disease, suggested no significant improvement in intention tremor or executive function (Seritan et al., 2014) and limited benefit for language and memory function (Hall et al., 2014; Yang, Niu, Simon, Chen, Seritan & Schneider, 2013b) compared to placebo. An open-label trial of the neurosteroid allopregnanolone (administered via intravenous infusions) also showed improvements in executive function and episodic memory, but with no significant impact on structural brain MRI outcomes (Wang et al., 2017). It has been suggested that other therapeutic modalities may improve motor, cognitive or psychiatric symptoms (Hagerman et al., 2008), although these have not been the subject of clinical trials. Potentially beneficial interventions include cholinesterase inhibitors, levodopa, antidepressants, antipsychotics, N-methyl-D-aspartate (NMDA) receptor antagonists, dietary supplements and aerobic exercise (ibid.). Current clinical best practice involves implementing individual treatment programs comprising a combination of these management strategies (Hagerman et al., 2009; Polussa, Schneider & Hagerman, 2014). A greater understanding of the pathogenic mechanisms of FXTAS (e.g. CGG expansion, mRNA toxicity, protein dysregulation) and their relationships to clinical manifestations is required to inform the development of targeted disease-modifying therapies.

Concluding remarks

Fragile X-associated tremor ataxia syndrome is an inherited neurodegenerative disorder affecting up to 45% of men and 8–16% of women who carry premutation expansions of the *FMR1* gene. Onset of symptoms is typically from the age of 50 years and the overall penetrance increases with advancing age. Motor, cognitive, and psychiatric signs are consistent with subcortical and white matter pathology seen on brain MRI. Several studies provide evidence of possible biological determinants of clinical features among PM carriers, including *FMR1*-related measures (e.g. longer CGG repeat length, elevated *FMR1* mRNA, depleted FMRP) and neural markers (e.g. structural and functional alterations in frontal, subcortical and cerebellar brain regions). Some of these markers have been observed in PM carriers prior to the onset of symptoms, suggesting potential utility as early markers of increased risk. Currently there are no disease-modifying therapies available for FXTAS but individualised treatment plans (incorporating multidisciplinary teams where appropriate) should be implemented to manage symptoms of concern. Further research is required to develop a greater understanding of the pathological mechanisms underlying the development of FXTAS, and to facilitate the identification of specific risk or protective factors related to symptom onset. This will inform the development of targeted treatments to slow the progression of FXTAS, or even to prevent onset in those at risk.

Abbreviations

ADLs	activities of daily living
FMR1	Fragile X Mental Retardation 1
FMRP	Fragile X Mental Retardation Protein
FXPOI	fragile X-associated primary ovarian insufficiency
FXS	fragile X syndrome
FXTAS	fragile X-associated tremor ataxia syndrome
MCP	middle cerebellar peduncles
NMDA	N-methyl-D-aspartate
PM	premutation
RNA	ribonucleic acid

Further reading

Birch, R. C., Cornish, K. M., Hocking, D. R. & Trollor, J. N. (2014) Understanding the neuropsychiatric phenotype of fragile X-associated tremor ataxia syndrome: A systematic review. *Neuropsychology Review, 24,* 491–513.

Hagerman, R. & Hagerman, P. (2013) Advances in clinical and molecular understanding of the *FMR1* premutation and fragile X-associated tremor/ataxia syndrome. *Lancet Neurology, 12,* 786–798.

Hall, D. A., Robertson, E., Shelton, A. L., Losh, M. C., Mila, M., Moreno, E. G., . . . O'Keefe, J. (2016) Update on the clinical, radiographic, and neurobehavioral manifestations in FXTAS and *FMR1* premutation carriers. *The Cerebellum, 15,* 578–586.

Robertson, E. E., Hall, D. A., McAsey, A. R. & O'Keefe, J. (2016) Fragile X-associated tremor/ataxia syndrome: Phenotypic comparisons with other movement disorders. *The Clinical Neuropsychologist, 30,* 849–900.

Wang, J. Y., Hessl, D., Hagerman, R. J., Simon, T. J., Tasone, F., Ferrer, E. & Rivera, S. M. (2017) Abnormal trajectories in cerebellum and brainstem volumes in carriers of the fragile X premutation. *Neurobiology of Aging, 55,* 11–19.

References

Adams, J. S., Adams, P. E., Nguyen, D., Brunberg, J. A., Tassone, F., Zhang, W., . . . Hagerman, R. J. (2007). Volumetric brain changes in females with fragile X-associated tremor/ataxia syndrome (FXTAS). *Neurology, 69*(9), 851–859.

Adams, P. E., Adams, J. S., Nguyen, D. V., Hessl, D., Brunberg, J. A., Tassone, F., . . . Hagerman, R. J. (2010). Psychological symptoms correlate with reduced hippocampal volume in fragile X premutation carriers. *American Journal of Medical Genetics Part B-Neuropsychiatric Genetics, 153B*(3), 775–785. doi:10.1002/ajmg.b.31046

Allen, E. G., Juncos, J., Letz, R., Rusin, M., Hamilton, D., Novak, G., . . . Sherman, S. L. (2008). Detection of early FXTAS motor symptoms using the CATSYS computerised neuromotor test battery. *Journal of Medical Genetics, 45*(5), 290–297. doi:10.1136/jmg.2007.054676

Allingham-Hawkins, D. J., Babul-Hirji, R., Chitayat, D., Holden, J. J. A., Yang, K. T., Lee, C., . . . Vieri, F. (1999). Fragile X premutation is a significant risk factor for premature ovarian failure: The international collaborative POF in fragile X study—preliminary data. *American Journal of Medical Genetics, 83*(4), 322–325. doi:10.1002/(SICI)1096-8628(19990402)83:4<322::AID-AJMG17>3.0.CO;2-B

Alvarez-Mora, M. I., Rodriguez-Revenga, L., Feliu, A., Badenas, C., Madrigal, I. & Mila, M. (2016). Skewed X inactivation in women carrying the *FMR1* premutation and its relation with fragile-X-associated tremor/ataxia syndrome. *Neurodegenerative Diseases, 16*(3–4), 290–292. doi:10.1159/000441566

American Psychiatric Association. (2000). *Diagnostic and Statistical Manual of Mental Disorders* (4th ed., text rev.). Washington, DC: American Psychiatric Association.

Apartis, E., Blancher, A., Meissner, W., Guyant-Maréchal, L., Maltête, D., De Broucker, T., . . . Anheim, M. (2012). FXTAS: New insights and the need for revised diagnostic criteria. *Neurology, 79*(18), 1898–1907. doi:10.1212/WNL.0b013e318271f7ff

Bacalman, S., Farzin, F., Bourgeois, J. A., Cogswell, J., Goodlin-Jones, B. L., Gane, L. W., . . . Hagerman, R. J. (2006). Psychiatric phenotype of the fragile X-associated tremor/ataxia syndrome (FXTAS) in males: Newly described fronto-subcortical dementia. *Journal of Clinical Psychiatry, 67*(1), 87–94.

Battistella, G., Niederhauser, J., Fornari, E., Hippolyte, L., Perrin, A. G., Lesca, G., . . . Jacquemont, S. (2013). Brain structure in asymptomatic *FMR1* premutation carriers at risk for fragile X-associated tremor/ataxia syndrome. *Neurobiology of Aging, 34*(6), 1700–1707. doi:10.1016/j.neurobiolaging.2012.12.001

Berry-Kravis, E., Potanos, K., Weinberg, D., Zhou, L. L. & Goetz, C. G. (2005). Fragile X-associated tremor/ataxia syndrome in sisters related to X-inactivation. *Annals of Neurology, 57*(1), 144–147. doi:10.1002/ana.20360

Biancalana, V., Toft, M., Le Ber, I., Tison, F., Scherrer, E., Thibodeau, S., . . . Durr, A. (2005). FMR1 premutations associated with fragile X-associated tremor/ataxia syndrome in multiple system atrophy. *Archives of Neurology, 62*(6), 962–966.

Birch, R. C., Cornish, K. M., Hocking, D. R. & Trollor, J. N. (2014). Understanding the neuropsychiatric phenotype of fragile X-associated tremor ataxia syndrome: A systematic review. *Neuropsychology Review, 24*(4), 491–513. doi:10.1007/s11065-014-9262-9

Birch, R. C., Hocking, D. R., Cornish, K. M., Menant, J. C., Georgiou-Karistianis, N., Godler, D. E., . . . Trollor, J. N. (2015). Preliminary evidence of an effect of cerebellar volume on postural sway in *FMR1* premutation males. *Genes, Brain and Behavior, 14*(3), 251–259. doi:10.1111/gbb.12204

Birch, R. C., Hocking, D. R., Cornish, K. M., Menant, J. C., Lord, S. R., Georgiou-Karistianis, N., . . . Trollor, J. N. (2017). Selective subcortical contributions to gait impairments in males with the FMR1 premutation. *Journal of Neurology, Neurosurgery & Psychiatry, 88*, 188–190. doi:10.1136/jnnp-2016-313937

Bourgeois, J. A., Coffey, S. M., Rivera, S. M., Hessl, D., Gane, L. W., Tassone, F., . . . Hagerman, R. J. (2009). A review of fragile X premutation disorders: Expanding the psychiatric perspective. *Journal of Clinical Psychiatry, 70*(6), 852–862.

Bourgeois, J. A., Seritan, A. L., Casillas, M., Hessl, D., Schneider, A., Yang, Y., . . . Hagerman, R. J. (2011). Lifetime prevalence of mood and anxiety disorders in fragile X premutation carriers. *The Journal of Clinical Psychiatry, 72*(2), 175–182. doi:10.4088/JCP.09m05407blu

Brega, A. G., Goodrich, G., Bennett, R. E., Hessl, D., Engle, K., Leehey, M. A., . . . Grigsby, J. (2008). The primary cognitive deficit among males with fragile X-associated tremor/ataxia syndrome (FXTAS) is a dysexecutive syndrome. *Journal of Clinical and Experimental Neuropsychology, 30*(8), 853–869. doi:10.1080/13803390701819044

Brega, A. G., Reynolds, A., Bennett, R. E., Leehey, M. A., Bounds, L. S., Cogswell, J. B., . . . Grigsby, J. (2009). Functional status of men with the fragile X premutation, with and without the tremor/ataxia syndrome (FXTAS). *International Journal of Geriatric Psychiatry, 24*(10), 1101–1109. doi:10.1002/gps.2231

Brunberg, J. A., Jacquemont, S., Hagerman, R. J., Berry-Kravis, E. M., Grigsby, J., Leehey, M. A., . . . Hagerman, P. J. (2002). Fragile X premutation carriers: Characteristic MR imaging findings of adult male patients with progressive cerebellar and cognitive dysfunction. *American Journal of Neuroradiology, 23*(10), 1757–1766.

Cohen, S., Masyn, K., Adams, J., Hessl, D., Rivera, S., Tassone, F., . . . Hagerman, R. (2006). Molecular and imaging correlates of the fragile X-associated tremor/ataxia syndrome. *Neurology, 67*(8), 1426–1431.

Cornish, K. M., Hocking, D. R., Moss, S. A. & Kogan, C. S. (2011). Selective executive markers of at-risk profiles associated with the fragile X premutation. *Neurology, 77*(7), 618–622. doi:10.1212/WNL.0b013e3182299e59

Cornish, K. M., Kogan, C. S., Li, L. X., Turk, J., Jacquemont, S. & Hagerman, R. J. (2009). Lifespan changes in working memory in fragile X premutation males. *Brain and Cognition, 69*(3), 551–558. doi:10.1016/j.bandc.2008.11.006

Cornish, K. M., Kraan, C. M., Bui, Q. M., Bellgrove, M. A., Metcalfe, S. A., Trollor, T., ... Godler, D. E. (2015). Novel methylation markers of the dysexecutive-psychiatric phenotype in FMR1 premutation females. *Neurology, 84*(16), 1631–1638.

Cornish, K. M., Li, L., Kogan, C. S., Jacquemont, S., Turk, J., Dalton, A., ... Hagerman, P. J. (2008). Age-dependent cognitive changes in carriers of the fragile X syndrome. *Cortex, 44*(6), 628–636.

Cronister, A., Schreiner, R., Wittenberger, M., Amiri, K., Harris, K. & Hagerman, R. J. (1991). Heterozygous fragile X female: Historical, physical, cognitive, and cytogenetic features. *American Journal of Medical Genetics, 38*(2–3), 269–274.

Filley, C. M. (2016). Fragile X tremor ataxia syndrome and white matter dementia. *Clinical Neuropsychologist, 30*(6), 901–912. doi:10.1080/13854046.2016.1165805

Filley, C. M., Brown, M. S., Onderko, K., Ray, M., Bennett, R., Berry-Kravis, E. & Grigsby, J. (2015). White matter disease and cognitive impairment in *FMR1* premutation carriers. *Neurology, 84*, 1–7.

Gallego, P., Burris, J. & Rivera, S. (2014). Visual motion processing deficits in infants with the fragile X premutation. *Journal of Neurodevelopmental Disorders, 6*(1), 29. doi:10.1186/1866-1955-6-29

Galloway, J. N. & Nelson, D. L. (2009). Evidence for RNA-mediated toxicity in the fragile X-associated tremor/ataxia syndrome. *Future Neurology, 4*(6), 785–798. doi:10.2217/fnl.09.44

Gokden, M., Al-Hinti, J. T. & Harik, S. I. (2009). Peripheral nervous system pathology in fragile X tremor/ataxia syndrome (FXTAS). *Neuropathology, 29*(3), 280–284. doi:10.1111/j.1440-1789.2008.00948.x

Goodrich-Hunsaker, N. J., Wong, L. M., McLennan, Y., Srivastava, S., Tassone, F., Harvey, D., ... Simon, T. J. (2011). Young adult female fragile X premutation carriers show age- and genetically-modulated cognitive impairments. *Brain and Cognition, 75*(3), 255–260. doi:10.1016/j.bandc.2011.01.001

Greco, C. M., Berman, R. F., Martin, R. M., Tassone, F., Schwartz, P. H., Chang, A., ... Hagerman, P. J. (2006). Neuropathology of fragile X-associated tremor/ataxia syndrome (FXTAS). *Brain, 129*, 243–255. doi:10.1093/brain/awh683

Greco, C. M., Hagerman, R. J., Tassone, F., Chudley, A. E., Del Bigio, M. R., Jacquemont, S., ... Hagerman, P. J. (2002). Neuronal intranuclear inclusions in a new cerebellar tremor/ataxia syndrome among fragile X carriers. *Brain, 125*, 1760–1771. doi:10.1093/brain/awf184

Greco, C. M., Soontrapornchai, K., Wirojanan, J., Gould, J. E., Hagerman, P. J. & Hagerman, R. J. (2007). Testicular and pituitary inclusion formation in fragile X associated tremor/ataxia syndrome. *Journal of Urology, 177*(4), 1434–1437. doi:10.1016/j.juro.2006.11.097

Grigsby, J., Brega, A. G., Bennett, R. E., Bourgeois, J. A., Seritan, A. L., Goodrich, G. K. & Hagerman, R. J. (2016). Clinically significant psychiatric symptoms among male carriers of the fragile X premutation, with and without FXTAS, and the mediating influence of executive functioning. *Clinical Neuropsychologist, 30*(6), 944–959. doi:10.1080/13854046.2016.1185100

Grigsby, J., Brega, A. G., Engle, K., Leehey, M. A., Hagerman, R. J., Tassone, F., ... Reynolds, A. (2008). Cognitive profile of fragile X premutation carriers with and without fragile X-associated tremor/ataxia syndrome. *Neuropsychology, 22*(1), 48–60. doi:10.1037/0894-4105.22.1.48

Grigsby, J., Brega, A. G., Jacquemont, S., Loesch, D. Z., Leehey, M. A., Goodrich, G. K., ... Hagerman, P. J. (2006). Impairment in the cognitive functioning of men with fragile X-associated tremor/ataxia syndrome (FXTAS). *Journal of the Neurological Sciences, 248*(1–2), 227–233. doi:10.1016/j.jns.2006.05.016

Grigsby, J., Brega, A. G., Leehey, M. A., Goodrich, G. K., Jacquemont, S., Loesch, D. Z., . . . Hagerman, R. J. (2007). Impairment of executive cognitive functioning in males with fragile X-associated tremor/ataxia syndrome. *Movement Disorders, 22*(5), 645–650.

Hagerman, P. J. (2012). Current gaps in understanding the molecular basis of FXTAS. *Tremor and Other Hyperkinetic Movements, 2.* doi:10.7916/D80C4TH0

Hagerman, P. J. & Hagerman, R. J. (2004). The fragile-X premutation: A maturing perspective. *American Journal of Human Genetics, 74*(5), 805–816. doi:10.1086/386296

Hagerman, R. J., Berry-Kravis, E., Kaufmann, W. E., Ono, M. Y., Tartaglia, N., Lachiewicz, A., . . . Tranfaglia, M. (2009). Advances in the treatment of fragile X syndrome. *Pediatrics, 123*(1), 378–390. doi:10.1542/peds.2008-0317

Hagerman, R. J., Hall, D. A., Coffey, S., Leehey, M., Bourgeois, J., Gould, J., . . . Hagerman, P. J. (2008). Treatment of fragile X-associated tremor ataxia syndrome (FXTAS) and related neurological problems. *Clinical Interventions in Aging, 3*(2), 251–262.

Hagerman, R. J., Leavitt, B. R., Farzin, F., Jacquemont, S., Greco, C. M., Brunberg, J. A., . . . Hagerman, P. J. (2004). Fragile-X-associated tremor/ataxia syndrome (FXTAS) in females with the *FMR1* premutation. *American Journal of Human Genetics, 74*(5), 1051–1056.

Hagerman, R. J., Leehey, M., Heinrichs, W., Tassone, F., Wilson, R., Hills, J., . . . Hagerman, P. J. (2001). Intention tremor, parkinsonism, and generalized brain atrophy in male carriers of fragile X. *Neurology, 57*(1), 127–130.

Hall, D. A., Berry-Kravis, E., Hagerman, R. J., Hagerman, P. J., Rice, C. D. & Leehey, M. A. (2006). Symptomatic treatment in the fragile X-associated tremor/ataxia syndrome. *Movement Disorders, 21*(10), 1741–1744. doi:10.1002/mds.21001

Hall, D. A., Berry-Kravis, E., Zhang, W., Tassone, F., Spector, E., Zerbe, G., . . . Leehey, M. A. (2011). *FMR1* gray-zone alleles: Association with Parkinson's disease in women? *Movement Disorders, 26*(10), 1900–1906. doi:10.1002/mds.23755

Hall, D. A., Birch, R. C., Anheim, M., Jonch, A. E., Pintado, E., O'Keefe, J., . . . Leehey, M. A. (2014). Emerging topics in FXTAS. *Journal of Neurodevelopmental Disorders, 6*(31). doi:10.1186/1866-1955-6-31

Hashimoto, R., Backer, K. C., Tassone, F., Hagerman, R. J. & Rivera, S. M. (2011a). An fMRI study of the prefrontal activity during the performance of a working memory task in premutation carriers of the fragile X mental retardation 1 gene with and without fragile X-associated tremor/ataxia syndrome (FXTAS). *Journal of Psychiatric Research, 45*(1), 36–43. doi:10.1016/j.jpsychires.2010.04.030

Hashimoto, R., Javan, A. K., Tassone, F., Hagerman, R. J. & Rivera, S. M. (2011b). A voxel-based morphometry study of grey matter loss in fragile X-associated tremor/ataxia syndrome. *Brain, 134*(3), 863–878. doi:10.1093/brain/awq368

Hashimoto, R., Srivastava, S., Tassone, F., Hagerman, R. J. & Rivera, S. M. (2011c). Diffusion tensor imaging in male premutation carriers of the fragile X mental retardation gene. *Movement Disorders, 26*(7), 1329–1336. doi:10.1002/mds.23646

Hessl, D., Rivera, S., Koldewyn, K., Cordeiro, L., Adams, J., Tassone, F., . . . Hagerman, R. J. (2007). Amygdala dysfunction in men with the fragile X premutation. *Brain, 130,* 404–416. doi:10.1093/brain/awl338

Hessl, D., Tassone, F., Loesch, D. Z., Berry-Kravis, E., Leehey, M. A., Gane, L. W., . . . Hagerman, R. J. (2005). Abnormal elevation of *FMR1* mRNA is associated with psychological symptoms in individuals with the fragile X premutation. *American Journal of Medical Genetics Part B: Neuropsychiatric Genetics, 139B*(1), 115–121.

Hessl, D., Wang, J. M., Schneider, A., Koldewyn, K., Le, L., Iwahashi, C., . . . Rivera, S. M. (2011). Decreased fragile X mental retardation protein expression underlies amygdala dysfunction in carriers of the fragile X premutation. *Biological Psychiatry, 70*(9), 859–865. doi:10.1016/j.biopsych.2011.05.033

Hippolyte, L., Battistella, G., Perrin, A. G., Fornari, E., Cornish, K. M., Beckmann, J. S., . . . Jacquemont, S. (2014). Investigation of memory, executive functions, and anatomic correlates in asymptomatic *FMR1* premutation carriers. *Neurobiology of Aging, 35*(8), 1939–1946. doi:10.1016/j.neurobiolaging.2014.01.150

Hocking, D. R., Birch, R. C., Bui, Q. M., Menant, J. C., Lord, S. R., Georgiou-Karistianis, N., . . . Trollor, J. N. (2017). Cerebellar volume mediates the relationship between FMR1 mRNA levels and voluntary step initiation in males with the premutation. *Neurobiology of Aging, 50*, 5–12. doi:10.1016/j.neurobiolaging.2016.10.017

Hocking, D. R., Kogan, C. S. & Cornish, K. M. (2012). Selective spatial processing deficits in an at-risk subgroup of the fragile X premutation. *Brain and Cognition, 79*(1), 39–44. doi:10.1016/j.bandc.2012.02.005

Hocking, D. R., Kraan, C. M., Godler, D. E., Bui, Q. M., Li, X., Bradshaw, J. L., . . . Cornish, K. M. (2015). Evidence linking *FMR1* mRNA and attentional demands of stepping and postural control in women with the premutation. *Neurobiology of Aging, 36*(3), 1400–1408. doi:10.1016/j.neurobiolaging.2014.11.012

Horvath, J., Burkhard, P. R., Morris, M., Bottani, A., Moix, I. & Delavelle, J. (2007). Expanding the phenotype of fragile x-associated tremor/ataxia syndrome: A new female case. *Movement Disorders, 22*(11), 1677–1678. doi:10.1002/mds.21571

Huber, K. M., Gallagher, S. M., Warren, S. T. & Bear, M. F. (2002). Altered synaptic plasticity in a mouse model of fragile X mental retardation. *Proceedings of the National Academy of Sciences, 99*(11), 7746–7750. doi:10.1073/pnas.122205699

Human Genetics Society of Australasia. (2012). *Best Practice Fragile X Testing and Analysis Guidelines for Australiasian Laboratories.* Sydney, NSW: Human Genetics Society of Australasia. Retrieved from www.hgsa.org.au/2011/12/draft-best-practice-fragile-x-testing-and-analysis-guidelines-for-australasian-laboratories/

Hunsaker, M. R., Greco, C. M., Spath, M. A., Smits, A. P. T., Navarro, C. S., Tassone, F., . . . Hukema, R. K. (2011). Widespread non-central nervous system organ pathology in fragile X premutation carriers with fragile X-associated tremor/ataxia syndrome and CGG knock-in mice. *Acta Neuropathologica, 122*(4), 467–479. doi:10.1007/s00401-011-0860-9

Iwahashi, C. K., Yasui, D. H., An, H. J., Greco, C. M., Tassone, F., Nannen, K., . . . Hagerman, P. J. (2006). Protein composition of the intranuclear inclusions of FXTAS. *Brain, 129*, 256–271. doi:10.1093/brain/awh650

Jacquemont, S., Hagerman, R. J., Leehey, M., Grigsby, J., Zhang, L., Brunberg, J. A., . . . Hagerman, P. J. (2003). Fragile X premutation tremor/ataxia syndrome: Molecular, clinical, and neuroimaging correlates. *The American Journal of Human Genetics, 72*(4), 869–878. doi:10.1086/374321

Jacquemont, S., Hagerman, R. J., Leehey, M. A., Hall, D. A., Levine, R. A., Brunberg, J. A., . . . Hagerman, P. J. (2004). Penetrance of the fragile X-associated tremor/ataxia syndrome in a premutation carrier population. *Journal of the American Medical Association, 291*(4), 460–469.

Jacquemont, S., Orrico, A., Galli, L., Sahota, P. K., Brunberg, J. A., Anichini, C., . . . Tassone, F. (2005). Spastic paraparesis, cerebellar ataxia, and intention tremor: A severe variant of FXTAS? *Journal of Medical Genetics, 42*(2), e14. doi:10.1136/jmg.2004.024190

Jin, P., Duan, R., Qurashi, A., Qin, Y., Tian, D., Rosser, T. C., . . . Warren, S. T. (2007). Pur α binds to rCGG repeats and modulates repeat-mediated neurodegeneration in a *Drosophila* model of fragile X tremor/ataxia syndrome. *Neuron, 55*(4), 556–564. doi:10.1016/j.neuron.2007.07.020

Juncos, J., Lazarus, J., Graves-Allen, E., Shubeck, L., Rusin, M., Novak, G., . . . Sherman, S. (2011). New clinical findings in the fragile X-associated tremor ataxia syndrome (FXTAS). *Neurogenetics, 12*(2), 123–135. doi:10.1007/s10048-010-0270-5

Kenneson, A., Zhang, F., Hagedorn, C. H. & Warren, S. T. (2001). Reduced FMRP and increased *FMR1* transcription is proportionally associated with CGG repeat number in intermediate-length and premutation carriers. *Human Molecular Genetics, 10*(14), 1449–1454. doi:10.1093/hmg/10.14.1449

Kogan, C. S. & Cornish, K. M. (2010). Mapping self-reports of working memory deficits to executive dysfunction in Fragile X Mental Retardation 1 (*FMR1*) gene premutation carriers asymptomatic for FXTAS. *Brain and Cognition, 73*(3), 236–243. doi:10.1016/j.bandc.2010.05.008

Koldewyn, K., Hessl, D., Adams, J., Tassone, F., Hagerman, P. J., Hagerman, R. J. & Rivera, S. M. (2008). Reduced hippocampal activation during recall is associated with elevated *FMR1* mRNA and psychiatric symptoms in men with the fragile X premutation. *Brain Imaging and Behavior, 2*(2), 105–116. doi:10.1007/s11682-008-9020-9

Kraan, C. M., Hocking, D. R., Georgiou-Karistianis, N., Metcalfe, S. A., Archibald, A. D., Fielding, J., . . . Cornish, K. M. (2013). Cognitive-motor interference during postural control indicates at-risk cerebellar profiles in females with the *FMR1* premutation. *Behavioural Brain Research, 253*, 329–336. doi:10.1016/j.bbr.2013.07.033

Kraan, C. M., Hocking, D. R., Georgiou-Karistianis, N., Metcalfe, S. A., Archibald, A. D., Fielding, J., . . . Cornish, K. M. (2014a). Impaired response inhibition is associated with self-reported symptoms of depression, anxiety, and ADHD in female *FMR1* premutation carriers. *American Journal of Medical Genetics Part B: Neuropsychiatric Genetics, 165*(1), 41–51. doi:10.1002/ajmg.b.32203

Kraan, C. M., Hocking, D. R., Georgiou-Karistianis, N., Metcalfe, S. A., Archibald, A. D., Fielding, J., . . . Cornish, K. M. (2014b). Age and CGG-repeat length are associated with neuromotor impairments in at-risk females with the *FMR1* premutation. *Neurobiology of Aging, 35*(9), 2179.e2177–2113. doi:10.1016/j.neurobiolaging.2014.03.018

Kurz, M. W., Schlitter, A. M., Klenk, Y., Mueller, T., Larsen, J. P., Aarsland, D. & Dekomien, G. (2007). FMR1 alleles in Parkinson's disease: Relation to cognitive decline and hallucinations, a longitudinal study. *Journal of Geriatric Psychiatry and Neurology, 20*(2), 89–92. doi:10.1177/0891988706297737

Leehey, M. A., Berry-Kravis, E., Goetz, C. G., Zhang, L., Hall, D. A., Li, L., . . . Hagerman, P. J. (2008). *FMR1* CGG repeat length predicts motor dysfunction in premutation carriers. *Neurology, 70*(16), 1397–1402.

Leehey, M. A., Hall, D., Rice, C., Jacquemont, S., Zhang, L., Grigsby, J., . . . Hagerman, P. J. (2005). Preliminary study of the natural history of the fragile X associated tremor/ataxia syndrome (FXTAS). *Neurology, 64*(6), A93.

Leow, A., Harvey, D., Goodrich-Hunsaker, N. J., Gadelkarim, J., Kumar, A., Zhan, L., . . . Simon, T. J. (2014). Altered structural brain connectome in young adult fragile X premutation carriers. *Human Brain Mapping, 35*(9), 4518–4530. doi:10.1002/hbm.22491

Loesch, D. Z., Khaniani, M. S., Slater, H. R., Rubio, J. P., Bui, Q. M., Kotschet, K., . . . Horne, M. (2009). Small CGG repeat expansion alleles of FMR1 gene are associated with parkinsonism. *Clinical Genetics, 76*(5), 471–476. doi:10.1111/j.1399-0004.2009.01275.x

Louis, E., Moskowitz, C., Friez, M., Amaya, M. & Vonsattel, J. P. G. (2006). Parkinsonism, dysautonomia, and intranuclear inclusions in a fragile X carrier: A clinical-pathological study. *Movement Disorders, 21*(3), 420–425. doi:10.1002/mds.20753

Moore, C. J., Daly, E. M., Tassone, F., Tysoe, C., Schmitz, N., Ng, V., . . . Murphy, D. G. M. (2004). The effect of pre-mutation of X chromosome CGG trinucleotide repeats on brain anatomy. *Brain, 127*(12), 2672–2681. doi:10.1093/brain/awh256

Nolin, S. L., Brown, W. T., Glicksman, A., Houck, J. G. E., Gargano, A. D., Sullivan, A., . . . Sherman, S. L. (2003). Expansion of the fragile X CGG repeat in females with premutation or intermediate alleles. *The American Journal of Human Genetics, 72*(2), 454–464.

O'Keefe, J. A., Robertson-Dick, E., Dunn, E. J., Li, Y., Deng, Y., Fiutko, A. N., . . . Hall, D. A. (2015). Characterization and early detection of balance deficits in fragile X premutation carriers with and without fragile X-associated tremor/ataxia syndrome (FXTAS). *The Cerebellum, 14*(6), 650–662. doi:10.1007/s12311-015-0659-7

Oh, S. Y., He, F., Krans, A., Frazer, M., Taylor, J. P., Paulson, H. L. & Todd, P. K. (2015). RAN translation at CGG repeats induces ubiquitin proteasome system impairment in models of fragile X-associated tremor ataxia syndrome. *Human Molecular Genetics, 24*(15), 4317–4326. doi:http://dx.doi.org/10.1093/hmg/ddv165

Peprah, E. (2012). Fragile X syndrome: The *FMR1* CGG repeat distribution among world populations. *Annals of Human Genetics, 76*(2), 178–191. doi:10.1111/j.1469-1809.2011.00694.x

Polussa, J., Schneider, A. & Hagerman, R. (2014). Molecular advances leading to treatment implications for fragile X premutation carriers. *Brain Disorders & Therapy, 3*(119). doi:10.4172/2168-975X.1000119

Reis, A. H. O., Ferreira, A. C. S., Gomes, K. B., Aguiar, M. J. B., Fonseca, C. G., Cardoso, F. E., . . . Carvalho, M. R. S. (2008). Frequency of FMR1 premutation in individuals with ataxia and/or tremor and/or parkinsonism. *Genetics and Molecular Research, 7*(1), 74–84.

Renaud, M., Perriard, J., Coudray, S., Sévin-Allouet, M., Marcel, C., Meissner, W., . . . Anheim, M. (2015). Relevance of corpus callosum splenium versus middle cerebellar peduncle hyperintensity for FXTAS diagnosis in clinical practice. *Journal of Neurology, 262*(2), 435–442. doi:10.1007/s00415-014-7557-7

Rodriguez-Revenga, L., Madrigal, I., Pagonabarraga, J., Xuncla, M., Badenas, C., Kulisevsky, J., . . . Mila, M. (2009). Penetrance of *FMR1* premutation associated pathologies in fragile X syndrome families. *European Journal of Human Genetics, 17*(10), 1359–1362. doi:10.1038/ejhg.2009.51

Schneider, A., Ballinger, E., Chavez, A., Tassone, F., Hagerman, R. J. & Hessl, D. (2011). Prepulse inhibition in patients with fragile X-associated tremor ataxia syndrome. *Neurobiology of Aging, 33*(6), 1045–1053. doi:10.1016/j.neurobiolaging.2010.09.002

Schwartz, C. E., Dean, J., Howard-Peebles, P. N., Bugge, M., Mikkelsen, M., Tommerup, N., . . . Stevenson, R. E. (1994). Obstetrical and gynecological complications in fragile X carriers: A multicenter study. *American Journal of Medical Genetics, 51*(4), 400–402. doi:10.1002/ajmg.1320510419

Sellier, C., Freyermuth, F., Tabet, R., Tran, T., He, F., Ruffenach, F., . . . Charlet-Berguerand, N. (2013). Sequestration of DROSHA and DGCR8 by expanded CGG RNA repeats alters microRNA processing in fragile X-associated tremor/ataxia syndrome. *Cell Reports, 3*(3), 869–880. doi:10.1016/j.celrep.2013.02.004

Sellier, C., Rau, F., Liu, Y., Tassone, F., Hukema, R. K., Gattoni, R., . . . Charlet-Berguerand, N. (2010). Sam68 sequestration and partial loss of function are associated with splicing alterations in FXTAS patients. *The EMBO Journal, 29*(7), 1248–1261. doi:10.1038/emboj.2010.21

Seritan, A. L., Kim, K., Benjamin, I., Seritan, I. & Hagerman, R. J. (2016). Risk factors for cognitive impairment in fragile X-associated tremor/ataxia syndrome. *Journal of Geriatric Psychiatry and Neurology.* doi:10.1177/0891988716666379

Seritan, A. L., Nguyen, D. V., Farias, S. T., Hinton, L., Grigsby, J., Bourgeois, J. A. & Hagerman, R. J. (2008). Dementia in fragile X-associated tremor/ataxia syndrome

(FXTAS): Comparison with Alzheimer's disease. *American Journal of Medical Genetics Part B: Neuropsychiatric Genetics, 147B*(7), 1138–1144. doi:10.1002/ajmg.b.30732

Seritan, A. L., Nguyen, D. V., Mu, Y., Tassone, F., Bourgeois, J. A., Schneider, A., . . . Hagerman, R. J. (2014). Memantine for fragile X-associated tremor/ataxia syndrome: A randomized, double-blind, placebo-controlled trial. *Journal of Clinical Psychiatry, 75*(3), 264–271. doi:10.4088/JCP.13m08546

Sevin, M., Kutalik, Z., Bergman, S., Vercelletto, M., Renou, P., Lamy, E., . . . Jacquemont, S. (2009). Penetrance of marked cognitive impairment in older male carriers of the *FMR1* gene premutation. *Journal of Medical Genetics, 46*(12), 818–824. doi:10.1136/jmg.2008.065953

Shelton, A. L., Cornish, K. M., Godler, D., Bui, Q. M., Kolbe, S. & Fielding, J. (2017). White matter microstructure, cognition, and molecular markers in fragile X premutation females. *Neurology, 88*(22), 2080–2088.

Shickman, R., Famula, J., Tassone, F., Leehey, M., Ferrer, E., Rivera, S. M. & Hessl, D. (2018). Age- and CGG repeat-related slowing of manual movement in fragile X carriers: A prodrome of fragile X-associated tremor ataxia syndrome? *Movement Disorders, 33*(4), 628–636. doi:10.1002/mds.27314

Sofola, O. A., Jin, P., Qin, Y., Duan, R., Liu, H., de Haro, M., . . . Botas, J. (2007). RNA binding proteins hnRNP A2/B1 and CUGBP1 suppress fragile X CGG premutation repeat-induced neurodegeneration in a *Drosophila* model of FXTAS. *Neuron, 55*(4), 565–571. doi:10.1016/j.neuron.2007.07.021

Tassone, F., Adams, J., Berry-Kravis, E. M., Cohen, S. S., Brusco, A., Leehey, M. A., . . . Hagerman, P. J. (2007). CGG repeat length correlates with age of onset of motor signs of the fragile X-associated tremor/ataxia syndrome (FXTAS). *American Journal of Medical Genetics Part B: Neuropsychiatric Genetics, 144B*(4), 566–569. doi:10.1002/ajmg.b.30482

Tassone, F., Hagerman, R. J., Taylor, A. K., Gane, L. W., Godfrey, T. E. & Hagerman, P. J. (2000). Elevated levels of *FMR1* mRNA in carrier males: A new mechanism of involvement in the fragile-X syndrome. *The American Journal of Human Genetics, 66*(1), 6–15.

Tassone, F., Iong, K. P., Tong, T., Lo, J., Gane, L. W., Berry-Kravis, E., . . . Hagerman, R. J. (2012). *FMR1* CGG allele size and prevalence ascertained through newborn screening in the United States. *Genome Medicine, 4*(12), 100. doi:10.1186/gm401

Tassone, F., Iwahashi, C. & Hagerman, P. J. (2004). *FMR1* RNA within the intranuclear inclusions of fragile X-associated tremor/ataxia syndrome (FXTAS). *RNA Biology, 1*(2), 103–105. doi:10.4161/rna.1.2.1035

Todd, P. K., Oh, S. Y., Krans, A., He, F., Sellier, C., Frazer, M., . . . Paulson, H. L. (2013). CGG repeat-associated translation mediates neurodegeneration in fragile X tremor ataxia syndrome. *Neuron, 78*(3), 440–455. doi:10.1016/j.neuron.2013.03.026

Verkerk, A. J. M. H., Pieretti, M., Sutcliffe, J. S., Fu, Y. H., Kuhl, D. P. A., Pizzuti, A., . . . Warren, S. T. (1991). Identification of a gene (FMR-1) containing a CGG repeat coincident with a breakpoint cluster region exhibiting length variation in fragile X syndrome. *Cell, 65*(5), 905–914. doi:10.1016/0092-8674(91)90397-H

Wang, J., Hessl, D., Schneider, A., Tassone, F. & Hagerman, R. J. (2013a). Fragile X associated tremor/ataxia syndrome: Influence of the *FMR1* gene on motor fiber tracts in males with normal and premutation alleles. *JAMA Neurology, 70*(8), 1022–1029. doi:10.1001/jamaneurol.2013.2934

Wang, J. Y., Hagerman, R. J. & Rivera, S. (2013b). A multimodal imaging analysis of subcortical gray matter in fragile X premutation carriers. *Movement Disorders, 28*(9), 1278–1284. doi:10.1002/mds.25473

Wang, J. Y., Trivedi, A. M., Carrillo, N. R., Yang, J., Schneider, A., Giulivi, C., . . . Hagerman, R. J. (2017). Open-label allopregnanolone treatment of men with fragile X-associated tremor/ataxia syndrome. *Neurotherapeutics, 14*(4), 1073–1083. doi:10.1007/ s13311-017-0555-6

Wong, L. M., Goodrich-Hunsaker, N. J., McLennan, Y., Tassone, F., Harvey, D., Rivera, S. M. & Simon, T. J. (2012). Young adult male carriers of the fragile X premutation exhibit genetically modulated impairments in visuospatial tasks controlled for psychomotor speed. *Journal of Neurodevelopmental Disorders, 4*(26). doi:10.1186/1866-1955-4-26

Yang, J., Chan, S., Khan, S., Schneider, A., Nanakul, R., Teichholtz, S., . . . Olichney, J. M. (2013a). Neural substrates of executive dysfunction in fragile X-associated tremor/ ataxia syndrome (FXTAS): A brain potential study. *Cerebral Cortex, 23*(11), 2657–2666. doi:10.1093/cercor/bhs251

Yang, J., Niu, Y. Q., Simon, C., Chen, L., Seritan, A. L. & Schneider, A. (2013b). Effects of Memantine on language/memory-related brain potentials in fragile X-associated tremor/ataxia syndrome (FXTAS). Paper presented at the 1st International Conference on the *FMR1* Premutation: Basic Mechanisms and Clinical Involvement, Perugia, Italy.

Yang, J. C., Simon, C., Niu, Y.-Q., Bogost, M., Schneider, A., Tassone, F., . . . Olichney, J. M. (2013c). Phenotypes of hypofrontality in older female fragile X premutation carriers. *Annals of Neurology, 74*(2), 257–283. doi:10.1002/ana.23933

Zalfa, F. & Bagni, C. (2004). Molecular insights into mental retardation: Multiple functions for the fragile X mental retardation protein? *Current Issues in Molecular Biology, 6*, 73–88.

Zhang, L., Sukharev, D., Schneider, A., Olichney, J. M., Seritan, A. & Hagerman, R. J. (2014). Case report: Dystonia in a fragile X carrier. *Movement Disorders, 29*(7), E4–E5. doi:10.1002/mds.23600

Zhang, X., Zhuang, X., Gan, S., Wu, Z., Chen, W., Hu, Y. & Wang, N. (2012). Screening for *FMR1* expanded alleles in patients with parkinsonism in mainland China. *Neuroscience Letters, 514*(1), 16–21.

7

MULTIPLE SCLEROSIS

Joanne Fielding and Meaghan Clough

Introduction

Our understanding of multiple sclerosis (MS) has advanced significantly since Charcot delivered his 1868 lectures on *la sclérose en plaque disséminée* at the Salpetriere (Charcot, 1877; Murray, 2005). While certainly not the first description of the disease, this was the first time the disease was framed and given a name (Murray, 2005), dissociating it from the myriad of other disorders previously lumped together as paraplegia. Building on these earlier descriptions, the last half century has witnessed an explosion of interest in the disease, corresponding with major advances in medical science and technology. Despite this, the highly heterogenous nature of the disease still poses significant challenges, with respect to fully understanding its complex pathophysiology and developing treatment strategies that encompass all aspects of the disease.

Preliminary considerations

Multiple sclerosis is an immune-mediated neurodegenerative disease of the central nervous system (CNS), and is the most common cause of non-traumatic neurological disability in young adults (Feigin et al., 2017). For most patients the disease course is one punctuated by fully or partially reversible episodes of neurological disability, which typically last days or weeks. The characteristics of these episodes can be highly variable depending on the CNS region(s) implicated in the disease process, but may include visual disturbances, cognitive changes, muscle weakness or paralysis, fatigue and sensory symptoms (Brownlee, Hardy, Fazekas & Miller, 2017). As the disease advances, patients often transition into a more progressive clinical course, leading to greater physical impairment and more profound cognitive changes. A relatively small proportion of patients experience a more progressive course from onset. At present there are 12 Therapeutic Goods Administration-approved disease-modifying medications available that target immune-mediated disease processes, subsequently reducing the frequency of episodes, or relapses. However, no medication fully prevents or reverses progressive neurological deterioration in MS, and whether any can delay clinical progression is yet to be determined (Cree et al., 2016; Signori et al., 2016; Zhang et al., 2015).

Epidemiology

MS affects approximately 2.5 million individuals worldwide. The prevalence of MS varies considerably across the world, the highest prevalence being in North America (140 per 100,000 population) and Europe (108 per 100,000), and lowest in East Asia (2.2 per 100,000 population) and sub-Saharan Africa (2.1 per 100,000). Further, prevalence increases with latitude, north and south of the equator (Leray, Moreau, Fromont & Edan, 2016). This geographic distribution has been proposed to be a consequence of environmental factors, as well as genetic susceptibility among populations. Women are affected more commonly than men, with the female-to-male ratio varying between 1.5:1 and 2.5:1 (Koch-Henriksen & Sorensen, 2010). Age at onset is relatively uniform across populations, with a low incidence in childhood, rapidly increasing to a peak between 25 and 35 years, followed by a slow decline (Ascherio & Munger, 2016).

Etiology

While the specific cause(s) of MS are still largely unknown, they likely involve a complex interaction of genetic and environmental factors. A genetic contribution is evident in studies involving informative cohorts, like twins and conjugal pairs and adoptees. Individuals with an affected first-degree relative have a 2–4% risk of developing MS, compared to a 0.1% risk in the general population. Concordance in monozygotic twins is between 30% and 50%, compared to 5% in dizygotic twins (Leray et al., 2016). Genome-wide association studies have identified over 200 gene variants that increase the risk of MS, the most significant being variations in the genes encoding human leukocyte antigens (HLAs) within the major histocompatibility complex. HLAs are the mechanism by which the immune system differentiates between self and foreign bodies. The main risk allele is HLA DRB1*1501, with an odds ratio of approximately 3 (Stephen, 2011). However, there are also a large number of variants including interleukin 7 receptor (IL7R) and interleukin 2 receptor A gene (IL-2RA), CD58, and CLEC16A (Beyeen et al., 2010). IL7, for example, is a cytokine essential to the development and homeostatic maintenance of T and B lymphocytes, both of which are implicated in the MS pathological process.

Although genetic susceptibility explains the within family clustering of MS, it does not explain the variations in MS frequency as a function of geographic location, the increasing prevalence over time, or the changes in risk that occur with migration. These strongly support the action of environmental factors. Of the many factors proposed, infection with Epstein–Barr virus (EBV), vitamin D status, and cigarette smoking are the most consistent environmental predictors of MS risk (Ascherio & Munger, 2016). Arguably the strongest of these is infection with EBV. The risk of developing MS is around 15 times higher for those infected with EBV in childhood compared with non-infected individuals, with the risk elevated to about 30 times higher among those infected with EBV in adolescence or later in life. Although the mechanisms are unclear, primary EBV infection early on in life is usually asymptomatic, but primary EBV infection later in life often manifests as infectious mononucleosis. Mononucleosis has been associated with a two- to threefold increased risk of developing MS (Ascherio & Munger, 2010).

For most individuals, the major source of vitamin D is sunlight exposure (ultra-violet B radiation). As duration and intensity of sunlight are strongly linked to latitude, the higher incidence of MS at higher latitudes has been proposed to reflect vitamin D deficiency. Certainly, epidemiological studies support a protective role of vitamin D in reducing MS risk, especially in childhood and adolescence, and there is also evidence that correcting vitamin D insufficiency in MS has a positive effect on clinical outcomes. While the mechanisms underlying these effects are unclear, there is accumulating evidence of a role for vitamin D in increasing IL-17 and induction of regulatory T cells (Hayes et al., 2015). A recent meta-analysis has also demonstrated a significant association between smoking and MS (Handel et al., 2011), however, the mechanisms behind the association are especially uncertain as are the interactions between smoking and other established risk factors. Overall, the mechanisms by which genetic polymorphisms and environmental factors raise the risk of MS are the subject of intense investigation.

Neuropathology

MS is characterised by the complex interplay of immunological and neurodegenerative processes, culminating in heterogeneity in the clinical course and symptom expression. The hallmark of the disease process, immune-mediated inflammation, is most evident within white matter, resulting in demyelination, and eventual axonal loss, leading to disruption to nerve conduction. Inflammatory processes, a distinguishing feature of early disease, activate inflammatory perivascular infiltrates (e.g. myelin-specific CD4+ autoreactive T cells, CD8+ T cells, and B cells secreting myelin-directed antibodies and cytokines), that attack the myelin sheath that surrounds axons, as well as oligodendrocytes, the cells responsible for the creation of myelin (Frohman, Racke & Raine, 2006; Lassmann, 2013).

As a consequence of these attacks, active inflammatory lesions are formed (for an elegant description of the mechanisms of plaque pathogenesis see Meltzer, Costello, Frohman & Frohman, 2018). These lesions demonstrate a predilection for peri-ventricular and peri-aqueductal areas, corpus callosum, chiasm and the brainstem, resulting in the stereotypical lesion distribution pattern often observed in MS patients (Frohman et al., 2006). In the early stages of the disease, remyelination helps to restore axonal conduction, with oligodendrocyte progenitor cells re-ensheathing demyelinated axons. However, repetitive attacks lead to successively less effective remyelination and degradation of axons, resulting in the formation of gliotic scar tissue and permanent, irreversible neurological damage (Lassmann, 2013).

Axonal degeneration also occurs early in the disease, beginning in active lesions. Because of the brain's capacity to compensate for this loss, this does not initially lead to permanent clinical disability. However, accumulated axonal loss contributes significantly to brain atrophy, reflected by change in brain parenchymal fraction and brain volume, and leading to more permanent neurological disability. Although the cause of axonal damage is unknown in MS, proposed elements include oxidative activation of microglia/macrophages, mitochondria and energy failure, hypoxia, Wallerian degeneration, iron accumulation, meningeal inflammation and activation of astrocytes (Kawachi & Lassmann, 2017).

In the past decade, the concept of MS as purely a disease of white matter has been reconsidered. The relevance of cortical pathology, in the form of both focal (grey matter lesions) and diffuse injury of normal-appearing white and grey matter, has led to a more inclusive idea of MS as a disease that affects the entire central nervous system. Cortical pathology is a frequent phenomenon in MS, and observed in all stages of the disease (Filippi et al., 2010).

Neurodegeneration is a recognised and important neuropathological component of MS. Although generally poorly understood, neurodegenerative changes have been identified early on in the disease, including at disease inception, becoming increasingly prominent as the disease progresses (Lassmann, 2012; Lucchinetti et al., 2011). Whether neurodegeneration is a consequence of inflammatory axonal degeneration, a concomitant process, a parallel process, or an initiating event is unclear. However, evidence suggesting a segregation between neurodegenerative and inflammatory processes is evident from the partial efficacy of anti-inflammatory and immunomodulatory treatments in early stages, and the modest or absence of any real benefit during progressive stages of the disease (Kawachi & Lassmann, 2017).

Presently, there is little understanding of the earliest pathological changes occurring in MS. Although not conclusive, it appears that the earliest pathological changes are concerned with widespread neurodegenerative changes affecting the functionality of neural networks. Indeed, there is some evidence to suggest that these changes predate explicit lesion formation (Calabrese et al., 2007).

Clinical presentation

Driven by this complex interplay of overlapping and interconnected inflammatory and degenerative changes, the clinical features of MS vary considerably, both at disease onset as well as throughout the course of the disease. Symptoms may be mild to debilitating, evolving over time as a function of the localisation of neuropathology. Characteristic symptoms seen in MS often reflect disruption to sensory, motor, bladder, bowel, sexual, cerebellar, brainstem, optic nerve, and cognitive functions. While there are no symptoms that are unique to MS, there are a number of key features that help differentiate MS from other diseases of the CNS. These include:

1   episodic symptoms, which evolve gradually, last for weeks, and then remit to some degree;
2   fatigability that is exacerbated by heat;
3   mild cognitive changes;
4   bizarre sensory perceptions;
5   bladder urgency or retention;
6   internuclear ophthalmoplegia (or other mild/subclinical ocular motor signs);
7   muscle weakness, especially of the fingers and pelvis;
8   gait ataxia; and
9   reduced vibration at toes.

For most patients, symptoms of an attack arise over hours to days, and typically last between 2 and 6 weeks. Symptoms remit, sometimes completely, but can result in long-lasting deficits (Lublin, Baier & Cutter, 2003). Symptoms may also reappear transiently, especially during infections, exercise, stress, menses, or heat.

Common presentations

Motor symptoms are especially common in MS, with some degree of muscle weakness experienced by almost 90% of patients at some point (Swingler & Compston, 1992). Paraparesis is the most common initial presentation, with weakness potentially occurring in a single limb (monoparesis), or all four limbs (quadriparesis). Weakness of the limbs is typically a consequence of corticospinal tract involvement and, as such, is often accompanied by symptoms of upper motor neuron dysfunction such as hyperreflexia, an extensor plantar response, and spasticity. Spasticity can be profoundly disabling even leading to permanent contractures of the muscle. It may manifest as increase in tone at rest (rigidity), slow contraction of antagonistic muscles (dystonia), tendon hyper-reflexivity, and myoclonia, which may occur independently or together. Tonic seizures are often seen when the spinal cord or brainstem is implicated in the disease process. Involuntary contractions of the affected limb, confined to one side of the body, can last up to a minute, and occur several times a day.

Eye movement abnormalities are also common in MS, and may profoundly affect patients' level of disability and prognostic future (Derwenskus et al., 2005). The most common eye movement disorder observed in MS is internuclear ophthalmoparesis (INO), a consequence of demyelination and axonal damage to the medial longitudinal fasciculus within the pons (ventral to the fourth ventricle), or midbrain (ventral to the cerebral aqueduct). In INO conjugacy is disrupted, with slowing of the adducting eye during horizontal saccades (adduction lag), and a corresponding nystagmus of the abducting eye. Patients with INO may also present with diplopia or blurred vision and visual confusion during head turns due to a transient break in binocular fusion (Mills et al., 2008).

After INO, gaze instability is the next most common disorder seen in MS (Serra, Derwenskus, Downey & Leigh, 2003), a consequence of disruption to the gaze controlling brainstem-cerebellar networks involved in neural integration and maintenance of gaze (Tilikete et al., 2011). Several forms of nystagmus are reported, including gaze-evoked nystagmus, a coarse to-and-fro eye oscillation, and downbeat nystagmus, a spontaneous vertical eye oscillation with upward slow phases. However, the most common form of nystagmus seen in MS is acquired pendular nystagmus (APN), or slow-phase eye movements in the horizontal, vertical, and torsional planes that form elliptical waveforms. APN causes significant disability. MS patients may also suffer disabling oscillopsia arising from saccadic intrusions and oscillations, such as square-wave jerks, macro square-wave jerks, and macrosaccadic oscillations.

Optic neuritis (ON) is inflammation of the *optic* nerve. Almost half of all MS patients experience an episode of ON at some point, and for approximately 20% of patients, it is the earliest or presenting symptom (Balcer, 2006). ON initially manifests as acute or subacute eye pain that is exacerbated by moving the eye, followed by a degree of visual disturbance (blurring or loss) that primarily affects central vision (Optic Neuritis Study Group, 1991). Colour vision, in particular red desaturation, and low-contrast vision are most affected. Although most patients regain normal vision over two to six months, desaturation of bright colours, or nonspecific dimming often persists. Once inflammation subsides, most patients exhibit some permanent loss of retinal nerve fibre layer, which can be quantified using retinal optical coherence tomography (Costello et al., 2006).

Incoordination, often a consequence of cerebellar pathology, is reflected in gait imbalance, difficulty performing coordinated actions, and slurred speech. Dysmetria and hypotonia, usually in the upper extremities, are also prevalent. In more severe MS, patients may be unable to stand, use their arms due to severe tremor, or produce comprehensible speech.

Sensory impairments such as numbness and paresthesias are also common in MS, and can be some of the most distressing symptoms. Common sensations experienced are akin to distorted perceptions of everyday stimuli and range from tingling, crawling or prickling sensations to burning pain. They may be transient, but can also last many hours and even days. Up to 87% of patients experience sensory changes at some point in the disease, and are a presenting syndrome in over one third of patients (Swingler & Compston, 1992). Pain and other unpleasant sensations, often have neuropathic features like electrical or sharp sensations. An example of this is Lhermitte's symptom, where electrical-shock-like sensations run down the spine when the neck is flexed, a consequence of involvement of the posterior column in the cervical or upper thoracic spinal cord.

Brainstem syndromes often manifest as double vision (lesion involving cranial nerves III, IV, VI), INO, facial weakness or muscle contractions (cranial nerve VII), vertigo (cranial nerve VIII), or bulbar (medullary) symptoms like dysphagia and dysarthria (cranial nerves IX, X, XII). Sensory impairments of the face may also arise from a brainstem lesion (cranial nerve V).

Depressive disorder is proposed to affect almost half of all MS patients, approximately three times the prevalence in the general population (Jones et al., 2012). The pathogenesis of depression in MS is complex, and most likely multifactorial, including psychological, social, neurobiological, immunologic, and genetic factors (Gold & Irwin, 2006). While depression may be reactive in nature, a consequence of living with a chronic illness with an uncertain prognosis and no known cure, it may also be related to disease-specific processes such as pathological changes in frontotemporal networks, or in immune processes. Further, patients must often manage a range of comorbid conditions including pain, anxiety, fatigue, substance abuse, and cognitive impairment.

Fatigue is considered one of the disease's most debilitating symptoms, reported in up to 83% of patients (Minden et al., 2006). MS-related fatigue can occur daily, with many patients complaining of feeling exhausted on waking, despite adequate sleep. Fatigue is often aggravated by heat and humidity, a potential consequence of slowing of neuronal conduction with increased body temperature. Often, fatigue is associated with an acute attack, preceding the onset of neurological symptoms, and persisting long after the attack has abated (Carnicka et al., 2015). While fatigue has been shown to correlate with degree of axonal injury, there is a poor correlation between fatigue and overall disease severity or presence of a particular symptom (Tartaglia et al., 2004).

Pain associated with MS can arise from neuropathological changes and may be paroxysmal, persistent or episodic, or may be caused by paralysis, immobility, or spasticity.

Bladder dysfunction and lower urinary tract impairment is a significant cause of disability in MS (Fowler et al., 2009), and attributable to detrusor hyperreflexia, or overactive bladder. Contraction of the detrusor muscle normally coincides with relaxation of the urethral sphincter. Usually, the detrusor reflex is inhibited voluntarily, with loss of this inhibition leading to over-activation of the reflex and the experience of urinary urgency, frequency, and incontinence. A less common symptom is detrusor-sphincter dysynergia, arising from the loss of coordination between the detrusor and sphincter muscles. This leads to urinary hesitancy, interruptions of the urinary stream, and incomplete emptying. Recurrent urinary tract infections are also common.

Cognitive impairment is now considered a primary deficit of the disease, affecting 40–70% of patients (Chiaravalloti & DeLuca, 2008), manifesting at all disease stages, including onset, and in all subtypes (Amato, Ponziani, Siracusa & Sorbi, 2001; Potagas et al., 2008). Although the disseminated and variable nature of MS pathology means that a range of cognitive domains can be affected, changes to information processing speed (IPS), attention and memory (particularly episodic) are most prominent, with executive deficits and verbal fluency less frequently reported; basic language abilities usually remain intact, even at more advanced stages of the disease (Amato et al., 2010; Chiaravalloti & DeLuca, 2008).

Once established, cognitive deficits appear to worsen with advancing disease, with the number of domains implicated usually extending (Amato et al., 2001). Overt dementia as seen in other progressive neurological disorders (e.g. Alzheimer's disease) is rare (Defer & Branger, 2015), with the more common presentation remaining domain specific and comparatively subtle. Despite this, cognitive deficits have a huge impact on a patient's quality of life, with those affected engaging in fewer vocational and social activities, and reporting higher levels of depressive symptomology (Ruet et al., 2013).

IPS is generally viewed as the efficiency with which information is processed and integrated with other cognitive processes, resulting in the formulation of a behavioural response. In MS, slowed IPS is prominent and has been shown to predict future cognitive decline (Bergendal, Fredrikson & Almkvist, 2007; Costa, Genova, DeLuca & Chiaravalloti, 2017; DeLuca, Chelune, Tulsky, Lengenfelder & Chiaravalloti, 2004). IPS deficits rarely appear in isolation and are usually related to deficits in other cognitive domains, specifically, executive function, memory and attention (Covey, Zivadinov, Shucard & Shucard, 2011; Drew, Starkey & Isler, 2009; Owens, Denney & Lynch, 2013; Roth, Denney & Lynch, 2015). This has led to the suggestion that slowed IPS underlies deficits in other cognitive domains: relative consequence model (DeLuca et al., 2004). Indeed, several studies have shown that, once time is removed as a task constraint, MS patients do not perform differently to healthy controls on measures of working memory, attention and executive function (Covey et al., 2011; DeLuca et al., 2004; Genova, DeLuca, Chiaravalloti & Wylie, 2013; Leavitt et al., 2014; Owens et al., 2013). Although compelling, IPS and other cognitive processes are also highly correlated in healthy individuals. This makes conclusions about a direct link between decline in IPS and other cognitive domain performance in MS, independent of premorbid ability or pathological measures of disease, contentious.

Memory deficits largely relate to long-term memory, or the ability to learn new information and to recall that information at a later date. Affecting up to approximately 60% of patients, evidence now suggests that MS patients have a primary deficit in the initial learning or consolidation of information, not retrieval as previously thought (Benedict et al., 2006; DeLuca, Gaudino, Diamond, Christodoulou & Engel, 1998; Thornton & Raz, 1997). Behaviourally, this type of deficit manifests as requiring increased repetition of new information to achieve memory consolidation; however, once consolidation has occurred, recall and recognition are no different to healthy individuals (DeLuca, Barbieri-Berger & Johnson, 1994; DeLuca et al., 1998). In patients with very early disease, deficits are more commonly associated with working memory, a limited capacity, temporary storage system that enables the active maintenance and integration of information (Fuso, Callegaro, Pompeia & Bueno, 2010; Panou, Mastorodemos, Papadaki, Simos & Plaitakis, 2012; Pelosi, Geesken, Holly, Hayward & Blumhardt, 1997).

Attention is a central cognitive process that facilitates the processing of relevant information and the inhibition or filtering of irrelevant information. In MS, deficits purportedly affect functions associated with sustaining, selecting, dividing and alternating between attentional sets, with simpler functions largely preserved (Amato et al., 2010; Beatty, Paul, Blanco, Hames & Wilbanks, 1995; McCarthy, Beaumont, Thompson & Peacock, 2005; Paul, Beatty, Schneider, Blanco & Hames, 1998). Attentional deficits are present even at the earliest stages of the disease, and are reportedly the most detrimental to normal functioning (Bobholz & Rao, 2003). Due to the ubiquitous nature of attention to functioning of other cognitive abilities, deficits in attentional processes are often associated with memory (maintenance and consolidation) and IPS in MS (Chiaravalloti & DeLuca, 2008; Kujala, Portin, Revonsuo & Ruutiainen, 1995).

Executive function is a general term referring to a set of cognitive abilities required for complex goal-directed and adaptive behaviour. Although occurring with much less frequency than the aforementioned deficits, changes to abstract and conceptual reasoning, fluency and planning have been reported in MS (Arnett et al., 1997; Foong et al., 1997; Hanssen, Beiske, Landro & Hessen, 2014; Joly, Cohen & Lebrun, 2014; Muhlert et al., 2014; Owens et al., 2013). In particular, changes to both phonemeic and semantic fluency, that is, the spontaneous production of words under restricted conditions, has been reported (Drew, Tippett, Starkey & Isler, 2008; Henry & Beatty, 2006). In addition, perseveration of errors is common, suggesting deficits within behavioural monitoring systems that may also be present (Parmenter, Zivadinov et al., 2007; Rao, Hammeke & Speech, 1987). However, executive deficits are rarely prominent or represent a complete loss of function within a specific ability (Defer & Branger, 2015). Indeed, as noted previously, performance on executive tests is highly correlated with other, more ubiquitous cognitive functions (namely, IPS and attention), as well as level of depressive symptomology; when these processes are controlled for, deficits are no longer demonstrable (Genova et al., 2013; Leavitt et al., 2014; Owens et al., 2013).

Despite the prevalence of cognitive deficits, routine cognitive assessment does not form part of standard clinical management. This is largely due to the absence of reliable and accepted neuropsychological measures specific to MS, as well as the time and expertise required to administer and interpret test performance. Of the range of neuropsychological tests used, the Symbol Digit Modalities Test (SDMT), Brief Visuospatial Memory Test–Revised (BVMT-R: visuospatial memory), and California Verbal Learning Test–II (CVLT-II: verbal memory) have been identified as particularly informative (Sumowski et al., 2018). The Paced Auditory Serial Addition Test (PASAT), a complex test of working memory and information processing speed, has historically been widely used in MS, particularly in clinical trials. However, its poor tolerability by patients and reliability has seen its use decline (Benedict et al., 2017), with the SDMT now considered the most sensitive in terms of screening for cognitive change and monitoring (Benedict et al., 2008, 2017; Parmenter, Weinstock-Guttman, Garg, Munschauer & Benedict, 2007). Attempts have been made to formulate brief and repeatable cognitive assessment batteries, to screen for and monitor cognitive changes. However, the capacity of neuropsychological tests generally, to detect subtle cognitive changes, a hallmark of MS and in particular early disease where neural compensatory mechanisms reduce or mask

TABLE 7.1 Overview of cognitive tests included in common MS cognitive batteries. SMDT: Symbol Digit Modalities Test; CVLT: California Verbal Learning Test; BVMT-R: Brief Visuospatial Memory Test–Revised; SRT: Selective Reminding Test; 10/36 SPART: Spatial Recall Test; COWAT: Controlled Oral Word Association Test; D-KEFS sorting test: Delis-Kaplan executive function system; JOLO: Judge of Line Orientation Test.

Measure	Cognitive process(es)	Batteries
SDMT	Information, processing speed, memory, visual scanning	MACFIMS BRB-N BICAMS
CVLT-II	Verbal memory	MACFIMS BICAMS
BVMT-R	Visuospatial memory	MACFIMS BICAMS
PASAT	Information processing speed, working memory, math ability	MACFIMS BRB-N
SRT	Verbal memory	BRB-N
10/36 SPART	Visual spatial memory	BRB-N
COWAT	Verbal fluency	MACFIMS BRB-N
D-KEFS sorting test	Executive function	MACFIMS
JOLO	Visual spatial processing	MACFIMS

deficits (Audoin et al., 2003; Forn et al., 2007; Staffen et al., 2002), is limited. This has led to the investigation of other novel methods for measuring cognition.

For example, ocular motor assessment, a recognised methodology for assessing subtle and disseminated damage to cognitive networks, has demonstrated utility in MS. Importantly, patients with early or mild disease, including those who have had only a single MS related episode (CIS), demonstrate significantly worse performance on cognitive ocular motor measures than healthy individuals, and despite comparable neuropsychological test performance (Clough, Millist et al., 2015; Clough, Mitchell et al., 2015; Fielding, Kilpatrick, Millist, Clough & White, 2012; Fielding, Kilpatrick, Millist & White, 2009a, 2009b, 2009c).

The pathophysiology underlying cognitive changes in MS is not well understood, and appears to be a consequence of focal as well as disseminated changes within gray and white matter. Many studies have reported an association with brain T2 hyperintense and T1 hypointense lesion volume. In particular, lesions within cognitive regions and white matter tracts, most notably the frontal lobe, have been found to be related to poorer cognitive performance (see Rocca et al., 2015, for a review of these studies). However, these associations are often weak and non-reproducible across different cohorts and measures. Indeed, the relative contribution of gray and white matter lesions to cognitive performance appears to only partially explain cognitive changes, with damage to normal appearing white matter and diffuse gray matter damage not only found to be associated with cognitive performance but also to be predictive of future decline (Rocca et al., 2015). Further, damage to certain gray matter structures, in particular the thalamus, has been found to provide a surrogate marker of cognitive change, particularly early cognitive change (Houtchens et al., 2007; Pinter et al., 2015; Schoonheim et al., 2012). However, it is currently unclear whether changes to these structures are directly accountable for deficits, or simply represent good measures of general cerebral damage that indirectly mediate changes in cognitive ability.

Diagnosis

The clinical presentation of MS poses a number of diagnostic challenges. Firstly, there are no symptoms that are pathognomonic for MS. Secondly, there is no test that is universally diagnostic of MS. To complicate matters, MS presents with a variety of symptoms that are often transitory and not always readily detectable by a clinician. However, the diagnosis of MS is generally a clinical one, contingent on a distinctive pattern and evolution of symptoms, supported by a number of paraclinical investigations that provide added certainty. Paraclinical investigations include visualisation of disseminated CNS lesions using magnetic resonance imaging (MRI) of the brain and spinal cord, assessment of inflammation and immunologic dysfunction by examining cerebrospinal fluid (CSF), and assessment of altered conduction consistent with demyelination using evoked potentials.

In MS, lesions, or plaques, are distributed throughout the CNS, characteristically in periventricular, cortical or juxtacortical, and infratentorial brain regions, and the spinal cord. These lesions are discrete and usually ovoid in shape, with well-defined margins. Pathologically they comprise areas of demyelination, perivascular infiltration of lymphocytes, macrophages and plasma. Clinical MRI protocols used to visualise MS lesions currently include conventional sequences based on T1-weighted and T2-weighted imaging. Chronic lesions are best visualised on fluid-attenuated inversion recovery (FLAIR) sequences that sensitively detect T2 hyperintensities. More acute lesions are best detected using T1-weighted imaging following post gadolinium infusion, when the increased permeability of the blood-brain barrier results in contrast enhancement. Contrast enhancement may persist for over one month, allowing the dissociation between acute and chronic lesions. Further, T1 hypointensities, or 'black holes' are characteristic of many lesions at the time of contrast enhancement. While the number, size and distinctive locations of lesions helps distinguish MS from other neurological diseases such as ischemia, systemic lupus erythematosus, HIV and sarcoidosis, a negative MRI does not have sufficient sensitivity or negative predictive value to rule out a diagnosis of MS.

CSF obtained through lumbar puncture can reveal evidence of abnormal immunoreactivity within the CNS. In MS, abnormalities include elevated immunoglobulin (IgG) levels, increased IgG synthesis rate, and the presence of oligoclonal bands. It is important to note, however, that oligoclonal bands and elevated CSF IgG are not MS-specific, and may be present in a range of other neurological conditions. Evoked-potential tests detect delayed conduction, such as occurs with demyelination.

As the optic nerve is frequently affected in MS, either clinically (optic neuritis) or sub-clinically, visual evoked potentials (VEPs) contribute the most in the diagnosis of MS, demonstrating demyelination of the optic nerve.

Diagnostic criteria

The diagnostic criteria for MS have evolved over time, the most recent being the McDonald criteria developed in 2001 by an international expert panel. Subsequent revisions in 2005, 2010, and 2017 reflect the availability of new data, emerging technologies and evolving consensus. The 2017 criteria, outlined below, require

TABLE 7.2 Criteria for diagnosis of MS.

Clinical presentation	Additional data needed for a diagnosis of MS
≥2 attacks; objective clinical evidence of ≥2 lesions; objective clinical evidence of one lesion together with reasonable historical evidence of a previous attack	None.
≥2 attacks; objective clinical evidence of one lesion	Dissemination in space demonstrated by: ≥1 MRI detected lesions typical of MS **or** a further attack implicating a different CNS site.
One attack; objective clinical evidence of ≥2 lesions	Dissemination in time demonstrated by: MRI evidence showing both an active (current) and non-active (previous) lesion, **or** MRI evidence of a new lesion since a previous scan, **or** a further attack implicating a different CNS site, **or** CSF-specific oligoclonal bands (substitute requirement).
One attack; objective clinical evidence of one lesion ('clinically isolated syndrome')	Dissemination in space demonstrated by activity in another part of the CNS by: ≥1 MRI detected lesions typical of MS, **or** a further attack implicating a different CNS site, **or** CSF-specific oligoclonal bands.
	Dissemination in time demonstrated by: MRI evidence showing both an active (current) and non-active (previous) lesion, **or** MRI evidence of a new lesion since a previous scan, **or** a further attack implicating a different CNS site.
Insidious neurological progression suggestive of MS (typical for primary progressive MS)	Continued progression for one year, **plus any two of:** ≥1MRI detected lesions in the brain typical of MS, ≥2 MRI detected lesions in the spinal cord, and CSF-specific oligoclonal bands.

objective clinical evidence of accrued damage to the CNS both over time (at different points in time) and in space (at different parts of the CNS), and specify that an MS clinical episode, or attack, must last for at least 24 hours, and be separated by at least 30 days from any previous or subsequent attack (Thompson et al., 2017).

Radiologically, dissemination in space is demonstrated by one or more T2-hyperintense lesions that are characteristic of MS in two or more of four areas of the CNS: periventricular, cortical or juxtacortical, and infratentorial brain regions, and the spinal cord. Dissemination in time is demonstrated by the simultaneous presence of gadolinium-enhancing and non-enhancing lesions at any time or by a new T2-hyperintense or gadolinium-enhancing lesion on follow-up MRI, irrespective of the timing of a baseline MRI. Based on these criteria a diagnosis can be made of clinically definite MS (CDMS), clinically isolated syndrome (CIS) or primary progressive MS (PPMS).

Clinical course

The majority of MS patients (approximately 85%) present with unpredictable acute or sub-acute attacks or relapses (Ebers, 2001), a consequence of an inflammatory attack on myelin and nerve fibres causing lesions throughout the CNS. The specific behavioural manifestations of a relapse depend on the anatomical location(s) of the pathology. A relapse is typically followed by complete or partial remission, followed at a future date (months or years later) by another relapse, with symptoms implicating a different region of the CNS. This pattern of relapse and recovery is known as a relapsing/remitting MS (RRMS) disease course. The first attack is referred to as a clinically isolated syndrome (CIS), where the initial presentation shows characteristics of inflammatory demyelination that *could* be MS, but does not yet fulfil the diagnostic criteria. This requires clinical evidence of accrued damage to the CNS both over time (at different points in time) and in space (at different parts of the CNS). Approximately 65% of patients with RRMS subsequently develop what is known as secondary progressive MS (SPMS), a second phase of the disease that features fewer relapses but greater neurological deterioration. Relatively fewer patients (approximately 15%) present in the first instance with a gradually progressive disease course, without well-defined attacks. This is known as a primary progressive MS (PPMS) disease course. PPMS largely affects the nerves of the spinal cord, and patients tend to have fewer brain lesions.

Clinical vignette

Karen, a 30-year-old Caucasian woman, presented to her optometrist with visual changes and pain in her right eye that had persisted for approximately 3 days. Following a routine examination of her vision that did not reveal a cause for her symptoms, she was referred to a neurologist, and underwent optical coherence tomography (OCT) and MRI. Karen's MRI revealed multiple T2 hyperintense lesions in periventricular regions of her brain. OCT results indicated inflammation of the right optic nerve. She was diagnosed with optic neuritis and treated with a course of steroids to reduce the inflammation. Her visual symptoms resolved completely. The neurologist explained to Karen that ON was a common first symptom of MS and that given the presence of lesions on her MRI, she would need to be monitored. Approximately 18 months later, Karen presented to her neurologist complaining of numbness in her left leg that she described as 'creeping' up her leg. A subsequent MRI revealed a new T2 hyperintense lesion within her spinal cord. Karen was again treated with a course of steroids, and given a formal diagnosis of MS. Karen began treatment with a disease modifying medication. Since diagnosis, the numbness in Karen's leg has lessened but tends to worsen in hot weather. Although Karen's MS has remained relatively stable, she complains of being easily fatigued and finds it difficult to concentrate, so much so she now only works 3 days a week. Karen is also highly concerned and stressed about her future, and is currently being treated for depression and seeing a psychologist regularly to help her manage her illness.

Measures of disease status and progression

Given the heterogeneity of symptoms seen in MS, it is perhaps not surprising that no single measure can capture the whole MS experience. At present, three major types of measures are used to support a diagnosis of MS, provide an understanding of prognosis, and assist in monitoring the effects of therapy. These are frequency of relapses, physical disability status, and biological markers such as magnetic resonance imaging (MRI). Relapses clearly reflect fluctuations in disease symptomatology, and are central to the experience of relapsing MS patients. As the disease progresses, or for patients with a primary progressive disease course, other measures are necessary. The most widely used measure of physical disability in MS is the Expanded Disability Severity Scale (EDSS). EDSS scores range from 0 to 10 in 0.5 unit increments that represent higher levels of disability; 1 represents a normal neurological exam, and 10 represent death due to MS (Kurtzke, 1983). The scale measures impairment or limitations in activity, based on the examination of eight functional systems; pyramidal, cerebellar, brainstem, sensory, bowel and bladder, visual function, 'mental' functions, and other. Despite the widespread clinical reliance on the EDSS, its subjectivity, unequal steps, its bias towards motor function and, significantly, its relative exclusion of cognitive assessment, limit its usefulness as a comprehensive clinical measure.

The Multiple Sclerosis Functional Composite (MSFC) was developed as a more comprehensive method for assessing MS in clinical trials. A MSFC score combines a measure of lower limb function (timed walk), upper limb function (nine-hole peg test), and cognitive function by way of the paced serial addition task (Hobart et al., 2004). However, unlike the EDSS, the MSFC requires considerable time and a relatively high level of training to perform. As such, its adoption into routine clinical examination is low. Further, despite the inclusion of some cognitive measures, it does not completely assess the complete range of cognitive domains affected in MS, limiting its utility as a comprehensive assessment of cognitive function.

MRI plays a central role not only to the diagnosis of MS, but also as a means for monitoring progression. Acute-phase T2-hyperintense MRI lesions are commonly used to measure disease activity, although oedema, inflammation, gliosis, and axonal loss can all contribute to T2 lesion formation. Gadolinium enhanced T1-weighted sequences are used to demonstrate lesions associated with inflammation, reflecting recent activity, and chronic or persistent Tl-hypointense lesions (black holes) are used as markers of axonal loss and neuronal atrophy. Although not widely used, clinically, advanced MRI techniques, such as magnetisation transfer imaging, diffusion tensor imaging, magnetic resonance spectroscopy, and relaxometry, are beginning to enrich our understanding of the natural evolution of MS lesions.

A number of ancillary measures may assist in the clinical diagnosis and management of MS. These include assessment of cerebrospinal fluid oligoclonal bands as a measure of inflammation (see below), and optical coherence tomography and visual evoked potentials as a measure of the integrity of the optic nerve.

Treatment

New treatments have radically changed the course and survival rate of MS, resulting in progressively fewer relapses and hospitalisations and slower disease progression. However, despite major advances, all available treatments are only partially effective – there is currently no cure for MS. Treatments either target individual symptoms or aim to modify disease progression. Symptomatic treatments do not alter the course of the disease and vary both inter- and intra-individually depending on the presenting complaint(s) at a given point in time. These might include muscle relaxants such as baclofen to relieve painful or uncomfortable muscle stiffness or spasms, antidepressant medications such as fluoxetine to treat affective disorders, and physical therapies to assist in the performance of everyday activities. These are critical in the care of MS patients, enhancing quality of life, and capacity to work. Treatments for MS attacks, or relapses, focus on shortening the length of the relapse and hastening recovery. Oral (prednisone) and intravenous (methylprednisolone) corticosteroids are most commonly used, altering the immune response by reducing inflammation. In more severe cases plasmapheresis may be used, the replacement of the blood's plasma thought to remove the circulating antibodies active in MS.

Disease-modifying treatments, as the name suggests, aim to halt or slow down progression of the underlying disease. Over recent years these have progressed from broad spectrum immunosuppressants, to immunomodulators, to ill-defined immunostimulants, to more selective, continuous immunosuppressants. As of January 2018, the Therapeutic Goods Administration had approved 12 of these medications for use in RRMS in Australia. These are four preparations of interferon beta, which has been at the forefront of disease management in MS for more than 20 years, glatiramer acetate, the monoclonal antibodies natalizumab, alemtuzumab, and daclizumab, the first B-cell-targeted therapy, ocrelizumab, and the small-molecule oral agents fingolimod, dimethyl fumarate, and teriflunomide. All reduce, to varying degrees, the likelihood of the development of new lesions, relapses, and stepwise accumulation of disability. First-line treatments are usually interferon-beta, glatiramer acetate or teriflunomide. Escalation treatments (natalizumab, fingolimod and mitoxantrone) are more potent than first-line treatments, although have potentially serious side effects.

Currently, there are no specific pharmacological treatments for cognitive impairment in MS, and only limited and inconsistent evidence to suggest that disease modifying therapies have any influence on the development and progression of deficit (Niccolai, Goretti & Amato, 2017). An emerging field gathering considerable interest is cognitive rehabilitation, which aims to improve cognitive functioning through specifically designed training programs, or through teaching compensatory strategies to offset the impact of cognitive deficits on day-to-day life. However, the efficacy of cognitive rehabilitation approaches is currently questionable (Mitolo, Venneri, Wilkinson & Sharrack, 2015; Rosti-Otajarvi & Hamalainen, 2014), in part due to the lack of theoretical and physiological models of cognitive impairment in MS.

Concluding remarks

The last two decades have witnessed unprecedented activity and interest in MS. Yet MS remains among the most challenging of all neurologic disorders, with a largely unknown aetiology, and a highly heterogeneous and variable clinical course. While all approved drugs predominantly exert their effects on the inflammatory component of the disease, no drug so far significantly improves the degenerative disease process. The real breakthrough in the treatment of MS will therefore come with the identification and application of treatments that can also prevent neurodegeneration as well as support remyelination and repair of damaged tissue.

Abbreviations

APN	acquired pendular nystagmus
BVMT-R	Brief Visuospatial Memory Test–Revised
CDMS	clinically definite multiple sclerosis
CIS	clinically isolated syndrome
CNS	central nervous system
CSF	cerebrospinal fluid
CVLT-II	California Verbal Learning Test–II
EBV	Epstein–Barr virus
EDSS	Expanded Disability Severity Scale
HLA	human leukocyte antigens
IgG	immunoglobulin

IL-2RA	interleukin 2 receptor A
IL7R	interleukin 7 receptor
INO	internuclear ophthalmoparesis
MRI	magnetic resonance imaging
MS	multiple sclerosis
MSFC	multiple sclerosis functional composite
OCT	optical coherence tomography
ON	optic neuritis
PASAT	Paced Auditory Serial Addition Test
PPMS	primary progressive multiple sclerosis
SDMT	Symbol Digit Modalities Test
SPMS	secondary progressive multiple sclerosis
VEP	visual evoked potentials

Further reading

Benedict, R. H. B., DeLuca, J., Phillips, G., LaRocca, N., Hudson, L. D., Rudick, R. & Multiple Sclerosis Outcome Assessments Consortium. (2017). Validity of the Symbol Digit Modalities Test as a cognition performance outcome measure for multiple sclerosis. *Multiple Sclerosis Journal, 23*(5), 721–733.

Brownlee, W. J., Hardy, T. A., Fazekas, F. & Miller, D. H. (2017). Diagnosis of multiple sclerosis: progress and challenges. *Lancet, 389*(10076), 1336–1346.

Fielding, J., Clough, M., Millist, L., Beh, S., Sears D., Frohman, A., Renneker, R., Lim, J., Lizak, N., Frohman, T., White, O. & Frohman, E. (2015). Ocular motor pathophysiological signatures of cognitive dysfunction in multiple sclerosis. *Nature Reviews Neurology, 11*, 637–645.

Matthews, P. M., Roncaroli, F., Waldman, A., Sormani, M. P., De Stefano, N., Giovannoni, G. & Reynolds, R. (2016). A practical review of the neuropathology and neuroimaging of multiple sclerosis. *Practical Neurology, 16(4)*, 279–287.

Rocca, M. A., Amato, M. P., De Stefano, N., Enzinger, C., Geurts, J. J., Penner, I. K., . . . MAGNIMS Study Group. (2015). Clinical and imaging assessment of cognitive dysfunction in multiple sclerosis. *Lancet Neurology, 14*(3), 302–317.

References

Amato, M. P., Ponziani, G., Siracusa, G. & Sorbi, S. (2001). Cognitive dysfunction in early-onset multiple sclerosis: A reappraisal after 10 years. *Archives of Neurology, 58*(10), 1602–1606.

Amato, M. P., Portaccio, E., Goretti, B., Zipoli, V., Hakiki, B., Giannini, M., . . . Razzolini, L. (2010). Cognitive impairment in early stages of multiple sclerosis. *Neurological Sciences, 31*(Suppl 2), S211–214. doi:10.1007/s10072-010-0376-4

Arnett, P. A., Rao, S. M., Grafman, J., Bernardin, L., Luchetta, T., Binder, J. R. & Lobeck, L. (1997). Executive functions in multiple sclerosis: An analysis of temporal ordering, semantic encoding, and planning abilities. *Neuropsychology, 11*(4), 535–544.

Ascherio, A. & Munger, K. L. (2010). Epstein–Barr virus infection and multiple sclerosis: A review. *Journal of Neuroimmune Pharmacology, 5*(3), 271–277. doi:10.1007/s11481-010-9201-3

Ascherio, A. & Munger, K. L. (2016). Epidemiology of multiple sclerosis: From risk factors to prevention – an update. *Seminars in Neurology, 36*(2), 103–114. doi:10.1055/s-0036-1579693

Audoin, B., Ibarrola, D., Ranjeva, J. P., Confort-Gouny, S., Malikova, I., Ali-Cherif, A., . . . Cozzone, P. (2003). Compensatory cortical activation observed by fMRI during a cognitive task at the earliest stage of MS. *Human Brain Mapping, 20*(2), 51–58. doi:10.1002/hbm.10128

Balcer, L. J. (2006). Clinical practice: Optic neuritis. *New England Journal of Medicine, 354*(12), 1273–1280. doi:10.1056/NEJMcp053247

Beatty, W. W., Paul, R. H., Blanco, C. R., Hames, K. A. & Wilbanks, S. L. (1995). Attention in multiple sclerosis: Correlates of impairment on the WAIS-R Digit Span Test. *Applied Neuropsychology, 2*(3–4), 139–144. doi:10.1080/09084282.1995.9645351

Benedict, R. H., Cookfair, D., Gavett, R., Gunther, M., Munschauer, F., Garg, N. & Weinstock-Guttman, B. (2006). Validity of the minimal assessment of cognitive function in multiple sclerosis (MACFIMS). *Journal of the International Neuropsychological Society, 12*(4), 549–558.

Benedict, R. H. B., DeLuca, J., Phillips, G., LaRocca, N., Hudson, L. D., Rudick, R. & Multiple Sclerosis Outcome Assessments Consortium. (2017). Validity of the Symbol Digit Modalities Test as a cognition performance outcome measure for multiple sclerosis. *Multiple Sclerosis Journal, 23*(5), 721–733. doi:10.1177/1352458517690821

Benedict, R. H. B., Duquin, J. A., Jurgensen, S., Rudick, R. A., Feitcher, J., Munschauer, F. E., . . . Weinstock-Guttman, B. (2008). Repeated assessment of neuropsychological deficits in multiple sclerosis using the Symbol Digit Modalities Test and the MS Neuropsychological Screening Questionnaire. *Multiple Sclerosis, 14*(7), 940–946. doi:10.1177/1352458508090923

Bergendal, G., Fredrikson, S. & Almkvist, O. (2007). Selective decline in information processing in subgroups of multiple sclerosis: An 8-year longitudinal study. *European Neurology, 57*(4), 193–202. doi:10.1159/000099158

Beyeen, A. D., Adzemovic, M. Z., Ockinger, J., Stridh, P., Becanovic, K., Laaksonen, H., . . . Olsson, T. (2010). IL-22RA2 associates with multiple sclerosis and macrophage effector mechanisms in experimental neuroinflammation. *Journal of Immunology, 185*(11), 6883–6890. doi:10.4049/jimmunol.1001392

Bobholz, J. A. & Rao, S. G. (2003). Cognitive dysfunction in multiple sclerosis: A review of recent developments. *Current Opinions in Neurology, 16*, 283–288.

Brownlee, W. J., Hardy, T. A., Fazekas, F. & Miller, D. H. (2017). Diagnosis of multiple sclerosis: Progress and challenges. *Lancet, 389*(10076), 1336–1346. doi:10.1016/S0140-6736(16)30959-X

Calabrese, M., Atzori, M., Bernardi, V., Morra, A., Romualdi, C., Rinaldi, L., . . . Gallo, P. (2007). Cortical atrophy is relevant in multiple sclerosis at clinical onset. *Journal of Neurology, 254*(9), 1212–1220. doi:10.1007/s00415-006-0503-6

Carnicka, Z., Kollar, B., Siarnik, P., Krizova, L., Klobucnikova, K. & Turcani, P. (2015). Sleep disorders in patients with multiple sclerosis. *Journal of Clinical Sleep Medicine, 11*(5), 553–557. doi:10.5664/jcsm.4702

Charcot, J. M. (1877). *Lectures on the Diseases of the Nervous System: Delivered at La Salpêtrière.* London: New Sydenham Society.

Chiaravalloti, N. D. & DeLuca, J. (2008). Cognitive impairment in multiple sclerosis. *Lancet Neurology, 7*(12), 1139–1151. doi:10.1016/S1474-4422(08)70259-X

Clough, M., Millist, L., Lizak, N., Beh, S., Frohman, T. C., Frohman, E. M., . . . Fielding, J. (2015). Ocular motor measures of cognitive dysfunction in multiple sclerosis

I: Inhibitory control. *Journal of Neurology, 262*(5), 1130–1137. doi:10.1007/s00415-015-7645-3

Clough, M., Mitchell, L., Millist, L., Lizak, N., Beh, S., Frohman, T. C., . . . Fielding, J. (2015). Ocular motor measures of cognitive dysfunction in multiple sclerosis II: Working memory. *Journal of Neurology, 262*(5), 1138–1147. doi:10.1007/s00415-015-7644-4

Costa, S. L., Genova, H. M., DeLuca, J. & Chiaravalloti, N. D. (2017). Information processing speed in multiple sclerosis: Past, present, and future. *Multiple Sclerosis Journal, 23*(6), 772–789. doi:10.1177/1352458516645869

Costello, F., Coupland, S., Hodge, W., Lorello, G. R., Koroluk, J., Pan, Y. I., . . . Kardon, R. H. (2006). Quantifying axonal loss after optic neuritis with optical coherence tomography. *Annals of Neurology, 59*(6), 963–969. doi:10.1002/ana.20851

Covey, T. J., Zivadinov, R., Shucard, J. L. & Shucard, D. W. (2011). Information processing speed, neural efficiency, and working memory performance in multiple sclerosis: Differential relationships with structural magnetic resonance imaging. *Journal of Clinical and Experimental Neuropsychology, 33*(10), 1129–1145. doi:10.1080/138033 95.2011.614597

Cree, B. A. C., Gourraud, P. A., Oksenberg, J. R., Bevan, C., Crabtree-Hartman, E., Gelfand, J. M., . . . Calif, U. (2016). Long-term evolution of multiple sclerosis disability in the treatment era. *Annals of Neurology, 80*(4), 499–510. doi:10.1002/ana. 24747

Defer, G. & Branger, P. (2015). Dementia in multiple sclerosis. In B. Brochet (Ed.), *Neuropsychiatric Symptoms of Inflammatory Demyelinating Diseases* (pp. 257–269). Cham: Springer International Publishing.

DeLuca, J., Barbieri-Berger, S. & Johnson, S. K. (1994). The nature of memory impairments in multiple sclerosis: Acquisition versus retrieval. *Journal of Clinical and Experimental Neuropsychology, 16*(2), 183–189. doi:10.1080/01688639408402629

DeLuca, J., Chelune, G. J., Tulsky, D. S., Lengenfelder, J. & Chiaravalloti, N. D. (2004). Is speed of processing or working memory the primary information processing deficit in multiple sclerosis? *Journal of Clinical and Experimental Neuropsychology, 26*(4), 550–562. doi:10.1080/13803390490496641

DeLuca, J., Gaudino, E. A., Diamond, B. J., Christodoulou, C. & Engel, R. A. (1998). Acquisition and storage deficits in multiple sclerosis. *Journal of Clinical and Experimental Neuropsychology, 20*(3), 376–390.

Derwenskus, J., Rucker, J. C., Serra, A., Stahl, J. S., Downey, D. L., Adams, N. L. & Leigh, R. J. (2005). Abnormal eye movements predict disability in MS: Two-year follow-up. *Annals of the New York Academy of Sciences, 1039*, 521–523. doi:10.1196/annals.1325.058

Drew, M. A., Starkey, N. J. & Isler, R. B. (2009). Examining the link between information processing speed and executive functioning in multiple sclerosis. *Archives of Clinical Neuropsychology, 24*(1), 47–58. doi:10.1093/arclin/acp007

Drew, M., Tippett, L. J., Starkey, N. J. & Isler, R. B. (2008). Executive dysfunction and cognitive impairment in a large community-based sample with multiple sclerosis from New Zealand: A descriptive study. *Archives of Clinical Neuropsychology, 23*(1), 1–19. doi:10.1016/j.acn.2007.09.005

Ebers, G. C. (2001). Natural history of multiple sclerosis. *Journal of Neurology Neurosurgery and Psychiatry, 71 Suppl 2*, ii16–19.

Feigin, V. L., Abajobir, A. A., Abate, K. H., Abd-Allah, F., Abdulle, A. M., Abera, S. F., . . . Disorders, G. N. (2017). Global, regional, and national burden of neurological disorders during 1990–2015: A systematic analysis for the Global Burden of Disease Study 2015. *Lancet Neurology, 16*(11), 877–897. doi:10.1016/S1474-4422(17)30299-5

Fielding, J., Kilpatrick, T., Millist, L., Clough, M. & White, O. (2012). Longitudinal assessment of antisaccades in patients with multiple sclerosis. *Plos One, 7*(2). doi:ARTN e3047510.1371/journal.pone.0030475

Fielding, J., Kilpatrick, T., Millist, L. & White, O. (2009a). Antisaccade performance in patients with multiple sclerosis. *Cortex, 45*(7), 900–903. doi:10.1016/j.cortex.2009.02.016

Fielding, J., Kilpatrick, T., Millist, L. & White, O. (2009b). Control of visually guided saccades in multiple sclerosis: Disruption to higher-order processes. *Neuropsychologia, 47*(7), 1647–1653. doi:10.1016/j.neuropsychologia.2009.01.040

Fielding, J., Kilpatrick, T., Millist, L. & White, O. (2009c). Multiple sclerosis: Cognition and saccadic eye movements. *Journal of the Neurological Sciences, 277*(1–2), 32–36. doi:10.1016/j.jns.2008.10.001

Filippi, M., Rocca, M. A., Calabrese, M., Sormani, M. P., Rinaldi, F., Perini, P., . . . Gallo, P. (2010). Intracortical lesions: Relevance for new MRI diagnostic criteria for multiple sclerosis. *Neurology, 75*(22), 1988–1994. doi:10.1212/WNL.0b013e3181ff96f6

Foong, J., Rozewicz, L., Quaghebeur, G., Davie, C. A., Kartsounis, L. D., Thompson, A. J., . . . Ron, M. A. (1997). Executive function in multiple sclerosis. The role of frontal lobe pathology. *Brain, 120*(Pt 1), 15–26.

Forn, C., Barros-Loscertales, A., Escudero, J., Benlloch, V., Campos, S., Antonia Parcet, M. & Avila, C. (2007). Compensatory activations in patients with multiple sclerosis during preserved performance on the auditory N-back task. *Human Brain Mapping, 28*(5), 424–430. doi:10.1002/hbm.20284

Fowler, C. J., Panicker, J. N., Drake, M., Harris, C., Harrison, S. C. W., Kirby, M., . . . Wells, M. (2009). A UK consensus on the management of the bladder in multiple sclerosis. *Journal of Neurology Neurosurgery and Psychiatry, 80*(5), 470–477. doi:10.1136/jnnp.2008.159178

Frohman, E., Racke, M. & Raine, C. S. (2006). Multiple sclerosis: The plaque and its pathogenesis. *New England Journal of Medicine, 354*, 942–955. doi:10.1056/NEJMra052130

Fuso, S. F., Callegaro, D., Pompeia, S. & Bueno, O. F. (2010). Working memory impairment in multiple sclerosis relapsing-remitting patients with episodic memory deficits. *Arq Neuropsiquiatr, 68*(2), 205–211.

Genova, H. M., DeLuca, J., Chiaravalloti, N. & Wylie, G. (2013). The relationship between executive functioning, processing speed, and white matter integrity in multiple sclerosis. *Journal of Clinical and Experimental Neuropsychology, 35*(6), 631–641. doi:10.1080/13803 395.2013.806649

Gold, S. M. & Irwin, M. R. (2006). Depression and immunity: Inflammation and depressive symptoms in multiple sclerosis. *Neurologic Clinics, 24*(3), 507–519. doi:10.1016/j.ncl.2006.03.007

Handel, A. E., Williamson, A. J., Disanto, G., Dobson, R., Giovannoni, G. & Ramagopalan, S. V. (2011). Smoking and multiple sclerosis: An updated meta-analysis. *PLoS One, 6*(1), e16149. doi:10.1371/journal.pone.0016149

Hanssen, K. T., Beiske, A. G., Landro, N. I. & Hessen, E. (2014). Predictors of executive complaints and executive deficits in multiple sclerosis. *Acta Neurologica Scandinavica, 129*(4), 234–242. doi:10.1111/ane.12177

Hayes, C. E., Hubler, S. L., Moore, J. R., Barta, L. E., Praska, C. E. & Nashold, F. E. (2015). Vitamin D actions on CD4(+) T cells in autoimmune disease. *Frontiers in Immunology, 6*, 100. doi:10.3389/fimmu.2015.00100

Henry, J. D. & Beatty, W. W. (2006). Verbal fluency deficits in multiple sclerosis. *Neuropsychologia, 44*(7), 1166–1174. doi:10.1016/j.neuropsychologia.2005.10.006

Hobart, J., Kalkers, N., Barkhof, F., Uitdehaag, B., Polman, C. & Thompson, A. (2004). Outcome measures for multiple sclerosis clinical trials: Relative measurement precision of the Expanded Disability Status Scale and Multiple Sclerosis Functional Composite. *Multiple Sclerosis, 10*(1), 41–46. doi:10.1191/1352458504ms983oa

Houtchens, M. K., Benedict, R. H. B., Killiany, R., Sharina, J., Jaisani, Z., Singh, B., . . . Bakshi, R. (2007). Thalamic atrophy and cognition in multiple sclerosis. *Neurology, 69*(12), 1213–1223. doi:10.1212/01.wnl.0000276992.17011.b5

Joly, H., Cohen, M. & Lebrun, C. (2014). Demonstration of a lexical access deficit in relapsing-remitting and secondary progressive forms of multiple sclerosis. *Revue Neurologique (Paris), 170*(8–9), 527–530. doi:10.1016/j.neurol.2014.05.003

Jones, K. H., Ford, D. V., Jones, P. A., John, A., Middleton, R. M., Lockhart-Jones, H., . . . Noble, J. G. (2012). A large-scale study of anxiety and depression in people with Multiple Sclerosis: A survey via the web portal of the UK MS Register. *PLoS One, 7*(7), e41910. doi:10.1371/journal.pone.0041910

Kawachi, I. & Lassmann, H. (2017). Neurodegeneration in multiple sclerosis and neuromyelitis optica. *Journal of Neurology Neurosurgery and Psychiatry, 88*(2), 137–145. doi:10.1136/jnnp-2016-313300

Koch-Henriksen, N. & Sorensen, P. S. (2010). The changing demographic pattern of multiple sclerosis epidemiology. *Lancet Neurology, 9*(5), 520–532. doi:10.1016/S1474-4422(10)70064-8

Kujala, P., Portin, R., Revonsuo, A. & Ruutiainen, J. (1995). Attention related performance in two cognitively different subgroups of patients with multiple sclerosis. *Journal of Neurology Neurosurgery and Psychiatry, 59*(1), 77–82.

Kurtzke, J. F. (1983). Rating neurologic impairment in multiple sclerosis: An expanded disability status scale (EDSS). *Neurology, 33*(11), 1444–1452.

Lassmann, H. (2012). Cortical lesions in multiple sclerosis: Inflammation versus neurodegeneration. *Brain, 135*(Pt 10), 2904–2905. doi:10.1093/brain/aws260

Lassmann, H. (2013). Pathology and disease mechanisms in different stages of multiple sclerosis. *Journal of the Neurological Sciences, 333*(1–2), 1–4. doi:10.1016/j.jns.2013.05.010

Leavitt, V. M., Wylie, G., Krch, D., Chiaravalloti, N., DeLuca, J. & Sumowski, J. F. (2014). Does slowed processing speed account for executive deficits in multiple sclerosis? Evidence from neuropsychological performance and structural neuroimaging. *Rehabilition Psychology, 59*(4), 422–428. doi:10.1037/a0037517

Leray, E., Moreau, T., Fromont, A. & Edan, G. (2016). Epidemiology of multiple sclerosis. *Revue Neurologique (Paris), 172*(1), 3–13. doi:10.1016/j.neurol.2015.10.006

Lublin, F. D., Baier, M. & Cutter, G. (2003). Effect of relapses on development of residual deficit in multiple sclerosis. *Neurology, 61*(11), 1528–1532.

Lucchinetti, C. F., Popescu, B. F. G., Bunyan, R. F., Moll, N. M., Roemer, S. F., Lassmann, H., . . . Ransohoff, R. M. (2011). Inflammatory cortical demyelination in early multiple sclerosis. *New England Journal of Medicine, 365*(23), 2188–2197. doi:10.1056/NEJMoa1100648

McCarthy, M., Beaumont, J. G., Thompson, R. & Peacock, S. (2005). Modality-specific aspects of sustained and divided attentional performance in multiple sclerosis. *Archives of Clinical Neuropsychology, 20*(6), 705–718. doi:10.1016/j.acn.2005.04.007

Meltzer, E. I., Costello, F. E., Frohman, E. M. & Frohman, T. C. (2018). New ways of 'seeing' the mechanistic heterogeneity of multiple sclerosis plaque pathogenesis. *Journal of Neuroophthalmology, 38*(1), 91–100. doi:10.1097/WNO.0000000000000633

Mills, D. A., Frohman, T. C., Davis, S. L., Salter, A. R., McClure, S., Beatty, I., . . . Frohman, E. M. (2008). Break in binocular fusion during head turning in MS patients with INO. *Neurology, 71*(6), 458–460. doi:10.1212/01.wnl.0000324423.08538.dd

Minden, S. L., Frankel, D., Hadden, L., Perloffp, J., Srinath, K. P. & Hoaglin, D. C. (2006). The Sonya Slifka Longitudinal Multiple Sclerosis Study: Methods and sample characteristics. *Multiple Sclerosis, 12*(1), 24–38. doi:10.1191/135248506ms1262oa

Mitolo, M., Venneri, A., Wilkinson, I. D. & Sharrack, B. (2015). Cognitive rehabilitation in multiple sclerosis: A systematic review. *Journal of the Neurological Sciences, 354*(1–2), 1–9. doi:10.1016/j.jns.2015.05.004

Muhlert, N., Sethi, V., Cipolotti, L., Haroon, H., Parker, G. J., Yousry, T., . . . Chard, D. (2014). The grey matter correlates of impaired decision-making in multiple sclerosis. *Journal of Neurology Neurosurgery and Psychiatry, 86*(5), 530. doi:10.1136/jnnp-2014-308169

Murray, T. J. (2005). *Multiple Sclerosis: The History of a Disease.* New York: Demos Medical Pub.

Niccolai, C., Goretti, B. & Amato, M. P. (2017). Disease modifying treatments and symptomatic drugs for cognitive impairment in multiple sclerosis: Where do we stand? *Multiple Sclerosis and Demyelinating Disorders, 2*(1), 8. doi:10.1186/s40893-017-0025-3

Optic Neuritis Study Group. (1991). The clinical profile of optic neuritis: Experience of the Optic Neuritis Treatment Trial. *Archives of Ophthalmology, 109*(12), 1673–1678.

Owens, E. M., Denney, D. R. & Lynch, S. G. (2013). Difficulties in planning among patients with multiple sclerosis: A relative consequence of deficits in information processing speed. *Journal of the International Neuropsychological Society, 19*(5), 613–620. doi:10.1017/S1355617713000155

Panou, T., Mastorodemos, V., Papadaki, E., Simos, P. G. & Plaitakis, A. (2012). Early signs of memory impairment among multiple sclerosis patients with clinically isolated syndrome. *Behavioural Neurology, 25*(4), 311–326. doi:10.3233/BEN-2012-110201

Parmenter, B. A., Weinstock-Guttman, B., Garg, N., Munschauer, F. & Benedict, R. H. B. (2007). Screening for cognitive impairment in multiple sclerosis using the Symbol Digit Modalities Test. *Multiple Sclerosis, 13*(1), 52–57. doi:10.1177/1352458506070750

Parmenter, B. A., Zivadinov, R., Kerenyi, L., Gavett, R., Weinstock-Guttman, B., Dwyer, M. G., . . . Benedict, R. H. (2007). Validity of the Wisconsin Card Sorting and Delis-Kaplan Executive Function System (DKEFS) Sorting Tests in multiple sclerosis. *Journal of Clinical and Experimental Neuropsychology, 29*(2), 215–223. doi:10.1080/13803390600672163

Paul, R. H., Beatty, W. W., Schneider, R., Blanco, C. & Hames, K. (1998). Impairments of attention in individuals with multiple sclerosis. *Multiple Sclerosis, 4*(5), 433–439.

Pelosi, L., Geesken, J. M., Holly, M., Hayward, M. & Blumhardt, L. D. (1997). Working memory impairment in early multiple sclerosis: Evidence from an event-related potential study of patients with clinically isolated myelopathy. *Brain, 120*(Pt 11), 2039–2058.

Pinter, D., Khalil, M., Pichler, A., Langkammer, C., Ropele, S., Marschik, P. B., . . . Enzinger, C. (2015). Predictive value of different conventional and non-conventional MRI-parameters for specific domains of cognitive function in multiple sclerosis. *Neuroimage-Clinical, 7,* 715–720. doi:10.1016/j.nicl.2015.02.023

Potagas, C., Giogkaraki, E., Koutsis, G., Mandellos, D., Tsirempolou, E., Sfagos, C. & Vassilopoulos, D. (2008). Cognitive impairment in different MS subtypes and clinically isolated syndromes. *Journal of the Neurological Sciences, 267*(1–2), 100–106. doi:10.1016/j.jns.2007.10.002

Rao, S. M., Hammeke, T. A. & Speech, T. J. (1987). Wisconsin Card Sorting Test: Performance in relapsing remitting and chronic progressive multiple-sclerosis. *Journal of Consulting and Clinical Psychology, 55*(2), 263–265. doi:10.1037/0022-006x.55.2.263

Rocca, M. A., Amato, M. P., De Stefano, N., Enzinger, C., Geurts, J. J., Penner, I. K., . . . MAGNIMS Study Group. (2015). Clinical and imaging assessment of cognitive dysfunction in multiple sclerosis. *Lancet Neurology, 14*(3), 302–317. doi:10.1016/S1474-4422(14)70250-9

Rosti-Otajarvi, E. M. & Hamalainen, P. I. (2014). Neuropsychological rehabilitation for multiple sclerosis. *Cochrane Database of Systematic Reviews, 2,* article CD009131.

Roth, A. K., Denney, D. R. & Lynch, S. G. (2015). Information processing speed and attention in multiple sclerosis: Reconsidering the Attention Network Test (ANT). *Journal of Clinical and Experimental Neuropsychology, 37*(5), 518–529. doi:10.1080/1380 3395.2015.1037252

Ruet, A., Deloire, M., Hamel, D., Ouallet, J. C., Petry, K. & Brochet, B. (2013). Cognitive impairment, health-related quality of life and vocational status at early stages of multiple sclerosis: A 7-year longitudinal study. *Journal of Neurology, 260*(3), 776–784. doi:10.1007/s00415-012-6705-1

Schoonheim, M. M., Popescu, V., Lopes, F. C. R., Wiebenga, O. T., Vrenken, H., Douw, L., . . . Barkhof, F. (2012). Subcortical atrophy and cognition: Sex effects in multiple sclerosis. *Neurology, 79*(17), 1754–1761. doi:10.1212/WNL.0b013e3182703f46

Serra, A., Derwenskus, J., Downey, D. L. & Leigh, R. J. (2003). Role of eye movement examination and subjective visual vertical in clinical evaluation of multiple sclerosis. *Journal of Neurology, 250*(5), 569–575. doi:10.1007/s00415-003-1038-8

Signori, A., Gallo, F., Bovis, F., Di Tullio, N., Maietta, I. & Sormani, M. P. (2016). Long-term impact of interferon or Glatiramer acetate in multiple sclerosis: A systematic review and meta-analysis. *Multiple Sclerosis and Related Disorders, 6*, 57–63. doi:10.1016/j.msard.2016.01.007

Staffen, W., Mair, A., Zauner, H., Unterrainer, J., Niederhofer, H., Kutzelnigg, A., . . . Ladurner, G. (2002). Cognitive function and fMRI in patients with multiple sclerosis: Evidence for compensatory cortical activation during an attention task. *Brain, 125* (Pt 6), 1275–1282.

Stephen, S. (2011). The major cause of multiple sclerosis is environmental: Genetics has a minor role. *Multiple Sclerosis Journal, 17*(10), 1174–1175. doi:10.1177/1352458511421106

Sumowski, J. F., Benedict, R., Enzinger, C., Filippi, M., Geurts, J. J., Hamalainen, P., . . . Rao, S. (2018). Cognition in multiple sclerosis. *State of the Field and Priorities for the Future, 90*(6), 278–288. doi:10.1212/wnl.0000000000004977

Swingler, R. J. & Compston, D. A. (1992). The morbidity of multiple sclerosis. *Quarterly Journal of Medicine, 83*(300), 325–337.

Tartaglia, M. C., Narayanan, S., Francis, S. J., Santos, A. C., De Stefano, N., Lapierre, Y. & Arnold, D. L. (2004). The relationship between diffuse axonal damage and fatigue in multiple sclerosis. *Archives of Neurology, 61*(2), 201–207. doi:DOI 10.1001/archneur.61.2.201

Thompson, A. J., Banwell, B. L., Barkhof, F., Carroll, W. M., Coetzee, T., Comi, G., . . . Cohen, J. A. (2017). Diagnosis of multiple sclerosis: 2017 revisions of the McDonald criteria. *Lancet Neurology, 17*(2), 162–173. doi:10.1016/S1474-4422(17)30470-2

Thornton, A. & Raz, N. (1997). Memory impairment in multiple sclerosis: A quantitative review. *Neuropsychology, 11*(3), 357–366.

Tilikete, C., Jasse, L., Pelisson, D., Vukusic, S., Durand-Dubief, F., Urquizar, C. & Vighetto, A. (2011). Acquired pendular nystagmus in multiple sclerosis and oculopalatal tremor. *Neurology, 76*(19), 1650–1657. doi:10.1212/WNL.0b013e318219fa9c

Zhang, T., Shirani, A., Zhao, Y., Karim, M. E., Gustafson, P., Petkau, J., . . . Neurologists, B. M. C. (2015). Beta-interferon exposure and onset of secondary progressive multiple sclerosis. *European Journal of Neurology, 22*(6), 990–1000. doi:10.1111/ene.12698

8

DEMENTIA WITH LEWY BODIES

Olivia Salthouse, Jenny Bradshaw and Michael Saling

Introduction

As the first and second most prevalent causes of dementia, Alzheimer disease dementia (ADD) and dementia with Lewy bodies (DLB) lie at opposite ends of what can be called, for want of a better term, a temperamental spectrum. ADD, at least in its earlier stages, is a quiet dementia. Patients present with a muted complaint of memory difficulties, tending to withdraw and listen when conversation demands more of their failing memory and language than they are able to retrieve. As the condition progresses, the scene is one of devastating cognitive loss, without overt and predominating excessive states or behaviours. Sensation and movement are preserved well beyond the advent of memory failure. Its underlying pathology, tauopathy in particular, causes massive neuronal loss and cerebral atrophy.

DLB, on the other hand, is a tumultuous condition. Its presentation is peppered with fluctuations that can range from inaccessibility, through to confusion, to muddlement, with hallucinations, delusional constructs, misrecognition of family members and friends, and sleep disturbances in which dreams are floridly acted out. Movement can be affected by fragments of what was once called *paralysis agitans*, in other words, parkinsonism. Sometimes there is a transient loss of consciousness, falling, and syncope. Memory loss is not an early feature, and while it progresses, it does not reach the relatively early amnestic proportions seen in ADD. Neuronal loss and cerebral atrophy are not as severe as that seen in ADD, but metabolic ups and downs go a long way to explain the clinical picture.

In this chapter, we explore the fluctuating nature of DLB as it manifests across multiple systems, with a particular emphasis on the relationship between sleep and wakefulness as a basis for aspects of the symptomatic landscape.

A brief epidemiology of dementia with Lewy bodies

Dementia with Lewy bodies (DLB) is considered to be the second most common form of dementia after dementia of the Alzheimer's type (DAT; Bonanni et al., 2008; Cromarty et al., 2016; Terzaghi et al., 2013). While some parallels can be drawn between DLB and DAT, the cardinal clinical and pathologic features of DLB are largely distinct (McKeith, 2002). DLB was initially conceptualised as a Lewy body variant (LBV) of DAT (McKeith, 1998, 2002; McKeith, Perry, Fairbairn, Jabeen & Perry, 1992), but continued research and clinical work within this area has, over recent decades, established DLB as a separate and distinct diagnostic entity (McKeith et al., 1996, 2005). It has been estimated that in older populations, DLB accounts for 10–15% of all dementias (McKeith, 2006); some estimates are as high as 25% (Mayo & Bordelon, 2014).

While early reports of Lewy body pathology date back to 1912 (McKeith, 1998), DLB has been recognised as a specific and distinct dementia subtype for just over two decades. The first operational criteria were published in 1992 (McKeith et al., 1992), followed shortly thereafter by the first diagnostic criteria (McKeith et al., 1996). These have been updated more recently to incorporate ongoing research, an increased evidence base, and a greater clinical understanding of the disease (McKeith et al., 2005, 2017).

Neuropathology

Pathologically, DLB is characterised by the presence of Lewy bodies (Kaplan, Ratner & Haas, 2003; McKeith, 2002). Lewy bodies, a hallmark feature, are distributed throughout the cortex, typically in temporal, frontal (with an emphasis on the cingulate region), parietal, and occipital cortices (Usman, Oskouian, Loukas & Tubbs, 2017). They are also found in the brain stem and autonomic structures. α-synuclein is the core constituent of Lewy bodies, uniting DLB with Parkinson's disease (PD), Parkinson's disease dementia (PDD), and multiple system atrophy (MSA) (the α-synucleinopathies) at a molecular level (Spillantini et al., 1997). A neuritic pathology has also been implicated (McKeith et al., 2004), along with a significant acetylcholine deficit (ibid.), the latter being more severe than that documented in Alzheimer's disease (AD). Neuritic features are common in the hippocampus (predominantly in the CA 2 and CA 3 regions, anatomically unlike the pattern of tau deposition in AD), parahippocampal gyrus and amygdala (Usman et al., 2017).

Foguem and Manckoundia (2018) have postulated a spectrum ranging from the α-synucleinopathies to the tauopathies (such as Alzheimer's disease and frontotemporal dementia), because of the extent to which these proteinaceous misaggregations overlap. In most cases with a clinical diagnosis of DLB, the Lewy body and neuritic pathology is accompanied by sparse Alzheimer pathology, which does not declare itself as an Alzheimer-type dementia at a clinical level, but might have an independent effect on cognition in DLB. Molecular neuroimaging points increasingly to the heterogeneity of DLB pathology, as well as to the possibility that α-synucleinopathy and Aβ-amyloidopathy, despite its low levels, might interact synergistically to increase dysfunction (Bohnen, Muller & Frey, 2017; Sarro et al., 2016). Cases with 'pure' Lewy pathology are rare (Gurd et al., 2000).

Cortical atrophy is generally less severe and extensive in DLB than in AD (Watson, O'Brien, Barber & Blamire, 2011). Grey matter atrophy in DLB is predominantly found in temporal, parietal, occipital, and subcortical structures relative to normal controls, and there is less mesial temporal atrophy than is typically found in AD (Watson et al., 2011). Occipital grey matter atrophy is less pronounced than it is in other parts of the cerebral hemisphere. Glucose uptake in the medial and lateral occipital lobes (despite the *relative* scarcity of occipital Lewy bodies) is significantly lower than in AD, but posterior cingulate uptake is higher (Lim et al., 2009), resulting in the 'cingulate island sign' on FDG PET (ibid.). This is characterised by a visually prominent posterior cingulate region against a background of low bilateral medial occipital uptake, and is highly sensitive and specific in differentiating DLB from typical onset AD (Lim et al., 2009; Sawyer & Kuo, 2018). It is worth emphasising the fact that the severe occipital metabolic defect in DLB is not accompanied by a commensurate degree of atrophy (Iaccarino et al., 2018), because it relates to the special role that metabolic factors and synaptic dysfunction play in DLB symptoms, and ultimately, early detection.

Clinical syndrome

Unlike its nearest epidemiological neighbour, AD, DLB is a more florid condition, characterised by neurological, neuropsychiatric, neurocognitive, and autonomic features (Marti, Campdelacreu & Tolosa, 2006).

Fluctuating cognitions

A core feature of the clinical presentation is a multidimensional functional instability that plays itself out over a highly variable time-frame, ranging from minute-to-minute changes, to larger scale fluctuations over hours, days, or weeks. This characteristic has been captured in the notion of 'fluctuating cognition' (FC), which has long been considered the quintessential symptomatic picture (Bradshaw, Saling, Hopwood, Anderson & Brodtmann, 2004; McKeith et al., 1992, 2005, 2017). Fluctuations might present at a fundamental level as shifts in alertness and arousal, orientation and attention, memory, or periods of profound unresponsiveness, varying from fleeting to profound. Alternatively, fluctuations might manifest as variations in higher cortical domains such as language, spatial awareness, or executive control. They also tend to involve distortions in conscious state (McKeith et al., 2017). There is no specific pattern in their periodicity (ibid., p. 2) and there can be substantial variability in their duration between and within patients (ibid.; McKeith et al., 1996).

Fluctuating cognitions occur more frequently than hallucinations or parkinsonism in early stage DLB (Byrne, Lennox, Lowe & Godwin-Austen, 1989; McKeith et al., 1992), but perhaps because of the extent of their sweep across the behavioural landscape, and the fact that fluctuation in one form or another is intrinsic to other dementias (Ballard et al., 2001), it has been a difficult phenomenon to pin-point clinically (Bradshaw et al., 2004; McKeith et al., 1996, 2005; Walker et al., 2000a). In a bid to clarify uncertainties surrounding the recognition of FC's, Bradshaw et al. (2004) investigated the comparative nature and quality of fluctuations in DLB and AD, as described by caregivers. Clinically significant FC was reported in 77% of the DLB sample. These typically took the form of momentary lapses in attention and awareness, with disengagement from inter-personal activity. These lapses appeared to be unprompted by, and unrelated to the setting, suggesting that they were internally driven (ibid.). In contrast, 'fluctuations' in the AD group were situationally specific, emerging as a result of patients' inability to manage the cognitive demands of the situation or task at hand, and for the most part were related to impaired memory function, the hallmark feature of AD (ibid.). EEG slowing and variability, which is greater in DLB than in patients with AD, shows a DLB-specific relationship with FC (Walker et al., 2000b, 2000c). The intrinsic and excessive variability of DLB, relative to AD, also expresses itself in the context of a multi-trial reaction time paradigm (Bradshaw, Saling, Anderson, Hopwood & Brodtmann, 2006; McKeith et al., 1996, 2017; Walker et al., 2000b, 2000c). It is highly probable that electroencephalographic slowing in DLB is influenced more by α-synucleinopathy and cholinergic deficit than by tauopathy or β-amyloidopathy (van der Zande et al., 2018).

Visual hallucinations

Well-formed and recurrent visual hallucinations occur frequently in DLB and are considered to be 'one of the most useful signposts to a clinical diagnosis' (McKeith et al., 2005, p. 1865). They are present in up to 80% of patients and occur early in the course of the disease (Donaghy et al., 2017; McKeith et al., 2005, 2017). Visual hallucinations are typically complex and animate in nature, usually involving people, children and/or animals, which are non-stationary (McKeith et al., 2017; Nagahama, Okina, Suzuki & Matsuda, 2010). While hallucinations are reacted to as if they are convincingly real encounters, their hallucinatory nature is accepted as the image begins to fade (Ffytche et al., 2017; McKeith et al., 2017). This insightful approach to hallucinations declines with progression of the disease and an increase in the severity of cognitive impairment (Ffytche et al., 2017). Reactions to hallucinations vary across patients, from an indifferent or philosophical approach to the experience, to an emotive and distressed reaction (Boeve, 2007).

REM sleep behaviour disorder

REM sleep behaviour disorder (RBD) is a sleep parasomnia that arises out of the rapid eye movement (REM) stage of sleep. The clinical symptom of RBD is dream enactment behaviour, in which an individual mimics scenarios that are playing out in dreams (Ferini-Strambi & Zucconi, 2000; Iranzo et al., 2013). This is made possible by the absence of muscle atonia, which is normally present during REM sleep (Ferini-Strambi & Zucconi, 2000; Gagnon, Petit, Latreille & Montplaisir, 2008). Dreams tend to be unusually vivid, and content is typically (although not always) distressing, often involving themes of being chased or fighting off an aggressor (Ferini-Strambi & Zucconi, 2000). As such, it is not uncommon for the dream enactment behaviours to result in injury to the affected individual or bed partner, often the circumstance that elicits clinical attention (ibid.). In the absence of a bed partner who witnesses the behaviour, RBD goes undetected. A diagnosis of RBD is made on the basis of witnessed recurrent dream enactment behaviour and polysomnographic recording that documents REM sleep without atonia (RWA; the electrophysiological correlate of RBD).

The association between RBD and DLB is relatively recent (Grace, Walker & McKeith, 2000), and RBD has only been recognised as a core (rather than supportive) disease feature since 2017 (McKeith et al., 2017). The first case report of co-occurring probable DLB and RBD was published in 1997 (Turner, Chervin, Frey, Minoshima & Kuhl, 1997). Subsequent longitudinal research has since reported striking conversion rates from idiopathic RBD to synucleinopathy-related disease of up to 82%, and further suggests that RBD onset can occur even decades prior to the onset of other disease features (Iranzo et al., 2013; Schenck, Boeve & Mahowald, 2013). While conversion to DLB, PD and MSA have all been documented, it is suggested that conversion to DLB is far more common than conversion to a primary movement or autonomic disorder (Boot et al., 2012). A recent study involving 78 DLB patients recorded RWA in 95% of their sample (Pao et al., 2013). Taken collectively, these findings suggest that the majority of people with idiopathic RBD go on to develop a Lewy body disease, and that RBD is more likely to be a prodromal, or even an early-stage manifestation of synucleinopathy-related neurodegenerative disease (Raggi, Neri & Ferri, 2015). This is now reflected in the most recent update of the diagnostic criteria, which recognise RBD as core to the clinical syndrome (McKeith et al., 2017).

Sleep in dementia with Lewy bodies

DLB has been associated with disordered sleep for more than a decade (Grace et al., 2000; McKeith et al., 2005). Specifically, there is a strong association with RBD (Gagnon et al., 2008; Iranzo et al., 2013; Schenck et al., 2013), with rates of conversion to synucleinopathy-related disease in as many as 82% of those diagnosed with idiopathic RBD (Iranzo et al., 2013; Schenck & Howell, 2013). In the face of these striking conversion rates, RBD has been the central focus in DLB-sleep research (as is also the case with PD and PDD). There has been a comparatively low level of interest in other aspects of sleep, including general sleep macrostructure and microstructure. Nevertheless, in the small body of research devoted to the whole spectrum of sleep from an electrophysiological perspective, EEG slowing during REM sleep (Iranzo et al., 2010), similar to that also reported during wakefulness in this population (Stylianou et al., 2018) is consistently found. REM sleep slowing in DLB is particularly pronounced in posterior cortical regions, but also occurs to a lesser extent across more widespread regions of the brain (Latreille et al., 2016), thereby showing a topographical pattern that is much the same as the characteristic pattern of hypometabolism in DLB (Petit, Gagnon, Fantini, Ferini-Strambi & Montplaisir, 2004). More specifically, there is a shift from alpha- to theta and delta power. Slowing has also been demonstrated in RBD, in the absence of dementia, and in PDD patients (Iranzo et al., 2010), unfolding the possibility that EEG slowing during REM sleep in PD patients might be an early marker of incipient dementia (Petit et al., 2004).

While RBD is the best characterised paroxysmal event in DLB, there is also evidence of other parasomnias emerging out of REM and non-rapid eye movement (NREM) sleep (Ratti et al., 2012, 2015). Are non-RBD parasomnias also markers of dementia? Ratti and colleagues (2012) found that arousal-related motor behavioural episodes (AMBE) arising out of REM and NREM sleep were significantly more frequent in those with dementia (either DLB or PDD), than in those with PD but no cognitive impairment. NREM parasomnia behaviours (NPBs) have also been detected in α-synucleinopathies (specifically PD and MSA) other than DLB (Ratti et al., 2015). These consisted of *elementary* behaviours that lacked purpose or coordination, or a *confusional* semiology involving interaction with a non-existent person or object. NPBs are selectively associated with a reduction in theta amplitude band in right frontal and central derivations. These are early findings and require replication, but they raise the hypothesis that the NPBs indicate 'a low performance state of the awaking cerebral cortex' (ibid., p. 11), in which there is a failure to integrate information from NREM sleep mentation with environmental sensory information (ibid.). This notion might constitute a starting point for considering the clinical implications of NREM parasomnias in the α-synucleinopathies, DLB in particular.

Severely disorganised sleep patterns have been identified (Vetrugno et al., 2009; Vetrugno & Montagna, 2011). These might represent an advanced development in synucleinopathy-related disease, beginning as RBD and progressing, within the context of incipient dementia, to state dissociation disorders (Antelmi et al., 2016), in which there is a blurring of the boundaries that separate sleep and wake, with elements of wake intruding into sleep and vice versa (ibid.). At their most severe, these abnormalities represent a *status dissociatus* (SD; Vetrugno & Montagna, 2011), in which there is almost continuous intrusion of different sleep and waking elements, making it impossible to distinguish the presence of any specific state of being (Antelmi et al., 2016; Schenck & Howell, 2013; Vetrugno & Montagna, 2011). Given the notion of progression from RBD to state dissociation, SD is presently considered to be an RBD subtype (Antelmi et al., 2016). These states are always symptomatic (Schenck & Howell, 2013), with clinical features of confusion, visual hallucinations, and abnormal motor and verbal behaviours (Antelmi et al., 2016; Vetrugno et al., 2009), seemingly analogous to the quintessential clinical characteristics of DLB (McKeith et al., 2005). A recent case series has documented two patients with a diagnosis of probable MSA, both of whom presented initially with RBD (Vetrugno et al., 2009). Over time, in both patients, autonomic dysfunction emerged, RBD episodes reduced, and sleep became severely disorganised. This was characterised clinically by motor and verbal abnormalities through the night and long awakenings with confusional features and animate visual hallucinations (ibid.). EEG recordings showed extensive disruption, with vague and ambiguous markers of sleep/wake, and complete absence of conventional sleep stages (ibid.). Terzaghi, Rustioni, and Manni (2010) have also published a cognate case study of a 76-year-old female who developed probable DLB. Prior to the emergence of DLB symptoms, insomnia and abnormal nocturnal behaviours were documented, progressing to a constellation of confusion, visual hallucinations, and night-time wanderings (ibid.) resembling that found in the MSA cases. The EEG record also revealed severely abnormal sleep incorporating elements of wakefulness, REM sleep and NREM sleep. Wakefulness was marked by fluctuating cognition, episodes of confusion and excessive daytime sleepiness, consistent with the clinical syndrome of DLB. These cases point towards the blurring of wake and sleep boundaries as a potential trigger of the more florid aspects of DLB symptomatology. Dissociated sleep characterised by concurrent elements of all three states of being has been described in a small number of DLB cases (ibid.). Whether or not dissociated, disorganised sleep is a feature of DLB over its natural course and is progressively associated with the tumultuous clinical presentation of the condition, remains a question still to be addressed.

Wakefulness in dementia with Lewy bodies

A striking feature of sleep research in α-synucleinopathies is the dissolution of electrophysiological boundaries between sleep stages (Antelmi et al., 2016; Ratti et al., 2015). Elements of waking activity intruding into sleep is of special interest in DLB (Terzaghi, Sartori, Rustioni & Manni, 2014; Terzaghi et al., 2009, 2012), since it appears that arousals and night-time behaviours (predominantly confusional in nature) during sleep are clinical expressions of such intrusions. The precise mechanism by which these intrusions occur is unclear, but the notion of dysfunctional switching, resulting in sleep instability seems reasonable. It is likely that defective switching spills over into daytime wakefulness, during which the DLB symptomatology of greatest diagnostic interest occurs.

In contrast to the sleep states in DLB, electrophysiological activity during wakefulness has received most attention (Cromarty et al., 2016; Gagnon et al., 2008; Petit et al., 2004). Slowing of dominant rhythms has been consistently demonstrated (Bonanni et al., 2015; Bonanni et al., 2008; Briel et al., 1999; Roks, Korf, van der Flier, Scheltens & Stam, 2008). More specifically, there are reductions in alpha and beta activity (both of which signal a waking state), and a significant shift towards increased delta and theta activity power (frequencies normally confined to NREM sleep) across frontal, temporal, parietal and occipital derivations (Andersson, Hansson, Minthon, Rosén & Londos, 2008; Cromarty et al., 2016; Gagnon et al., 2008; Iranzo et al., 2010). These findings could be conceptualised as elements of sleep intruding into the state of wakefulness, and that fluctuating cognition, attentional variability (Bradshaw et al., 2006), and visual hallucinations are the behavioural correlates that arise from this abnormal and confused underlying state.

Arnulf et al. (2000) have drawn attention to a historical case, originally studied by Pinelli (1959), of a 48-year-old woman with post-encephalitic PD and diurnal visual hallucinations. She underwent EEG monitoring before, during, and after the hallucinatory ictus on a number of separate occasions. The hallucinations were animate and well formed. By way of example, during one of her hallucinations she saw a horse, which was attempting to bite her, standing in the corner of the room. She was able to describe the image, and pointed to the position in which the horse was standing. When staff stood in the exact position she had pointed to, she reacted with perplexity, and finally interpreted the hallucinated horse as a dream. Of direct interest to our argument, the hallucination was preceded electroencephalographically by an alpha to theta band shift. Recordings during the hallucination were marred by artefact.

Visual hallucinations in DLB appear to be less the result of *occipital* grey matter atrophy and Lewy pathology, and more the result of an intra-occipital disconnection, and poor co-operation between distributed visual and attentional networks (Iaccarino et al., 2018). Nevertheless, the density of Lewy bodies in the amygdala and parahippocampal region is associated with visual hallucinations, possibly by increasing neuronal demands on metabolic resources for neuronal survival (Harding, Broe & Halliday, 2002).

Concluding remarks

In many ways DLB remains an enigmatic form of dementia. Boundaries are blurred between cloudiness and clarity of consciousness, situational contact and inaccessibility, stability and fluctuation, hallucination and reality, identification and delusions of duplication. In this chapter, we argue that there might also be an underlying and possibly explanatory dissolution of the boundaries of sleep states, and intermittent loss of the distinction between sleep and waking. To some extent, shades of this turmoil might characterise other α-synucleinopathies (Foguem & Manckoundia, 2018), but the exploration of sleep disruption as an explanatory mechanism is a promising road less taken, and DLB offers unique opportunities in this endeavour.

Abbreviations

AD	Alzheimer's disease
ADD	Alzheimer disease dementia
DAT	dementia of the Alzheimer's type
DLB	dementia with Lewy bodies

EEG	electroencephalogram
FC	fluctuating cognition
FDG–PET	fluorodeoxyglucose-positron emission tomography
LBV	Lewy body variant
MSA	multiple system atrophy
NPB	NREM parasomnia behaviours
NREM	non-rapid eye movement
PD	Parkinson's disease
PDD	Parkinson's disease dementia
RBD	REM sleep behaviour disorder
REM	rapid eye movement
RWA	REM sleep without atonia
SD	status dissociatus

Further reading

Dauvilliers, Y., Schenk, C. H., Postuma, R. B., Iranzo, A., Luppi, P. H., Plazzi, G., . . . Boeve, B. F. (2018). REM sleep behaviour disorder. *Nature Reviews/Disease Primers*, *4*, 1–16.

Fields, J. A. (2017). Cognitive and neuropsychiatric features in in Parkinson's and Lewy body dementias. *Archives of Clinical Neuropsychology*, *32*, 786–801.

Jellinger, K. A. (2018). Dementia with Lewy bodies and Parkinson's disease dementia: Current concepts and controversies. *Journal of Neural Transmission*, *125*, 615–650.

Marchand, D. G., Postuma, R. B., Escudier, F., De Roy, J., Pelletier, A., Montplaisir, J. & Gagnon, J. F. (2018). How does dementia with Lewy bodies start? Prodromal cognitive changes in REM sleep behaviour disorder. *Annals of Neurology*, *83*, 1016–1026.

References

Andersson, M., Hansson, O., Minthon, L., Rosén, I. & Londos, E. (2008). Electro-encephalogram variability in dementia with Lewy bodies, Alzheimer's disease and controls. *Dementia and Geriatric Cognitive Disorders*, *26*(3), 284–290. doi:10.1159/000160962

Antelmi, E., Ferri, R., Iranzo, A., Arnulf, I., Dauvilliers, Y., Bhatia, K. P., . . . Plazzi, G. (2016). From state dissociation to status dissociatus. *Sleep Medicine Reviews*, *28*, 5–17. doi:10.1016/j.smrv.2015.07.003

Arnulf, I., Bonnet, A. M., Damier, P., Bejjani, B. P., Seilhean, D., Derenne, J. P. & Agid, Y. (2000). Hallucinations, REM sleep, and Parkinson's disease: A medical hypothesis. *Neurology*, *55*(2), 281–288. doi:10.1212/WNL.55.2.281

Ballard, C., O'Brien, J. T., Gray, A., Cormack, F., Ayre, G. A., Rowan, E. N., . . . Tovee, M. (2001). Attention and fluctuating attention in patients with dementia with Lewy bodies and Alzheimer's disease. *Archives of Neurology*, *58*(6), 977–982. doi:10.1001/archneur.58.6.977

Boeve, B. (2007). Dementia with Lewy bodies. In A. Schapira (ed.), *Neurology and Clinical Neuroscience*. London: Elsevier Health Sciences.

Bohnen, N. I., Muller, M. L. T. M. & Frey, K. A. (2017). Molecular imaging and updated diagnostic criteria for Lewy body dementias. *Current Neurology and Neuroscience Reports*, *17*(10), 73–81. doi:10.1007/s11910-017-0789-z

Bonanni, L., Perfetti, B., Bifolchetti, S., Taylor, J. P., Franciotti, R., Parnetti, L., . . . Onofrj, M. (2015). Quantitative electroencephalogram utility in predicting conversion of mild cognitive impairment to dementia with Lewy bodies. *Neurobiology of Aging*, *36*(1), 434–445. doi:10.1016/j.neurobiolaging.2014.07.009

Bonanni, L., Thomas, A., Tiraboschi, P., Perfetti, B., Varanese, S. & Onofrj, M. (2008). EEG comparisons in Alzheimer's disease, dementia with Lewy bodies and Parkinson's disease with dementia patients with a 2-year follow-up. *Brain*, *131*(3), 690–705. doi:10.1093/brain/awm322

Boot, B. P., Boeve, B. F., Roberts, R. O., Ferman, T. J., Geda, Y. E., Pankratz, V. S., . . . Petersen, R. C. (2012). Probable rapid eye movement sleep behavior disorder increases risk for mild cognitive impairment and Parkinson disease: A population-based study. *Annals of Neurology*, *71*(1), 49–56. doi:10.1002/ana.22655

Bradshaw, J. M., Saling, M., Anderson, V., Hopwood, M. & Brodtmann, A. (2006). Higher cortical deficits influence attentional processing dementia with Lewy bodies, relative to patients with dementia of the Alzheimer's type and controls. *Journal of Neurology Neurosurgery and Psychiatry*, *77*(10), 1129–1135. doi:10.1136/jnnp.2006.090183

Bradshaw, J. M., Saling, M., Hopwood, M., Anderson, V. & Brodtmann, A. (2004). Fluctuating cognition in dementia with Lewy bodies and Alzheimer's disease is qualitatively distinct. *Journal of Neurology Neurosurgery and Psychiatry*, *75*(3), 382–387. doi:10.1136/jnnp.2002.002576

Briel, R. C. G., McKeith, I. G., Barker, W. A., Hewitt, Y., Perry, R. H., Ince, P. G. & Fairbairn, A. F. (1999). EEG findings in dementia with Lewy bodies and Alzheimer's disease. *Journal of Neurology Neurosurgery and Psychiatry*, *66*(3), 401–403. doi:10.1136/jnnp.66.3.401

Byrne, E., Lennox, G., Lowe, J. & Godwin-Austen, R. B. (1989). Diffuse Lewy body disease: Clinical features in 15 cases. *Journal of Neurology Neurosurgery and Psychiatry*, *52*(6), 709–717. doi:10.1136/jnnp.52.6.709

Cromarty, R. A., Elder, G. J., Graziadio, S., Baker, M., Bonanni, L., Onofrj, M., . . . Taylor, J. P. (2016). Neurophysiological biomarkers for Lewy body dementias. *Clinical Neurophysiology*, *127*(1), 349–359. doi:10.1016/j.clinph.2015.06.020

Donaghy, P. C., Barnett, N., Olsen, K., Taylor, J.-P., McKeith, I. G., O'Brien, J. T. & Thomas, A. (2017). Symptoms associated with Lewy body disease in mild cognitive impairment. *International Journal of Geriatric Psychiatry*, *32*(11), 1163–1171. doi:10.1002/gps.4742

Ferini-Strambi, L. & Zucconi, M. (2000). REM sleep behavior disorder. *Clinical Neurophysiology*, *11*(Supplement 2), S136–S140. doi:10.1016/S1388-2457(00)00414-4

Ffytche, D. H., Pereira, J. B., Ballard, C., Chaudhuri, K. R., Weintraub, D. & Aarsland, D. (2017). Risk factors for early psychosis in PD: Insights from the Parkinson's Progression Markers Initiative. *Journal of Neurology Neurosurgery and Psychiatry*, *88*(4), 325–221. doi:10.1136/jnnp-2016-314832

Foguem, C. & Manckoundia, P. (2018). Lewy body disease: Clinical and pathological 'overlap syndrome' between synucleinopathies (Parkinson disease) and tauopathies (Alzheimer disease). *Movement Disorders*, *18*(5), 1–9. doi:10.1007/s11910-018-0835-5

Gagnon, J. F., Petit, D., Latreille, V. & Montplaisir, J. (2008). Neurobiology of sleep disturbances in neurodegenerative disorders. *Current Pharmaceutical Design*, *14*(32), 3430–3445. doi:10.2174/138161208786549353

Grace, J. B., Walker, M. P. & McKeith, I. G. (2000). A comparison of sleep profiles in patients with dementia with Lewy bodies and Alzheimer's disease. *International Journal of Geriatric Psychiatry*, *15*(11), 1028–1033. doi:10.1002/1099-1166(200011)15:11<1028::AID-GPS227>3.0.CO;2-E

Gurd, J. M., Herzberg, L., Joachim, C., Marshall, J. C., Jobst, K., McShane, R. H., . . . King, E. E. (2000). Dementia with Lewy bodies: A pure case. *Brain and Cognition, 44*(3), 307–323. doi:10.1006/brcg.1999.1124

Harding, A. J., Broe, G. A. & Halliday, G. (2002). Visual hallucinations in Lewy body disease relate to Lewy bodies in the temporal lobe. *Brain, 125*(2), 391–403. doi:10.1093/brain/awf033

Iaccarino, L., Sala, A., Caminiti, S. P., Santangelo, R., Iannaccone, S., Magnani, G. & Perani, D. (2018). The brain metabolic signature of visual hallucinations in dementia with Lewy bodies. *Cortex, 108*, 13–24. doi:10.1016/j.cortex.2018.06.014

Iranzo, A., Isetta, V., Molinuevo, J. L., Serradell, M., Navajas, D., Farre, R. & Santamaria, J. (2010). Electroencephalographic slowing heralds mild cognitive impairment in idiopathic REM sleep behavior disorder. *Sleep Medicine, 11*(6), 534–539. doi:10.1016/j.sleep.2010.03.006

Iranzo, A., Tolosa, E., Gelpi, E., Molinuevo, J. L., Valldeoriola, F., Serradell, M., . . . Santamaria, J. (2013). Neurodegenerative disease status and post-mortem pathology in idiopathic rapid-eye-movement sleep behaviour disorder: An observational cohort study. *The Lancet Neurology, 12*(5), 443–453. doi:10.1016/S1474-4422(13)70056-5

Kaplan, B., Ratner, V. & Haas, E. (2003). α-Synuclein: Its biological function and role in neurodegenerative diseases. *Journal of Molecular Neuroscience, 20*(2), 83–92. doi:10.1385/JMN:20:2:83

Latreille, V., Carrier, J., Gaudet-Fex, B., Rodrigues-Brazete, J., Panisset, M., Chouinard, S., . . . Gagnon, J. F. (2016). Electroencephalographic prodromal markers of dementia across conscious states in Parkinson's disease. *Brain, 139*(4), 1189–1199. doi:10.1093/brain/aww018

Lim, S. M., Katsifis, A., Villemagne, V. L., Best, R., Jones, G., Saling, M., . . . Rowe, C. C. (2009). The ¹⁸F-FDG PET cingulate island sign and comparison to ¹²³I-B-CIT SPECT for diagnosis of dementia with Lewy bodies. *Journal of Nuclear Medicine, 50*(10), 1638–1645. doi:10.2967/jnumed.109.065870

Marti, M. J., Campdelacreu, J. & Tolosa, E. (2006). Clinical spectrum of Lewy body disease. In J. T. O'Brien, I. G. McKeith, D. Ames & E. Chiu (eds), *Dementia with Lewy Bodies and Parkinson's Disease Dementia*. London: Taylor and Francis.

Mayo, M. C. & Bordelon, Y. (2014). Dementia with Lewy bodies. *Seminars in Neurology, 34*(2), 182–188. doi:10.1055/s-0034-1381741

McKeith, I. G. (1998). Dementia with Lewy bodies: Clinical and pathological diagnosis. *Alzheimer's Reports, 1*(2), 83–87.

McKeith, I. G. (2002). Dementia with Lewy bodies. *British Journal of Psychiatry, 180*(2), 144–147. doi:10.1192/bjp.180.2.144

McKeith, I. G. (2006). Consensus guidelines for the clinical and pathologic diagnosis of dementia with Lewy bodies (DLB): Report of the consortium on DLB international workshop. *Journal of Alzheimer's Disease, 9*(3 Supplement), 417–423.

McKeith, I. G., Boeve, B. F., Dickson, D. W., Halliday, G., Taylor, J.-P., Weintraub, D., . . . Ballard, C. G. (2017). Diagnosis and management of dementia with Lewy bodies: Fourth consensus report of the DLB Consortium. *Neurology, 89*(1), 88–100. doi:10.1212/WNL.0000000000004058

McKeith, I. G., Dickson, D. W., Lowe, J., Emre, M., O'Brien, J. T., Feldman, H., . . . Yamada, M. (2005). Diagnosis and management of dementia with Lewy bodies: Third report of the DLB consortium. *Neurology, 65*(12), 1863–1872. doi:10.1212/01.wnl.0000187889.17253.b1

McKeith, I. G., Galasko, D., Kosaka, K., Perry, E. K., Dickson, D. W., Hansen, L. A., . . . Perry, R. H. (1996). Consensus guidelines for the clinical and pathologic diagnosis of dementia with Lewy bodies (DLB): Report of the consortium on DLB international workshop. *Neurology*, *47*(5), 1113–1124. doi:10.1212/WNL.47.5.1113

McKeith, I. G., Mintzer, J., Aarsland, D., Burn, D. J., Chiu, H., Cohen-Mansfield, J., . . . Reid, W. (2004). Dementia with Lewy bodies. *Lancet Neurology*, *3*(1), 19–28. doi:10.1016/S1474-4422(03)00619-7

McKeith, I. G., Perry, R. H., Fairbairn, A. F., Jabeen, S. & Perry, E. K. (1992). Operational criteria for senile dementia of Lewy body type (SDLT). *Psychological Medicine*, *22*(4), 911–922. doi:10.1017/S0033291700038484

Nagahama, Y., Okina, T., Suzuki, N. & Matsuda, M. (2010). Neural correlates of psychotic symptoms in dementia with Lewy bodies. *Brain*, *133*(2), 557–567. doi:10.1093/brain/awp295

Pao, W. C., Boeve, B. F., Ferman, T. J., Lin, S. C., Smith, G. E., Knopman, D. S., . . . Silber, M. H. (2013). Polysomnographic findings in dementia with Lewy bodies. *Neurologist*, *19*(1), 1–6. doi:10.1097/NRL.0b013e31827c6bdd

Petit, D., Gagnon, J. F., Fantini, M. L., Ferini-Strambi, L. & Montplaisir, J. (2004). Sleep and quantitative EEG in neurodegenerative disorders. *Journal of Psychosomatic Research*, *56*(5), 487–496. doi:10.1016/j.jpsychores.2004.02.001

Pinelli, P. (1959). La sindrome acinetico-ipertonica ed i disturbi narcolettici latenti nei parkinsoniani. *Casa editrice renzo cortina. Pavia*, 168–223.

Raggi, A., Neri, W. & Ferri, R. (2015). Sleep-related behaviours in Alzheimer's disease and dementia with Lewy bodies. *Reviews in the Neurosciences*, *26*(1), 31–38. doi:10.1515/revneuro-2014-0050

Ratti, P. L., Sierra-Peña, M., Manni, R., Simonetta-Moreau, M., Bastin, J., Mace, H., . . . David, O. (2015). Distinctive features of NREM parasomnia behaviours in Parkinson's disease and multiple system atrophy. *PLOS One*, *10*(3), 1–15. doi:10.1371.journal.pone.0120973

Ratti, P. L., Terzaghi, M., Minafra, B., Repetto, A., Pasotti, C., Zangaglia, R., . . . Manni, R. (2012). REM and NREM sleep enactment behaviors in Parkinson's disease, Parkinson's disease dementia, and dementia with Lewy bodies. *Sleep Medicine*, *13*(7), 926–932. doi:10.1016/j.sleep.2012.04.015

Roks, G., Korf, E. S. C., van der Flier, W. M., Scheltens, P. & Stam, C. J. (2008). The use of EEG in the diagnosis of dementia with Lewy bodies. *Journal of Neurology Neurosurgery and Psychiatry*, *79*(4), 370–380. doi:10.1136/jnnp.2007.125385

Sarro, L., Senjem, M. L., Lundt, E. S., Przybelski, S. A., Lesnick, T. G., Graff-Radford, J., . . . Kantarci, K. (2016). Amyloid-beta deposition and regional grey matter atrophy rates in dementia with Lewy bodies. *Brain*, *139*(10), 2740–2750. doi:10.1093/brain/aww193

Sawyer, D. M. & Kuo, P. H. (2018). 'Occipital tunnel' sign on FDG PET for differentiating dementias. *Clinical Nuclear Medicine*, *43*(2), 59. doi:10.1097//RLU.0000000000001925

Schenck, C. H., Boeve, B. F. & Mahowald, M. W. (2013). Delayed emergence of a parkinsonian disorder or dementia in 81% of older men initially diagnosed with idiopathic rapid eye movement sleep behavior disorder: A 16-year update on a previously reported series. *Sleep Medicine*, *14*(8), 744–748. doi:10.1016/j.sleep.2012.10.009

Schenck, C. H. & Howell, M. J. (2013). Spectrum of rapid eye movement sleep behavior disorder (overlap between rapid eye movement sleep behavior disorder and other parasomnias). *Sleep and Biological Rhythms*, *11*(S1), 27–34. doi:10.1111/j.1479-8425.2012.00548.x

Spillantini, M. G., Schimdt, M. L., Lee, V. M. Y., Trojanowski, J. Q., Jakes, R. & Goedert, M. (1997). α-synuclein in Lewy bodies. *Nature*, *388*(6645), 839–840.

Stylianou, M., Murphy, N., Peraza, L. R., Graziadio, S., Cromarty, R. A., Killen, A., . . . Taylor, J. P. (2018). Quantitative electroencephalography as a marker of fluctuations in dementia with Lewy bodies and an aid to differential diagnosis. *Clinical Neurophysiology*, *129*(6), 1209–1220. doi:10.1016/j.clinph.2018.03.013

Terzaghi, M., Arnaldi, D., Rizzetti, M. C., Minafra, B., Cremascoli, R., Rustioni, V., . . . Manni, R. (2013). Analysis of video-polysomnographic sleep findings in dementia with Lewy bodies. *Movement Disorders*, *28*(10), 1416–1423. doi:10.1002/mds.25523

Terzaghi, M., Rustioni, V. & Manni, R. (2010). Agrypnia with nocturnal confusional behaviors in dementia with Lewy bodies: Immediate efficicacy of Rivastigmine. *Movement Disorders*, *25*(5), 647–649. doi:10.1002/mds.22726

Terzaghi, M., Sartori, I., Rustioni, V. & Manni, R. (2014). Sleep disorders and acute nocturnal delirium in the elderly: A comorbidity not to be overlooked. *European Journal of Internal Medicine*, *25*(4), 350–355. doi:10.106/j.ejim.2014.02.008

Terzaghi, M., Sartori, I., Tassi, L., Didato, G., Rustioni, V., Lorusso, G., . . . Nobili, L. (2009). Evidence of dissociated arousal states during NREM parasomnia from an intracerebral neurophysiological study. *Sleep*, *32*(3), 409–412.

Terzaghi, M., Sartori, I., Tassi, L., Rustioni, V., Proserpio, P., Lorusso, G., . . . Nobili, L. (2012). Dissociated local arousal states underlying essential clinical features of non-rapid eye movement arousal parasomnia: A intracerebral stereo-encephalographic study. *Journal of Sleep Research*, *21*(5), 502–506. doi:10.1111/j.1365-2869.2012.01003.x

Turner, R. S., Chervin, R. D., Frey, K. A., Minoshima, S. & Kuhl, D. E. (1997). Probable diffuse Lewy body disease presenting as REM sleep behavior disorder. *Neurology*, *42*(2), 523–527. doi:10.1212/WNL.49.2.523

Usman, S., Oskouian, R. J., Loukas, M. & Tubbs, R. S. (2017). Clinical anatomy of the most common dementias. *Clinical Anatomy*, *30*(1), 53–57. doi:10.1002/ca.22784

van der Zande, J. J., Gouw, A. A., van Steenoven, I., Scheltens, P., Stam, C. J. & Lemstra, A. W. (2018). EEG characteristics of dementia with Lewy bodies, Alzheimer's disease and mixed pathology. *Front Aging Neurosci*, *10*, 190. doi:10.3389/fnagi.2018.00190.

Vetrugno, R., Alessandria, M., D'Angelo, R., Plazzi, G., Provini, F., Cortelli, P. & Montagna, P. (2009). Status dissociatus evolving from REM sleep behaviour disorder in multiple system atrophy. *Sleep Medicine*, *10*(2), 247–252. doi:10.1016/j.sleep.2008.01.009

Vetrugno, R. & Montagna, P. (2011). From REM sleep behaviour disorder to status dissociatus: Insights into the maze of states of being. *Sleep Medicine*, *12*, S68–S71. doi:10.1016/j.sleep.2011.10.015

Walker, M. P., Ayre, G. A., Cummings, J., Wesnes, K., McKeith, I. G., O'Brien, J. T. & Ballard, C. (2000a). The Clinician Assessment of Fluctuation and the One Day Fluctuation Assessment Scale: Two methods to assess fluctuating confusion in dementia. *British Journal of Psychiatry*, *177*(3), 252–256. doi:10.1192/bjp.177.2.252

Walker, M. P., Ayre, G. A., Cummings, J., Wesnes, K., McKeith, I. G., O'Brien, J. T. & Ballard, C. (2000b). Quantifying fluctuation in dementia with Lewy bodies, Alzheimer's disease, and vascular dementia. *Neurology*, *54*(8), 1616–1625. doi:10.1212/WNL.54.8.1616

Walker, M. P., Ayre, G. A., Perry, E. K., Wesnes, K., McKeith, I. G., Tovee, M., . . . Ballard, C. G. (2000c). Quantification and characterisation of fluctuating cognition in dementia with Lewy bodies and Alzheimer's disease. *Dementia and Geriatric Cognitive Disorders*, *11*(6), 327–335. doi:10.1159/000017262

Watson, R., O'Brien, J. T., Barber, R. & Blamire, A. M. (2011). Patterns of gray matter atrophy in dementia with Lewy bodies: A voxel-based morphometry study. *International Psychogeriatrics*, *24*(4), 532–540. doi:10.1017/S1041610211002171

9

MOTOR NEURON DISEASE

William Huynh, Thanuja Dharmadasa, Smriti Agarwal,
Jashelle Caga and Matthew C. Kiernan

Introduction

Motor neuron disease (MND) or amyotrophic lateral sclerosis (ALS) is a rapidly progressive and universally fatal neurodegenerative disorder of the human motor system that was first described in 1869 by Jean-Martin Charcot (Cleveland & Rothstein, 2001; Simon, Huynh, Vucic, Talbot & Kiernan, 2015). The condition is commonly referred to as Lou Gehrig's disease, in honour of the great New York Yankees baseball player who developed the disease in the 1930s (Kiernan & Turner, 2015) (Figure 9.1). MND is characterised by degeneration of motor neurons in the brain and spinal cord that usually begins insidiously with focal weakness and subsequent relentless progression to involve most muscles, including the diaphragm ultimately resulting in death due to respiratory paralysis (Al-Chalabi et al., 2016). The average overall survival is approximately 3–5 years but varies immensely depending on clinical phenotype and genetic factors, with approximately 10% of patients surviving more than 8 years (Brown & Al-Chalabi, 2017; Simon, Huynh, Vucic, Talbot & Kiernan, 2015). Although previously considered as a pure motor disorder, cumulative evidence from imaging, neuropathological and clinical studies now suggest that MND affects extra-motor systems, representative of a multisystems disease that extends beyond upper and lower motor neurons. In particular, a significant proportion (up to 50%) of patients with MND develop cognitive impairment and behavioural changes (van Es et al., 2017).

Clinical vignette

AC is a 64-year-old man who presented with progressive weakness in his limbs over the past 18 months. He first noticed wasting and weakness that started in his right hand which then over the pursuing 3 months spread to affect the left hand.

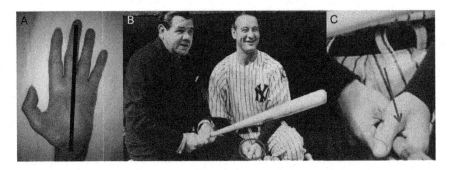

FIGURE 9.1 Lou Gehrig (1903–1941), the New York Yankees baseball player nicknamed 'the Iron Horse', began a streak of 2,130 consecutive games in June 1925 that ended when he developed left leg weakness 14 years later. (A) The ALS split-hand refers to preferential wasting of abductor pollicis brevis and first dorsal interosseous muscles, with relative preservation of the lateral abductor digit minimi. (B) A photograph of Gehrig (right) with teammate 'Babe' Ruth (left), on display at Yankee Stadium, confirms wasting of his left first dorsal interosseous (close-up shown in panel C). It developed after initial ipsilateral leg weakness, and this pattern of spread of symptoms to contiguous body regions is typical in MND.

Source: Kiernan & Turner (2015); reproduced with permission (copyright licence 4340721264708)

About 2 months later bulbar symptoms became apparent with dysphonia and dysarthria followed by mild dysphagia mainly for liquids. Respiratory symptoms have also become an issue in more recent times with dyspnoea upon minimal physical activity. There is no significant personal or family medical history and he does not drink alcohol nor smoke cigarettes.

On examination he was cachectic and there was prominent wasting with severe weakness of the intrinsic muscles bilaterally and a split-hand appearance (preferential thenar over hypothenar muscle wasting). There were frequent upper limb fasciculations. Tongue appeared mildly wasted and weak and jaw jerk was brisk. Facial muscle and neck strength were otherwise preserved. He had moderate dysphonia and mild flaccid dysarthria. Reflexes were globally brisk with spreading and there was unsustained ankle clonus bilaterally. He had moderate wrist weakness but preserved more proximally. In the lower limbs there was mild right ankle dorsiflexion weakness.

Brain and spinal cord MRI was normal. Nerve conduction studies (NCS) demonstrated normal sensory responses in the upper and lower limbs, but markedly reduced or absent distal motor responses in the upper and lower limbs associated with an abnormal split-hand index. Needle electromyography (EMG) showed widespread neurogenic changes with active denervation in all four limb muscles as well as denervation observed in the trapezius muscle.

Transcranial magnetic stimulation (TMS) studies to assess for cortical excitability demonstrated a reduction in short-interval cortical inhibition (SICI) in both motor cortices indicative of cortical hyperexcitability. He also underwent a cognitive assessment and he scored 86/100 on the Addenbrooke's Clinical Examination (normal range being >88), with his worst performance in measures of executive functioning.

The clinical presentation of AC together with the electrophysiological features was consistent with an upper limb onset MND with features to suggest early cognitive impairment with executive dysfunction. A positron emission tomography (PET) scan was arranged to exclude an underlying malignancy given his significant weight loss but did not reveal evidence of a neoplastic process. The brain images, however, did show reduction in glucose metabolism in the frontal and parietal lobes bilaterally as well as temporal regions.

Epidemiology

The incidence of MND is approximately 1–2.6 per 100,000 persons annually, while the worldwide prevalence is estimated to be 4–6 per 100,000 (Huynh & Kiernan, 2015; Talbott, Malek & Lacomis, 2016). The average age of onset of MND is currently 58–60 years but may vary depending on demographic factors such as geography with much younger age of onset observed in the Chinese population (Chen et al., 2015; Sabatelli, Conte & Zollino, 2013; Talbott, Malek & Lacomis, 2016). Sporadic MND (90–95%) constitutes the majority of cases, while the remaining 5–10% are hereditary, termed familial MND, although sporadic MND is postulated to involve genetic susceptibility to environmental risk factors (Huynh & Kiernan, 2015; Talbott, Malek & Lacomis, 2016). Age of onset appears to be slightly younger at 57–52 in familial cases (Kiernan et al., 2011), but clinical features are indistinguishable between sporadic and familial cases. Lifetime risk is higher in men (1 in 350) than for women (1 in 400), although the incidence between men and women is about the same in familial disease (Kiernan et al., 2011; van Es et al., 2017). There is evidence to suggest that the incidence and prevalence of MND is lower in populations of mixed ancestral origin than in European populations, with differences in age of onset in genetically heterogeneous populations (generally about 10 years earlier) (van Es et al., 2017). An onset in the late teenage or early adult years is suggestive of familial disease (Brown & Al-Chalabi, 2017).

Clinical presentation

MND is characterised by progressive motor deficits involving any voluntary muscle usually resulting in heterogeneous presentations that range from hand weakness to dysarthria to a foot drop depending on the initially involved region (Figure 9.2; see also Plate 2 in the colour section). Motor neurons in the oculomotor nuclei and in Onuf's nucleus however, appear to be resistant therefore sparing of eye movement and sphincter control is often observed (van Es et al., 2017). The classical

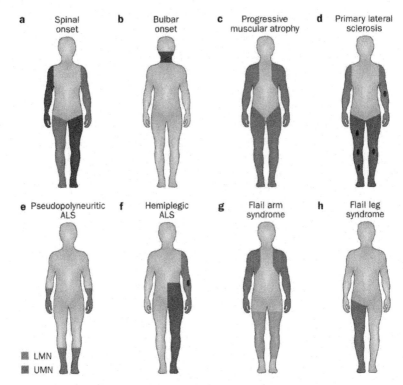

FIGURE 9.2 Pattern of motor involvement in different ALS phenotypes. A colour version of this image is shown as Plate 3 in the colour section, where red indicates LMN involvement and blue indicates UMN involvement. Darker shading indicates more severe involvement. (a) In spinal-onset ALS, patchy UMN and LMN involvement is observed in all limbs. (b) In bulbar-onset ALS, UMN and LMN involvement is observed in the bulbar muscles. (c) In progressive muscular atrophy, LMNs in arms and legs are involved, often proximally. (d) In primary lateral sclerosis, UMNs of arms and legs are primarily involved, but later in the disease, discrete LMN involvement can be detected. (e) In pseudopolyneuritic ALS, only LMNs restricted to the distal limbs are involved. (f) In hemiplegic ALS, unilateral UMN involvement with sparing of the face, and sometimes discrete LMN involvement, can be observed. (g) In flail arm syndrome, LMN involvement is restricted to the upper limbs, but mild UMN signs can be detected in the legs. (h) In flail leg syndrome, LMN involvement is restricted to the lower limbs, and is often asymmetric. ALS, amyotrophic lateral sclerosis; LMN, lower motor neuron; UMN, upper motor neuron.

Source: Swinnen & Robberecht (2014); reproduced with permission (copyright licence 4342890349018)

hallmark of MND is the presence of both upper and lower motor neuron signs involving brainstem and multiple spinal cord regions of innervation on neurological examination (Kiernan et al., 2011) with the onset of disease often being focal but with the eventual spread to other body regions. The progression and spread of the disease appears to be both local (within the same region for example distal to proximal in the one limb) and between neuroanatomically linked regions (contralateral or rostrocaudal) (van Es et al., 2017).

Upper motor neuron (UMN) disturbances involving the limbs result clinically in spasticity, weakness, and brisk deep tendon reflexes, while lower motor neuron (LMN) limb features include muscle wasting and weakness with fasciculations. Bulbar UMN dysfunction is evident by the presence of spastic dysarthria characterised by slow, laboured, and distorted speech with a nasal quality and associated with a brisk gag and jaw jerk. Bulbar LMN dysfunction is identified by tongue wasting, weakness, and fasciculations that is accompanied by flaccid dysarthria and dysphagia. Flaccid dysarthria results in nasal speech caused by palatal weakness, hoarseness, and a weak cough (Duffy, Peach & Strand, 2007; Kiernan et al., 2011).

The initial clinical presentations constituting 95% of all ALS, may be classified according to region: (1) limb-onset MND (70%); (2) bulbar onset MND (25%). Alternatively it may be sub-divided into much rarer extremes of LMN or UMN involvement: (1) progressive muscular atrophy (PMA), with pure LMN involvement, and typically limb-onset; or (2) primary lateral sclerosis (PLS), characterised by predominant UMN involvement, typically lower limb or bulbar in site of onset, both of which are rare (Huynh et al., 2016; Kiernan et al., 2011). Pathological and novel neuroimaging and electrophysiological studies, however, often disclose evidence of involvement in either UMN or LMNs that appear to be clinically unaffected in these variants and hence considered part of different ends of the MND clinical spectrum. Initial trunk or respiratory involvement is very rare (5%) and is associated with a very poor survival (Kiernan et al., 2011; Swinnen & Robberecht, 2014).

Early hand dysfunction in MND preferentially affects the 'thenar hand', which includes the abductor pollicis brevis and first dorsal interosseous muscles (Figures 9.1A and 9.3C). In contrast, there is relative sparing of the hypothenar muscles (abductor digiti minimi). This dissociated atrophy of the intrinsic hand muscles is virtually unique to MND and is explained by the marked vulnerability of the hand-corticomotoneuronal system. The muscles involved underlie pincer and precision grips (prehensility), which are dependent on the corticomotoneuronal system, a prime pathological target of the disease (Eisen et al., 2017).

Disease progression in MND is characterised by an organised process of non-random spread of symptoms from site of onset to subsequent body regions, with preferred and most rapid symptom development to the contralateral limb. The organised development of symptoms to contiguous anatomical regions appears to be consistent throughout the spectrum of MND (Simon, Huynh, Vucic, Talbot & Kiernan, 2015; Walhout, Verstraete, van den Heuvel, Veldink & van den Berg, 2018) (Figure 9.4; see also Plate 4 in the colour section).

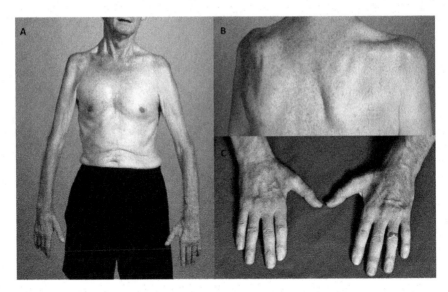

FIGURE 9.3 Clinical features of muscles wasting in a patient with MND. (A) Proximal and symmetrical upper limb wasting resulting in an inability to lift arms against gravity ('man–in–the–barrel' or flail arm variant MND). (B) Significant wasting of supraspinatus and infraspinatus muscles, as well as substantial loss of deltoid muscle. (C) Preferential wasting of the thenar muscles combined with the first dorsal interossei, the so-called 'split-hand', is a typical feature in MND.

PLS is characterised by slower progression and deterioration of function with sparing of respiratory function and less-severe weight loss than seen in classical MND. The diagnosis of PLS includes the presence of upper motor neuron dysfunction, in the absence of other neurological findings, or alternative explanations on diagnostic testing including familial causes such as hereditary spastic paraparesis (HSP), structural, metabolic, infectious and inflammatory aetiologies. Ultimately PLS is a diagnosis of exclusion (Statland, Barohn, Dimachkie, Floeter & Mitsumoto, 2015). Some patients may present with UMN-predominant MND at onset but may develop evidence of LMN involvement. For this reason, sufficient time is usually required to lapse before a definitive diagnosis of PLS is made – usually 3–5 years, depending on the criteria used (ibid.).

Upper motor neuron involvement can be asymmetrical with an extreme form being the hemiplegic variant called Mills syndrome or progressive hemiplegia. In this phenotype, unilateral upper motor neuron involvement usually starts in the lower limb, followed by slow progression to the ipsilateral upper limb and relative sparing of the face. After a variable time however, the disease spreads to the initially unaffected contralateral side (Swinnen & Robberecht, 2014). Patients may have lower motor neuron onset that remains limited to the upper limbs for at least 12 months, while the lower limbs are unaffected by weakness, although

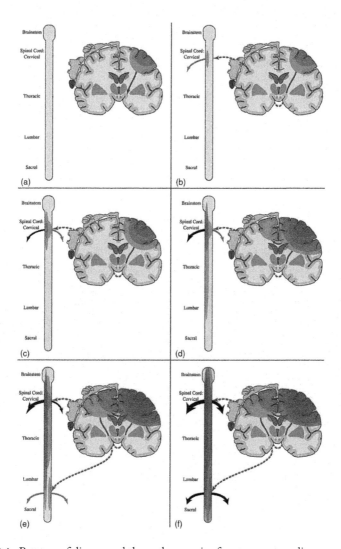

FIGURE 9.4 Patterns of disease and the pathogenesis of motor neuron disease.
(a) Representation of the hypothesis of contiguous cortical and spinal spread
as an explanation of clinical patterns of disease, with the focus of disease
onset in the motor cortex representing the right upper limb. (b) Pathology
may then spread within the ipsilateral motor cortex and involve the spinal
cord through the corticospinal tract. (c) Independently, pathology may
spread within the spinal cord both through contiguous anatomic spread
from the initial focus in the right cervical spinal cord. (d) Pathology may
continue to spread within the motor cortex involving the contralateral
hemisphere by spreading across the corpus callosum, and (e,f) through
ongoing descending transmission through the corticospinal tract. This
mechanism of spread may help explain the complex patterns of clinical
involvement and spread seen in amyotrophic lateral sclerosis patients.

Source: Simon, Huynh, Vucic, Talbot & Kiernan (2015); reproduced with permission (copyright licence 4340750880994)

some UMN features may be observed. This phenotype called flail arm syndrome (synonyms include scapulohumeral form of MND, man-in-a-barrel syndrome or brachial amyotrophic diplegia) has a male predominance (male-to-female ratio 4:1) (Figures 9.3A and 9.3B). Most patients with this syndrome however develop more widespread disease after a period of about 20 months. Other rarer variants include the flail leg and dropped head syndrome.

Prognosis

Although median survival of ALS (MND) is generally around 3 years from diagnosis, variability in survival is remarkable and reflects the variability in the rate of disease progression particularly among the different clinical phenotypes (Swinnen & Robberecht, 2014). Only a minority of ALS patients survive >5 years (up to 20%) (Fujimura-Kiyono et al., 2011) and >10 years (5–10%) (Chio et al., 2009). Older age at symptom onset, early respiratory muscle dysfunction, El Escorial category (see 'diagnosis' section), shorter interval between first symptoms and first examination, low score on the revised version of the ALS Functional Rating Scale (ALSFRS-R) and bulbar-onset disease are associated with reduced survival, whereas limb-onset disease, younger age at presentation, and longer diagnostic delay are independent predictors of prolonged survival (Fujimura-Kiyono et al., 2011; Kiernan et al., 2011). Lower limb onset may have a slightly better prognosis than upper limb onset (Fujimura-Kiyono et al., 2011) although this is not consistent (Chio et al., 2009). Furthermore, the involvement of two regions within one month of presentation or the progression from first symptom to second within 2–3 months is associated with the poorest prognosis (Fujimura-Kiyono et al., 2011). In the pure bulbar palsy phenotype that typically affects women older than 65 years of age and disease confined to oropharyngeal musculature with UMN features predominating, the prognosis varies from 2–4 years (Kiernan et al., 2011).

Patients with symptom onset before 40 years of age (majority being male) tend to have a longer survival that often exceeds 10 years while median survival among patients presenting after 80 years of age is less than two years (Chio et al., 2009).

Patients with PMA fare slightly better than patients with both UMN and LMN clinical involvement although novel electrophysiological and neuroimaging studies in these subsets of patients frequently unveil subclinical UMN dysfunction (Huynh et al., 2016). The flail limb variant of MND has a mean survival of 4 years and long-term survival of 17% (Swinnen & Robberecht, 2014). The average symptom duration for PLS has reported to range from 7.2 to 14.5 years and progression seemingly ceasing after several years, with varied levels of disability among patients (Statland, Barohn, Dimachkie, Floeter & Mitsumoto, 2015). The mean survival of UMN-predominant MND patients is around 6 years, with approximately 30% having longer-term (>10 years) survival and appears to lie between that of PLS and classic MND (Swinnen & Robberecht, 2014).

Genetic factors

Approximately 10% of MND cases are familial in nature (Renton, Chio & Traynor, 2014). Over recent years, rapid advances in the genetics of MND have led to the discovery of over 25 mutant genes (Brown & Al-Chalabi, 2017) with more than 120 genetic variants associated with a risk of MND (Chia, Chio & Traynor, 2018; Taylor, Brown & Cleveland, 2016). About 60–80% of familial cases can be attributed to mutations in C9ORF72 (40%), SOD1 (20%), TARDBP (1–5%), and FUS (1–5%) (Chio et al., 2014; Huynh & Kiernan, 2015; Turner et al., 2013; van Es et al., 2017). Genetic mutations are also responsible for up to 11% of apparently sporadic cases (Renton, Chio & Traynor, 2014) suggesting that genetic changes can act as rare disease determinants of major effect, as well as simple Mendelian alleles (Majounie et al., 2012). First degree relatives of patients with sporadic MND are at an eight-fold higher risk of developing the disease (Hanby et al., 2011). SOD1 was the first ALS gene to be identified in 1993 (Rosen, 1993). The most remarkable discovery was that of the C9ORF72 mutation which causes repeat expansion in the GGGGCC hexanucleotide sequence, present in about 40% and 7% of familial and sporadic cases, respectively (Konno et al., 2013). This suggests that both sporadic and familial forms of ALS share potentially similar molecular pathological mechanisms. This expansion is also found in approximately 25% of patients with familial frontotemporal dementia (FTD) and 6% of sporadic cases, providing the genetic basis for the overlap between MND and FTD, underscoring an MND–FTD spectrum of neurodegenerative disorders (Robberecht & Philips, 2013). Recent studies have demonstrated that the genetic architecture of MND in Asian populations is distinct from that in European populations. In particular, in European populations the most common mutations were the C9orf72 repeat expansions followed by SOD1, TARDBP and FUS mutations, while in Asian populations the most common were SOD1 mutations, followed by FUS, C9orf72 and TARDBP mutations (Zou et al., 2017).

Although familial MND is predominantly inherited in an autosomal dominant pattern, with X-linked and recessive forms being rare, increased knowledge of the variability in the penetrance of various mutations complicates genetic counselling in MND and makes it difficult to provide individualised risk evaluation for family members (Chio et al., 2014; Robberecht & Philips, 2013; Talbot, 2014). Additionally, the polygenic nature of MND, as well as the uncertainty relating to the precise pathogenicity of specific mutations, suggests that many cases are likely to be due to the involvement of multiple genetic and environmental factors for disease manifestation (Simon, Huynh, Vucic, Talbot & Kiernan, 2015). Furthermore, the heterogeneous phenotypical presentation observed from the same mutation even between affected individuals within the same family renders genetic analysis difficult based on the clinical picture of a single patient. An oligogenic model is consistent with the incomplete penetrance in many MND pedigrees, the reduced rate of MND in genetically heterogeneous populations, and the cosegregation of multiple MND-associated genes with disease in some kindreds (van Blitterswijk et al., 2012; van Es et al., 2017). Heritability can also be obscured in small pedigrees (death resulting from other causes before the onset of ALS, loss of contact, etc), causing familial cases to appear sporadic. To further complicate matters, a number of MND genes appear to be pleiotropic. The most obvious example would be C9orf72 mutation, which is clearly linked to MND and FTD but is also linked to Parkinsonism, Huntington phenocopies, Alzheimer's disease, corticobasal degeneration, schizophrenia, and bipolar disorder (Cooper-Knock, Shaw & Kirby, 2014).

Diagnosis

MND remains a clinical diagnosis and there is no single definitive diagnostic test (Turner & Talbot, 2012), with the diagnostic process critically involving a comprehensive clinical history and neurological examination identifying the combination of UMN and LMN signs in the same body region, often with serial assessments to confirm progression of symptoms and signs to other regions over time (Kiernan et al., 2011). This also holds true for the various clinical phenotypes as no biomarkers are available to distinguish them (Al-Chalabi et al., 2016) (Figure 9.5; see also Plate 5 in the colour section). Clinical assessments are supplemented by electrodiagnostic studies, looking for muscle denervation and to exclude alternative diagnoses, particularly inflammatory neuropathy. Imaging of the brain and spinal cord may exclude metabolic and structural central nervous system disorders. Conventional MRI has identified hypointensities over the motor cortices in patients with MND/ALS while hyperintense signalling was observed on T2-weighted images involving the corticospinal tracts (CST) (Agosta et al., 2010; Huynh et al., 2010; Peretti-Viton et al., 1999; Rocha & Maia Junior, 2012), but neither were specific to the disease itself being also present in other neurodegenerative disorders as well as older age controls (Huynh et al., 2016).

The El Escorial criteria were developed by the World Federation of Neurology Research Group on Motor Neuron Diseases to define research-based consensus diagnostic criteria and was published in 1994, which were subsequently revised as the Airlie House criteria and the Awaji-Shima criteria (Brooks, 1994; Brooks, Miller, Swash, Munsat & World Federation of Neurology Research Group on Motor Neuron, 2000; Carvalho & Swash, 2009; de Carvalho et al., 2008). The criteria use a combination of UMN and LMN signs to establish levels of diagnostic certainty. However, these criteria have poor sensitivity in the early stages of MND, often resulting in a long delay before a definitive diagnosis can be reached with the median time to diagnosis of about 14 months (Kiernan et al., 2011). The diagnosis of MND according to the El Escorial criteria depends on identification of upper and lower motor neuron signs within body regions defined as bulbar, cervical, thoracic, and lumbar. Furthermore, the El Escorial diagnostic criteria are based on the certainty for the more classical phenotype ALS as opposed to others such as PMA or PLS. For this reason, the terms possible, probable, and definite refer to the severity of clinical presentation as a result of the pathology involved, and not to the underlying diagnosis of MND, which often lead to confusion in communicating the diagnosis with patients using such diagnostic criteria (Al-Chalabi et al., 2016) (Table 9.1).

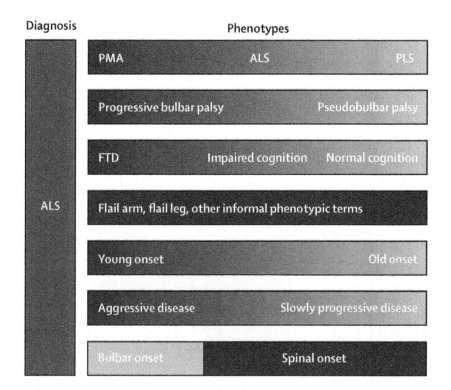

FIGURE 9.5 Diagnosis and phenotypes of motor neuron disease. The term amyotrophic lateral sclerosis (ALS) is an overarching diagnosis, and is used interchangeably with motor neuron disease in the UK and some other countries. The term ALS is also used to distinguish the ALS phenotype from progressive muscular atrophy (PMA), primary lateral sclerosis (PLS), and other clinical manifestations. Whether PLS and PMA should be regarded as phenotypes of ALS or as diseases in their own right is not clear. The terms bulbar palsy and pseudobulbar palsy are sometimes used as diagnoses, but they are actually phenotypes of ALS. Cognitive impairment presents as a continuum but criteria define a cut-off for the diagnosis of frontotemporal dementia (FTD). Whether ALS–FTD should be regarded as a phenotype of ALS or as a diagnosis is also not clear. Flail arm, flail leg, and other terms are used to describe specific patterns of symmetrical limb weakness that are seen fairly frequently. Cut-offs for other continuous variables, such as age of onset and disease progression, are not defined by existing criteria. Bulbar onset accounts for about 25% of cases of ALS; bulbar onset and spinal onset can occur simultaneously, and other sites of onset, such as respiratory muscles, are sometimes seen.

Source: Al-Chalabi, Hardiman, Kiernan, Chio, Rix-Brooks & van den Berg (2016); reproduced with permission (copyright licence 4353570431941)

TABLE 9.1 The El Escorial criteria and its revisions. LMN, lower motor neuron; UMN, upper motor neuron; ¥, components that are not part of the classification. Neuroimaging and clinical laboratory studies must be done to exclude alternative diagnoses. δ regions: bulbar, cervical (corresponding to neck, arm, hand, diaphragm, and cervical spinal cord-innervated muscles), thoracic (corresponding to back and abdomen muscles), and lumbar (corresponding to back, abdomen, leg, foot, and lumbosacral spinal cord-innervated muscles).

	Definite ALS	Probable ALS	Laboratory-supported probable ALS	Possible ALS	Suspected ALS
El Escorial criteria (1994)	UMN and LMN signs in three regions of the body δ	UMN and LMN signs in at least two regions, with some UMN signs rostral to LMN signs	¥	UMN and LMN signs in only one region, or UMN signs alone in two or more regions, or LMN signs rostral to UMN signs	LMN signs only
Airlie House criteria (2000)	UMN and LMN signs in the bulbar region and at least two spinal regions, or UMN and LMN signs in at least two spinal regions and LMN signs in three spinal regions	UMN and LMN signs in at least two regions, with some UMN signs rostral to LMN signs	Clinical evidence of UMN and LMN signs in only one region, or UMN signs alone in one region and electrophysiological evidence of LMN signs in at least two regions	UMN and LMN signs in only one region, or UMN signs alone in two or more regions, or LMN signs rostral to UMN signs	¥
Awaji-Shima criteria (2008)	Clinical or electrophysiological evidence of UMN and LMN signs in the bulbar region and at least two spinal regions, or UMN and LMN signs in three spinal regions	Clinical or electrophysiological evidence of UMN and LMN signs in at least two regions, with some UMN signs rostral to LMN signs	¥	Clinical or electrophysiological evidence of UMN and LMN signs in only one region, or UMN signs alone in two or more regions, or LMN signs rostral to UMN signs	¥

Source: Al-Chalabi, Hardiman, Kiernan, Chio, Rix-Brooks & van den Berg (2016); reproduced with permission (copyright licence 4353570431941)

Muscle biopsy samples can be of further diagnostic value for excluding unusual myopathies or for confirming the presence of MND by indicating atrophy of mixed-fibre types (Baloh, Rakowicz, Gardner & Pestronk, 2007). Electrodiagnostic studies (nerve conduction and electromyography; EMG) are useful in the work-up of patients with suspected MND. Nerve conduction studies typically show a pattern of normal sensory responses with reduced motor amplitudes. The median nerve compound muscle action potential (CMAP) was more commonly reduced in amplitude than the tibial and ulnar motor responses, which is consistent with the sensitivity of the median nerve to degeneration in MND (Simon, Lomen-Hoerth & Kiernan, 2014).

Neurophysiological evidence of the MND 'split-hand' (clinically observed as preferential thenar over hypothenar muscle wasting) was frequent and appeared to be independent of the clinical region of onset (Simon, Lomen-Hoerth & Kiernan, 2014). Needle EMG may uncover LMN changes (indicative of denervation) that were not apparent on clinical examination in keeping with the estimation that one-third of motor fibres may have degenerated before clinical weakness becomes apparent (Wohlfart, 1958). As such, recent diagnostic criteria have incorporated EMG as a surrogate marker of LMN involvement, and have in turn improved the sensitivity of 'definite' diagnostic categories (de Carvalho et al., 2008). When EMG changes were considered by region, there was a relatively uniform rate of detection of neurogenic abnormalities on EMG, including limbs without apparent clinical weakness (Simon, Lomen-Hoerth & Kiernan, 2014).

Novel diagnostic techniques

In the presence of progressive LMN weakness, features of UMN involvement are an important component supporting the diagnosis of MND (de Carvalho, 2012), but often clinical signs of UMN dysfunction may not be easily appreciated in a limb that is concurrently affected by LMN degeneration particularly in the early stages (Geevasinga, Menon, Yiannikas, Kiernan & Vucic, 2014; Swash, 2012). Clinical UMN signs are found to be initially absent in 7–10% of MND patients (Rocha & Maia Junior, 2012). However, the various components of the UMN syndrome reflect different physiological abnormalities in the descending motor system that is expressed by the intact LMN system, the latter being invariably affected in MND (Pierrot-Deseilligny & Burke, 2005; Swash, 2012). Furthermore, simultaneous alpha and gamma spinal motor neuron loss in conjunction with spinal interneuron degeneration has an effect on the expression of UMN signs (de Carvalho, 2012; Swash, 2012). As such, objective UMN markers are critical to the diagnosis, as purely LMN syndromes may be caused not only by MND (Simon, Turner et al., 2014), but mimics various motor neuropathies, including Kennedy's disease and adult-onset spinal muscular atrophy (SMA).

Importantly, autopsy reports have identified UMN degeneration in 50–75% patients without apparent clinical signs affecting the corticospinal tract (Ince et al., 2003; Kaufmann et al., 2004; Lawyer & Netsky, 1953). Failure to recognise UMN features in patients presenting with suspected MND consequently results in diagnostic uncertainty and thereby delay, which according to population studies is more than a year from symptom onset to diagnosis. This will inevitably delay the commencement of potentially disease modifying or neuroprotective therapy, most effective when started early in the disease course, in addition to adversely affecting enrolment into therapeutic trials (Hardiman, van den Berg & Kiernan, 2011; Turner et al., 2013).

An important focus in the development of a neurophysiological biomarker of MND/ALS has been the identification of cortical hyperexcitability and the quantification of UMN dysfunction (Turner, Kiernan, Leigh & Talbot, 2009). Transcranial magnetic stimulation (TMS) techniques have gained credibility as a clinical tool to investigate the integrity of the corticomotoneuronal system in MND. Single, paired, and triple-pulse TMS techniques have all been utilised, with such parameters as motor threshold (MT), central motor conduction time (CMCT), cortical silent period (CSP), and intracortical inhibition and facilitation, which are taken to reflect corticomotoneuronal function (Vucic & Kiernan, 2013). Features of cortical hyperexcitability were characterised by functional abnormalities, including reduced short-interval intracortical inhibition and CSP duration, as well as an increase in intracortical facilitation, along with inexcitability in the motor cortex (Grieve et al., 2015). Moreover, there were significant bilateral TMS abnormalities evident in the MND cohort at an early stage of the disease process, in keeping with previous studies reporting that functional abnormalities of the motor cortex are an early and specific feature of MND, preceding the development of LMN dysfunction (Geevasinga, Menon, Yiannikas, Kiernan & Vucic, 2014; Grieve et al., 2015; Menon, Kiernan & Vucic, 2015; Vucic & Kiernan, 2006; Vucic, Nicholson & Kiernan, 2008; Vucic, Ziemann, Eisen, Hallett & Kiernan, 2013) (Figure 9.6).

In recent times, advanced neuroimaging techniques have facilitated investigation of the central nervous system for atrophy and alterations in microstructure, biochemistry, neural networks, metabolism and neuronal receptors that may occur in patients with MND as means to identify an objective marker of UMN dysfunction especially at the earlier stages of disease (Foerster, Welsh & Feldman, 2013). Advanced MRI techniques based on high resolution T1 images such as voxel-based morphometry (VBM) measure relative grey and white matter volumes in specific brain regions, while surface-based morphometry (SBM) measure cortical thickness. Most VBM analyses have demonstrated widespread grey matter atrophy involving the motor cortex extending into the frontal and parietal regions in patients with MND while SBM show consistent reductions in cortical thickness in MND motor cortices with progressive thinning over time (Foerster et al., 2013; Zhu et al., 2015). Some studies have proposed such cortical thinning as a potential early biomarker of UMN dysfunction (Mezzapesa et al., 2013; Thorns et al., 2013; Verstraete et al., 2012; Walhout et al., 2015). Functional MRI (fMRI) is able to

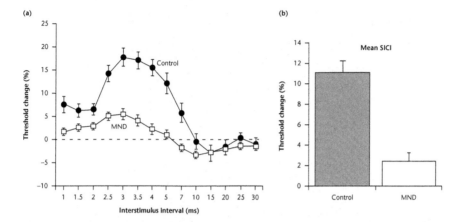

FIGURE 9.6 Cortical excitability in motor neuron disease (MND). Paired-pulse subthreshold conditioning transcranial magnetic stimulation demonstrating (a) reduction in short-interval intracortical inhibition (SICI; above dotted line) and intracortical facilitation (ICF; below dotted line) and (b) significant reductions in averaged SICI (between interstimulus intervals of 1–7 ms) in MND patients compared with controls.

Source: Simon, Huynh, Vucic, Talbot & Kiernan (2015); reproduced with permission (copyright licence 4340750880994)

assess physiological function of the upper motor neurons and provides high-resolution measures of neural activity that is reflected by changes in blood flow to local vasculature in response to activity. During index–thumb opposition in patients with MND of lower motor neuron onset, results were similar to normal controls revealing activation over M1 and some activation over the sensorimotor cortex. In MND patients with upper motor neuron signs the activation appeared more widespread, involving the supplementary motor, pre-motor, and sensory cortex (Agosta et al., 2010; Brooks, Bushara et al., 2000; Eisen & Weber, 2001), which was also observed on the contralateral hemisphere (Schoenfeld et al., 2005).

Positron emission tomography (PET) imaging allows qualitative and quantitative studies of brain metabolism in vivo (Kaufmann & Mitsumoto, 2002). In MND patients, frontal hypometabolism has been uniformly demonstrated using [18]FDG-PET in all patients. The most commonly reported regions with hypometabolism involved the perirolandic and frontal brain regions and appeared to be a sensitive marker of MND (Dalakas, Hatazawa, Brooks & Di Chiro, 1987; Foerster et al., 2013; Pagani et al., 2014; Shiozawa et al., 2000; Van Laere et al., 2014) (Figure 9.7, see also Plate 6 in the colour section), with a diagnostic accuracy of greater than 90% for differentiating MND patients from health controls (Chio & Traynor, 2015) and sensitivity and specificity greater than 90% and 80%

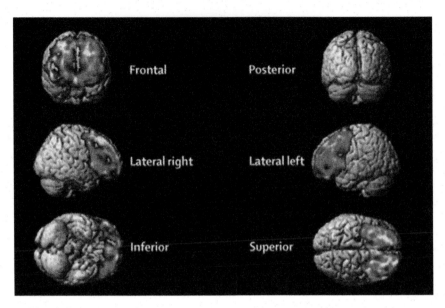

FIGURE 9.7 18F-fluorodeoxyglucose PET analysis in MND patients demonstrating hypometabolism. The images show three-dimensional rendering of the brain cortical surface of the clusters of voxels in which patients with MND show hypometabolism compared with healthy controls. Uptake is substantially impaired mainly in the frontal and anterior cingulate cortex.

Source: Chio, Pagani, Agosta, Calvo, Cistaro & Filippi (2014); reproduced with permission (copyright licence 4358050287769)

respectively (Pagani et al., 2014; Van Laere et al., 2014). Of relevance, patients clinically diagnosed with PMA also demonstrated a similar pattern of hypometabolism (Van Laere et al., 2014) that underscores the presence of subclinical corticomotoneuronal involvement as well as PMA being part of the MND clinical spectrum.

Cognitive and behavioural manifestations

While MND has been long considered a disorder primarily involving the motor system, cognitive and behavioural features appear in early descriptions of MND (Charcot & Joffroy, 1869). Within the last three decades, cognitive impairment in MND has been much discussed in the literature, with estimates suggesting up to 50% of patients with MND have a degree of cognitive impairment (Goldstein & Abrahams, 2013; Lillo & Hodges, 2010). Out of these 10–15% of cases meet the criteria for frontotemporal dementia (FTD) (Goldstein & Abrahams, 2013; Phukan et al., 2012). Bulbar onset ALS and lower educational attainment are recognised risk factors for the development of cognitive dysfunction (Gordon et al., 2011). Additionally, the presence of cognitive impairment, especially coexistence of FTD is a predictor of shorter survival (Elamin et al., 2011; Westeneng et al., 2018) and functional decline (Elamin et al., 2011) in MND.

The cognitive profile of MND includes deficits in executive function, verbal fluency, language, social cognition and verbal memory. Accounting for motor impairments, verbal fluency deficits are commonly observed in MND with a moderate effect size (0.56, range 0.43–0.70) compared to controls (Beeldman et al., 2016). Verbal fluency deficits occur early in the course of the disease (Abrahams, Leigh & Goldstein, 2005), and have been shown to correlate with abnormalities in the dorsolateral prefrontal cortex and inferior frontal gyri (Abrahams et al., 1996; Pettit et al., 2013) and white matter tracts including the corpus callosum and frontotemporal tracts (Abrahams, Goldstein et al., 2005; Agosta et al. 2016).

Social cognition deficits, such as impairments in emotion recognition and theory of mind, have also been increasingly recognised in MND, particularly in ALS–FTD overlap (Beeldman et al., 2016; Strong et al., 2017). Language deficits have been documented in up to 40% of patients with MND and coexistent cognitive impairment in the absence of frank dementia (Taylor et al., 2013). While there are diagnostic challenges in interpreting language deficits in the presence of executive function impairments, particularly with coexistent FTD (Strong et al., 2017), there is evidence that language impairment dissociates from executive function deficits and motor impairments (Bak & Hodges, 2004). Memory impairments, particularly those in verbal memory when compared to visual memory deficits, have been documented in MND (Beeldman et al., 2016) but do not appear in the current diagnostic criteria for cognitive impairment in MND (Strong et al., 2017) as they have not been consistently demonstrated and rarely occur in isolation.

Behavioural changes that do not meet the full criteria for FTD but are obvious deviations in premorbid behaviour are referred to as MND with behavioural impairment (Strong et al., 2017). Behavioural symptoms similar to those with behavioural-variant frontotemporal dementia (bvFTD) affect more than 50% of patients (ibid.), with approximately 5% to 22% meeting criteria for FTD (Lomen-Hoerth et al., 2003; Raaphorst, de Visser, Linssen, de Haan & Schmand, 2010). Behavioural symptoms include perseveration, disinhibition and most commonly apathy (Grossman, Woolley-Levine, Bradley & Miller, 2007; Lillo, Mioshi, Zoing, Kiernan & Hodges, 2011; Raaphorst, Beeldman, De Visser, De Haan & Schmand, 2012). There is increasing evidence that behavioural symptoms in MND carries a negative prognosis (Caga et al., 2016; Hu et al., 2013).

Furthermore, emerging research suggests that changes in personality and behaviour rather than cognitive impairment per se places a heavier burden on MND caregivers (Burke, Elamin, Galvin, Hardiman & Pender, 2015; Chio et al., 2010; Hsieh et al., 2016; Tremolizzo et al., 2016; Watermeyer et al., 2015). Caregivers must not only be able to cope with progressive physical deterioration, but also behavioural symptoms that require more supervision, prompting or taking over tasks for the patient (Radakovic et al., 2017), including greater accountability over treatment decision making (Hogden, Greenfield, Nugus & Kiernan, 2013) and adherence to life-sustaining interventions (Olney et al., 2005). Psychological support for caregivers of MND patients presenting with behavioural symptoms is often recommended to assist with management of these non-motor manifestations of the disease (Miller et al., 2009). However, little is actually known about what types of interventions are appropriate. Thus, while there is growing support for interventions to manage behavioural symptoms in MND there have been no interventions systematically tried to date (ibid.).

Based on the dementia literature, recommended strategies for caregivers of MND patients with behavioural symptoms mainly focus on educating and helping caregivers adjust their expectations about patients' reduced capacity to perform day-to-day tasks as well as environmental modifications to ensure patients safety (e.g, hide car keys from patient) (Merrilees, Klapper, Murphy, Lomen-Hoerth & Miller, 2010). However, there is a lack of information available on interventions that may be suitable and effective for MND patients with behavioural symptoms (Caga et al., 2018). Tailoring successful psychological interventions in dementia may be an important first step towards guiding and developing future management strategies for MND patients with behavioural symptoms and their caregivers.

Various screening tools have been developed to assess cognition, along with behavioural deficits in MND, including the Edinburgh Cognitive and Behavioural ALS screen (ECAS) (Niven et al., 2015), MND Cognitive and Behavioural Screen (ALS-CBS) (Woolley et al., 2010), modified version of the Addenbrooke's Cognitive examination (M-ACE) administered alongside the Motor Neuron Disease Behavioural Scale (MiND-B) (Hsieh et al., 2016).

The ALS–FTD continuum

It is now well established that the pure motor phenotype of MND and fronto-temporal dementia (FTD) lie on opposite ends of the frontal neurodegeneration continuum (Burrell et al., 2016), with concurrence of these two conditions in patients with the chromosome 9 open reading frame 72 (C9orf72 mutation) (DeJesus-Hernandez et al., 2011; Renton et al., 2011). Occurrence of TAR DNA binding protein-43 (TDP-43) pathology in both conditions (Neumann et al., 2006), alongside the cognitive and behavioural impairments in ALS (Goldstein & Abrahams, 2013; Lillo & Hodges, 2010) support this continuum theory of MND and FTD. Heterogeneity exists in clinical phenotypes along this spectrum and further refinement of clinical and pathological syndromes is needed.

Management and potential therapeutic strategies

The complex heterogenic profile of MND has made therapeutic targets difficult to identify, and there remains no cure for the disease. Although management is centered primarily around supportive and symptomatic care, recent advances in the understanding of this syndrome has identified several factors that have increased patient survival and quality of life, transforming the historically conservative approach to MND disease management and identifying critical treatment targets (Dharmadasa et al., 2016). Such interventions with known positive survival benefit include: (i) institution of disease-modifying therapy; (ii) management in a multidisciplinary care team (MDC) setting; (iii) early respiratory intervention; and (iv) weight management.

Disease-modifying therapies

Riluzole is as an inhibitor of glutamate release with wide-ranging, multimodal effects on neural activity in MND. It confers a modest survival benefit of 3–6 months and has an estimated increase in 1-year survival by 9% (Miller, Mitchell & Moore, 2012). Disease modulation has been postulated to occur at very early (Geevasinga et al., 2016) and late stages of the disease (Fang et al., 2018), suggesting different mechanisms of action occurring at different disease points (Dharmadasa & Kiernan, 2018). A second disease modifying drug, edaravone, has recently been approved by the FDA in Japan and the US for use in a subgroup of MND patients. As a free radical scavenger originally marketed for use after ischaemic stroke, a 2–3-month benefit from this intravenous medication was seen in MND patients who had relatively minimal disability, preserved respiratory function (estimated by a forced vital capacity of >80%), and were at a relatively early stage of disease (within 2 years of onset) (Abe et al., 2014).

Multidisciplinary care

Benefits of MDC in the management of MND is now well-recognised and recommended as standard of care for all patients, prolonging survival by 7–24 months and reducing the risk of death by 45% at 5 years (Van den Berg et al., 2005). To address the complex and dynamic care needs of the patient, such a setting involves medical, nursing and allied health professionals, as well as specialist input from a respiratory physician, gastroenterologist and palliative care physician (Figure 9.8; see also Plate 7 in the colour section) (Dharmadasa, Matamala & Kiernan, 2016). Care coordination and support is also given through various MND state-based associations. The MDC network delivers an anticipatory management model, providing proactive intervention in order to address medical issues early, minimise deterioration from functional disability, enhance quality of life and provide a framework for support for the treating clinicians as well as the caregivers (Dharmadasa et al., 2017).

Respiratory intervention

Almost all MND patients develop respiratory symptoms during the course of disease and respiratory failure represents the most common cause of death (Miller et al., 2009). Assessment of lung function is therefore of central importance in MND management, with measures such as forced vital capacity (FVC), maximal inspiratory pressure (MIP), maximal expiratory pressure, sniff nasal inspiratory pressure (SNIP), and arterial blood gases regularly evaluated. The early institution of non-invasive positive pressure ventilation (NIV) has been shown to extend survival by up to 13 months, improving quality of life and common secondary symptoms such as dyspnea, sleep disturbance, daytime somnolence, and early morning headache (Carratu et al., 2009). Invasive ventilatory options, such as tracheostomy, remain a consideration for patients not able to tolerate NIV or with deteriorating function.

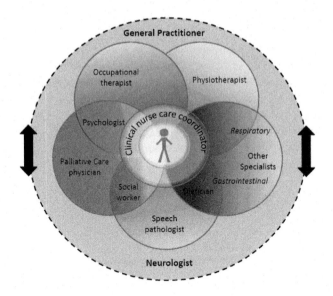

FIGURE 9.8 MND multidisciplinary care model. The multidisciplinary care model centres around the MND patient. It involves dynamic integration of medical, nursing and allied health professionals for optimal patient management. Care is often coordinated by the clinical nurse, with the neurologist and general practitioner overseeing all aspects of care.

However, despite providing respiratory support, this option remains controversial and is not widely adopted due to the significant risk of side effects such as infection, bleeding, and tracheoesophageal fistula formation (Sancho, Servera, Banuls & Marin, 2010). In addition, the ethical difficulty of instituting such invasive treatment for a progressive and terminal disease remains a challenging concept.

Nutrition and weight

Weight loss has a negative survival impact and is associated with more rapid disease progression (Desport et al., 2000). Cause is multifactorial, and commonly includes development of a hypermetabolic state, bulbar dysfunction, respiratory dysfunction, potential neuropsychiatric problems, and increasing barriers due to physical limitations from limb weakness. Management is thus driven by the MDC, with assessment of cause(s) and institution of any appropriate therapies, as required. Options for invasive nutritional intervention, such as enteral feeding, is considered when >10% baseline weight has been lost despite the above (Desport et al., 1999). Such nutritional support can be given via insertion of a nasogastric tube or, more commonly, gastrostomy (such as percutaneous endoscopic gastrostomy tubes), which will also bypass dysphagia and similar difficulties in patients requiring long-term ventilatory support (Spataro, Ficano, Piccoli & La Bella, 2011).

End-of-life management

Advanced care planning is a critical issue that requires appropriate discussion by the MDC, particularly the palliative care team, within a reasonable timeframe. This is often considered when introducing interventional options such as NIV or gastrostomy, but palliative care involvement remains inconsistent globally and poorly defined. Poor symptom control can cause significant distress to both patients and families and has been highlighted as the major cause of patient distress in the end stage of the disease, highlighting the critical need for sensitively structured implementation of end-of-life conversations (Connolly, Galvin & Hardiman, 2015).

Abbreviations

ALS	amyotrophic lateral sclerosis
C9orf72	chromosome 9 open reading frame 72
CSP	cortical silent period
EMG	electromyography
fMRI	functional magnetic resonance imaging
FTD	frontotemporal dementia
FUS	fused in sarcoma
FVC	forced vital capacity
ICF	intracortical facilitation
LMN	lower motor neuron
MND	motor neuron disease
MRI	magnetic resonance imaging
NCS	nerve conduction studies
NIV	non-invasive ventilation
PLS	primary lateral sclerosis
PMA	progressive muscular atrophy
RMT	resting motor threshold
SBM	surfaced-based morphometry
SICI	short-interval intracortical inhibition
SMA	spinal muscular atrophy
SOD-1	superoxide dismutase 1
TARDP	trans-activating response region DNA-binding protein
TMS	transcranial magnetic stimulation
UMN	upper motor neuron
VBM	volume-based morphometry

Further reading

Chio, A., Logroscino, G., Hardiman, O., et al. (2009) Prognostic factors in ALS: A critical review. *Amyotrophic Lateral Sclerosis, 10*(5–6), 310–323.

Dharmadasa, T., Henderson, R., Talman, P., et al. (2017) Motor neurone disease: Progress and challenges. *Medical Journal of Australia, 206*(8), 357–362.

Hardiman, O., van den Berg, L. H. & Kiernan, M. C. (2011) Clinical diagnosis and man-agement of amyotrophic lateral sclerosis. *Nature Reviews Neurology*, 7(11), 639–649.

Kiernan, M., Vucic, S., Cheah, B., et al. (2011) Amyotrophic lateral sclerosis. *Lancet*, *277*, 942–955.

Miller, R. G., Jackson, C. E., Kasarskis, E. J., et al. (2009) Practice parameter update: The care of the patient with amyotrophic lateral sclerosis: Multidisciplinary care, symptom management, and cognitive/behavioral impairment (an evidence-based review): Report of the Quality Standards Subcommittee of the American Academy of Neurology. *Neurology*, 73(15), 1227–1233.

Simon, N. G., Huynh, W., Vucic, S., Talbot, K. & Kiernan, M. C. (2015) Motor neuron dis-ease: Current management and future prospects. *Internal Medicine Journal*, *45*(10), 1005–1013.

References

Abe, K., Itoyama, Y., Sobue, G., Tsuji, S., Aoki, M., Doyu, M., . . . Yoshino, H. (2014). Confirmatory double-blind, parallel-group, placebo-controlled study of efficacy and safety of edaravone (MCI-186) in amyotrophic lateral sclerosis patients. *Amyotrophic Lateral Sclerosis and Frontotemporal Degeneration*, *15*, 610–617.

Abrahams, S., Goldstein, L. H., Kew, J. J., Brooks, D. J., Lloyd, C. M., Frith, C. D. & Leigh, P. N. (1996). Frontal lobe dysfunction in amyotrophic lateral sclerosis. A PET study. *Brain*, *119*(Pt 6), 2105–2120.

Abrahams, S., Goldstein, L. H., Suckling, J., Ng, V., Simmons, A., Chitnis, X., . . . Leigh, P. N. (2005). Frontotemporal white matter changes in amyotrophic lateral sclero-sis. *Journal of Neurology*, *252*(3), 321–331. doi:10.1007/s00415-005-0646-x

Abrahams, S., Leigh, P. N. & Goldstein, L. H. (2005). Cognitive change in ALS: A prospec-tive study. *Neurology*, *64*(7), 1222–1226. doi:10.1212/01.WNL.0000156519.41681.27

Agosta, F., Chio, A., Cosottini, M., De Stefano, N., Falini, A., Mascalchi, M., . . . Filippi, M. (2010). The present and the future of neuroimaging in amyotrophic lateral sclerosis. *American Journal of Neuroradiology*, *31*(10), 1769–1777. doi:10.3174/ajnr.A2043

Agosta, F., Ferraro, P. M., Riva, N., Spinelli, E. G., Chio, A., Canu, E., . . . Filippi, M. (2016). Structural brain correlates of cognitive and behavioral impairment in MND. *Human Brain Mapping*, *37*(4), 1614–1626. doi:10.1002/hbm.23124

Al-Chalabi, A., Hardiman, O., Kiernan, M. C., Chio, A., Rix-Brooks, B. & van den Berg, L. H. (2016). Amyotrophic lateral sclerosis: Moving towards a new classification system. *Lancet Neurology*, *15*(11), 1182–1194. doi:10.1016/S1474-4422(16)30199-5

Bak, T. H. & Hodges, J. R. (2004). The effects of motor neurone disease on language: Further evidence. *Brain and Language*, *89*(2), 354–361. doi:10.1016/S0093-934X(03)00357-2

Baloh, R. H., Rakowicz, W., Gardner, R. & Pestronk, A. (2007). Frequent atrophic groups with mixed-type myofibers is distinctive to motor neuron syndromes. *Muscle and Nerve*, *36*(1), 107–110. doi:10.1002/mus.20755

Beeldman, E., Raaphorst, J., Klein Twennaar, M., de Visser, M., Schmand, B. A. & de Haan, R. J. (2016). The cognitive profile of ALS: A systematic review and meta-analysis update. *Journal of Neurology, Neurosurgery & Psychiatry*, *87*(6), 611–619. doi:10. 1136/jnnp-2015-310734

Brooks, B. R. (1994). El Escorial World Federation of Neurology criteria for the diag-nosis of amyotrophic lateral sclerosis. Subcommittee on Motor Neuron Diseases/ Amyotrophic Lateral Sclerosis of the World Federation of Neurology Research Group on Neuromuscular Diseases and the El Escorial 'Clinical limits of amyotrophic lateral sclerosis' workshop contributors. *Journal of the Neurological Sciences*, *124*(Suppl), S96–107.

Brooks, B. R., Bushara, K., Khan, A., Hershberger, J., Wheat, J. O., Belden, D. & Henningsen, H. (2000). Functional magnetic resonance imaging (fMRI) clinical studies in ALS: Paradigms: Problems and promises. *Amyotrophic Lateral Sclerosis and Other Motor Neuron Disorders, 1 Suppl 2,* S23–32.

Brooks, B. R., Miller, R. G., Swash, M., Munsat, T. L. & World Federation of Neurology Research Group on Motor Neuron, Diseases. (2000). El Escorial revisited: Revised criteria for the diagnosis of amyotrophic lateral sclerosis. *Amyotrophic Lateral Sclerosis and Other Motor Neuron Disorders, 1*(5), 293–299.

Brown, R. H., Jr. & Al-Chalabi, A. (2017). Amyotrophic lateral sclerosis. *New England Journal of Medicine, 377*(16), 1602. doi:10.1056/NEJMc1710379

Burke, T., Elamin, M., Galvin, M., Hardiman, O. & Pender, N. (2015). Caregiver burden in amyotrophic lateral sclerosis: A cross-sectional investigation of predictors. *Journal of Neurology, 262*(6), 1526–1532. doi:10.1007/s00415-015-7746-z

Burrell, J. R., Halliday, G. M., Kril, J. J., Ittner, L. M., Gotz, J., Kiernan, M. C. & Hodges, J. R. (2016). The frontotemporal dementia-motor neuron disease continuum. *Lancet, 388*(10047), 919–931. doi:10.1016/S0140-6736(16)00737-6

Caga, J., Hsieh, S., Highton-Williamson, E., Zoing, M. C., Ramsey, E., Devenney, E., . . . Kiernan, M. C. (2018). Apathy and its impact on patient outcome in amyotrophic lateral sclerosis. *Journal of Neurology, 265*(1), 187–193. doi:10.1007/s00415-017-8688-4

Caga, J., Turner, M. R., Hsieh, S., Ahmed, R. M., Devenney, E., Ramsey, E., . . . Kiernan, M. C. (2016). Apathy is associated with poor prognosis in amyotrophic lateral sclerosis. *European Journal of Neurology, 23*(5), 891–897. doi:10.1111/ene.12959

Carratu, P., Spicuzza, L., Cassano, A., Maniscalco, M., Gadaleta, F., Lacedonia, D., . . . Resta, O. (2009). Early treatment with noninvasive positive pressure ventilation prolongs survival in Amyotrophic Lateral Sclerosis patients with nocturnal respiratory insufficiency. *Orphanet Journal of Rare Diseases, 4*(10).

Carvalho, M. D. & Swash, M. (2009). Awaji diagnostic algorithm increases sensitivity of El Escorial criteria for ALS diagnosis. *Amyotrophic Lateral Sclerosis, 10*(1), 53–57. doi:10.1080/17482960802521126

Charcot, J. M. & Joffroy, A. (1869). Deus cas d'atrophie musculaire progressive avec lesions de la substance grise et des faisceaux antéro-latérale. *Archives of Physiology, 2,* 354–367.

Chen, L., Zhang, B., Chen, R., Tang, L., Liu, R., Yang, Y., . . . Fan, D. (2015). Natural history and clinical features of sporadic amyotrophic lateral sclerosis in China. *Journal of Neurology Neurosurgery & Psychiatry, 86*(10), 1075–1081. doi:10.1136/jnnp-2015-310471

Chia, R., Chio, A. & Traynor, B. J. (2018). Novel genes associated with amyotrophic lateral sclerosis: Diagnostic and clinical implications. *Lancet Neurology, 17*(1), 94–102. doi:10.1016/S1474-4422(17)30401-5

Chio, A., Battistini, S., Calvo, A., Caponnetto, C., Conforti, F. L., Corbo, M., . . . Surbone, A. (2014). Genetic counselling in ALS: Facts, uncertainties and clinical suggestions. *Journal of Neurology Neurosurgery & Psychiatry, 85*(5), 478–485. doi:10.1136/jnnp-2013-305546

Chio, A., Logroscino, G., Hardiman, O., Swingler, R., Mitchell, D., Beghi, E., . . . Eurals Consortium. (2009). Prognostic factors in ALS: A critical review. *Amyotrophic Lateral Sclerosis, 10*(5–6), 310–323. doi:10.3109/17482960802566824

Chio, A., Pagani, M., Agosta, F., Calvo, A., Cistaro, A. & Filippi, M. (2014). Neuroimaging in amyotrophic lateral sclerosis: Insights into structural and functional changes. *Lancet Neurology, 13*(12), 1228–1240. doi:10.1016/S1474-4422(14)70167-X

Chio, A. & Traynor, B. J. (2015). Motor neuron disease in 2014. Biomarkers for ALS: In search of the Promised Land. *Nature Reviews Neurology, 11*(2), 72–74. doi:10.1038/nrneurol.2014.250

Chio, A., Vignola, A., Mastro, E., Giudici, A. D., Iazzolino, B., Calvo, A., . . . Montuschi, A. (2010). Neurobehavioral symptoms in ALS are negatively related to caregivers' burden and quality of life. *European Journal of Neurology, 17*(10), 1298–1303. doi:10.1111/j.1468-1331.2010.03016.x

Cleveland, D. W. & Rothstein, J. D. (2001). From Charcot to Lou Gehrig: Deciphering selective motor neuron death in ALS. *Nature Reviews Neuroscience, 2*(11), 806–819. doi:10.1038/35097565

Connolly, S., Galvin, M. & Hardiman, O. (2015). End of life management in patients with amyotrophic lateral sclerosis. *Lancet Neurology, 14,* 435–442.

Cooper-Knock, J., Shaw, P. J. & Kirby, J. (2014). The widening spectrum of C9ORF72-related disease: Genotype/phenotype correlations and potential modifiers of clinical phenotype. *Acta Neuropathologica, 127*(3), 333–345. doi:10.1007/s00401-014-1251-9

Dalakas, M. C., Hatazawa, J., Brooks, R. A. & Di Chiro, G. (1987). Lowered cerebral glucose utilization in amyotrophic lateral sclerosis. *Annals of Neurology, 22*(5), 580–586. doi:10.1002/ana.410220504

De Carvalho, M. (2012). Testing upper motor neuron function in amyotrophic lateral sclerosis: The most difficult task of neurophysiology. *Brain, 135*(Pt 9), 2581–2582. doi:10.1093/brain/aws228

De Carvalho, M., Dengler, R., Eisen, A., England, J. D., Kaji, R., Kimura, J., . . . Swash, M. (2008). Electrodiagnostic criteria for diagnosis of ALS. *Clinical Neurophysiology, 119*(3), 497–503. doi:10.1016/j.clinph.2007.09.143

DeJesus-Hernandez, M., Mackenzie, I. R., Boeve, B. F., Boxer, A. L., Baker, M., Rutherford, N. J., . . . Rademakers, R. (2011). Expanded GGGGCC hexanucleotide repeat in noncoding region of C9ORF72 causes chromosome 9p-linked FTD and ALS. *Neuron, 72*(2), 245–256. doi:10.1016/j.neuron.2011.09.011

Desport, J. C., Preux, P. M., Truong, C. T., Courat, L., Vallat, J. M. & Couratier, P. (2000). Nutritional assessment and survival in ALS patients. *Amyotrophic Lateral Sclerosis and Other Motor Neuron Disorders, 1*(2), 91–96.

Desport, J. C., Preux, P. M., Truong, T. C., Vallat, J. M., Sautereau, D. & Couratier, P. (1999). Nutritional status is a prognostic factor for survival in ALS patients. *Neurology, 53*(5), 1059–1063.

Dharmadasa, T., Henderson, R. D., Talman, P., Macdonell, R. A., Mathers, S., Schultz, D., . . . Kiernan, M. C. (2017). Motor neurone disease: Progress and challenges. *Medical Journal of Australia, 206*(8), 357–362.

Dharmadasa, T. & Kiernan, M. C. (2018). Riluzole, disease stage and survival in ALS. *Lancet Neurology, 17*(5), 385–386.

Dharmadasa, T., Matamala, J. M. & Kiernan, M. C. (2016). Treatment approaches in motor neurone disease. *Current Opinions in Neurology, 29*(5), 581–591. doi:10.1097/WCO.0000000000000369

Duffy, J. R., Peach, R. K. & Strand, E. A. (2007). Progressive apraxia of speech as a sign of motor neuron disease. *American Journal of Speech and Language Pathology, 16*(3), 198–208. doi:10.1044/1058-0360(2007/025)

Eisen, A., Braak, H., Del Tredici, K., Lemon, R., Ludolph, A. C. & Kiernan, M. C. (2017). Cortical influences drive amyotrophic lateral sclerosis. *Journal of Neurology, Neurosurgery & Psychiatry, 88*(11), 917–924. doi:10.1136/jnnp-2017-315573

Eisen, A. & Weber, M. (2001). The motor cortex and amyotrophic lateral sclerosis. *Muscle and Nerve, 24*(4), 564–573.

Elamin, M., Phukan, J., Bede, P., Jordan, N., Byrne, S., Pender, N. & Hardiman, O. (2011). Executive dysfunction is a negative prognostic indicator in patients with ALS without dementia. *Neurology, 76*(14), 1263–1269. doi:10.1212/WNL.0b013e318214359f

Fang, T., Ahmad, A. K., Meurgey, J. H., Jones, A., Leigh, P. N., Bensimon, G. & Al-Chalabi, A. (2018). Stage of prolonged survival with riluzole treatment in patients with amyotrophic lateral sclerosis: A retrospective analysis. *Lancet Neurology*. In press.

Foerster, B. R., Welsh, R. C. & Feldman, E. L. (2013). 25 years of neuroimaging in amyotrophic lateral sclerosis. *Nature Reviews Neurology*, *9*(9), 513–524. doi:10.1038/nrneurol.2013.153

Fujimura-Kiyono, C., Kimura, F., Ishida, S., Nakajima, H., Hosokawa, T., Sugino, M. & Hanafusa, T. (2011). Onset and spreading patterns of lower motor neuron involvements predict survival in sporadic amyotrophic lateral sclerosis. *Journal of Neurology Neurosurgery & Psychiatry*, *82*(11), 1244–1249. doi:10.1136/jnnp-2011-300141

Geevasinga, N., Menon, P., Ng, K., Van den Bos, M., Byth, K., Kiernan, M. C. & Vucic, S. (2016). Riluzole exerts transient modulating effects onf cortical and axonal hyperexcitability in ALS. *Amyotrophic Lateral Sclerosis and Frontotemporal Degeneration*, *17*, 580–588.

Geevasinga, N., Menon, P., Yiannikas, C., Kiernan, M. C. & Vucic, S. (2014). Diagnostic utility of cortical excitability studies in amyotrophic lateral sclerosis. *European Journal of Neurology*, *21*(12), 1451–1457. doi:10.1111/ene.12422

Goldstein, L. H. & Abrahams, S. (2013). Changes in cognition and behaviour in amyotrophic lateral sclerosis: Nature of impairment and implications for assessment. *Lancet Neurology*, *12*(4), 368–380. doi:10.1016/S1474-4422(13)70026-7

Gordon, P. H., Delgadillo, D., Piquard, A., Bruneteau, G., Pradat, P. F., Salachas, F., . . . Lacomblez, L. (2011). The range and clinical impact of cognitive impairment in French patients with ALS: A cross-sectional study of neuropsychological test performance. *Amyotrophic Lateral Sclerosis*, *12*(5), 372–378. doi:10.3109/17482968.2011.580847

Grieve, S. M., Menon, P., Korgaonkar, M. S., Gomes, L., Foster, S., Kiernan, M. C. & Vucic, S. (2015). Potential structural and functional biomarkers of upper motor neuron dysfunction in ALS. *Amyotrophic Lateral Sclerosis and Frontotemporal Degeneration*, *17*(1–2), 85–92. doi:10.3109/21678421.2015.1074707

Grossman, A. B., Woolley-Levine, S., Bradley, W. G. & Miller, R. G. (2007). Detecting neurobehavioral changes in amyotrophic lateral sclerosis. *Amyotrophis Lateral Sclerosis*, *8*(1), 56–61. doi:10.1080/17482960601044106

Hanby, M. F., Scott, K. M., Scotton, W., Wijesekera, L., Mole, T., Ellis, C. E., . . . Al-Chalabi, A. (2011). The risk to relatives of patients with sporadic amyotrophic lateral sclerosis. *Brain*, *134*(Pt 12), 3454–3457. doi:10.1093/brain/awr248

Hardiman, O., van den Berg, L. H. & Kiernan, M. C. (2011). Clinical diagnosis and management of amyotrophic lateral sclerosis. *Nature Reviews Neurology*, *7*(11), 639–649. doi:10.1038/nrneurol.2011.153

Hogden, A., Greenfield, D., Nugus, P. & Kiernan, M. C. (2013). What are the roles of carers in decision-making for amyotrophic lateral sclerosis multidisciplinary care? *Patient Preference and Adherence*, *7*, 171–181. doi:10.2147/PPA.S40783

Hsieh, S., Leyton, C. E., Caga, J., Flanagan, E., Kaizik, C., O'Connor, C. M., . . . Mioshi, E. (2016). The evolution of caregiver burden in frontotemporal dementia with and without amyotrophic lateral sclerosis. *Journal of Alzheimers Disease*, *49*(3), 875–885. doi:10.3233/JAD-150475

Hu, W. T., Shelnutt, M., Wilson, A., Yarab, N., Kelly, C., Grossman, M., . . . Glass, J. (2013). Behavior matters: Cognitive predictors of survival in amyotrophic lateral sclerosis. *PLoS One*, *8*(2), e57584. doi:10.1371/journal.pone.0057584

Huynh, W. & Kiernan, M. C. (2015). A unique account of ALS in China: Exploring ethnic heterogeneity. *Journal of Neurology Neurosurgery & Psychiatry*, *86*(10), 1051–1052. doi:10.1136/jnnp-2015-311293

Huynh, W., Lam, A., Vucic, S., Cheah, B. C., Clouston, P. & Kiernan, M. C. (2010). Corticospinal tract dysfunction and development of amyotrophic lateral sclerosis following electrical injury. *Muscle and Nerve, 42*(2), 288–292. doi:10.1002/mus.21681

Huynh, W., Simon, N. G., Grosskreutz, J., Turner, M. R., Vucic, S. & Kiernan, M. C. (2016). Assessment of the upper motor neuron in amyotrophic lateral sclerosis. *Clinical Neurophysiology, 127*(7), 2643–2660. doi:10.1016/j.clinph.2016.04.025

Ince, P. G., Evans, J., Knopp, M., Forster, G., Hamdalla, H. H., Wharton, S. B. & Shaw, P. J. (2003). Corticospinal tract degeneration in the progressive muscular atrophy variant of ALS. *Neurology, 60*(8), 1252–1258.

Kaufmann, P. & Mitsumoto, H. (2002). Amyotrophic lateral sclerosis: Objective upper motor neuron markers. *Current Neurology and Neuroscience Reports, 2*(1), 55–60.

Kaufmann, P., Pullman, S. L., Shungu, D. C., Chan, S., Hays, A. P., Del Bene, M. L., . . . Mitsumoto, H. (2004). Objective tests for upper motor neuron involvement in amyotrophic lateral sclerosis (ALS). *Neurology, 62*(10), 1753–1757.

Kiernan, M. C. & Turner, M. R. (2015). Lou Gehrig and the ALS split hand. *Neurology, 85*(22), 1995. doi:10.1212/WNL.0000000000002172

Kiernan, M. C., Vucic, S., Cheah, B. C., Turner, M. R., Eisen, A., Hardiman, O., . . . Zoing, M. C. (2011). Amyotrophic lateral sclerosis. *Lancet, 377*(9769), 942–955. doi:10.1016/S0140-6736(10)61156-7

Konno, T., Shiga, A., Tsujino, A., Sugai, A., Kato, T., Kanai, K., . . . Onodera, O. (2013). Japanese amyotrophic lateral sclerosis patients with GGGGCC hexanucleotide repeat expansion in C9ORF72. *Journal of Neurology Neurosurgery & Psychiatry, 84*(4), 398–401. doi:10.1136/jnnp-2012-302272

Lawyer, T., Jr. & Netsky, M. G. (1953). Amyotrophic lateral sclerosis. *AMA Arch Neurol Psychiatry, 69*(2), 171–192.

Lillo, P. & Hodges, J. R. (2010). Cognition and behaviour in motor neurone disease. *Current Opinions in Neurology, 23*(6), 638–642. doi:10.1097/WCO.0b013e3283400b41

Lillo, P., Mioshi, E., Zoing, M. C., Kiernan, M. C. & Hodges, J. R. (2011). How common are behavioural changes in amyotrophic lateral sclerosis? *Amyotrophic Lateral Sclerosis, 12*(1), 45–51. doi:10.3109/17482968.2010.520718

Lomen-Hoerth, C., Murphy, J., Langmore, S., Kramer, J. H., Olney, R. K. & Miller, B. (2003). Are amyotrophic lateral sclerosis patients cognitively normal? *Neurology, 60*(7), 1094–1097.

Majounie, E., Renton, A. E., Mok, K., Dopper, E. G., Waite, A., Rollinson, S., . . . Traynor, B. J. (2012). Frequency of the C9orf72 hexanucleotide repeat expansion in patients with amyotrophic lateral sclerosis and frontotemporal dementia: A cross-sectional study. *Lancet Neurology, 11*(4), 323–330. doi:10.1016/S1474-4422(12)70043-1

Menon, P., Kiernan, M. C. & Vucic, S. (2015). Cortical hyperexcitability precedes lower motor neuron dysfunction in ALS. *Clinical Neurophysiology, 126*(4), 803–809. doi:10.1016/j.clinph.2014.04.023

Merrilees, J., Klapper, J., Murphy, J., Lomen-Hoerth, C. & Miller, B. L. (2010). Cognitive and behavioral challenges in caring for patients with frontotemporal dementia and amyotrophic lateral sclerosis. *Amyotrophic Lateral Sclerosis, 11*(3), 298–302. doi:10.3109/17482961003605788

Mezzapesa, D. M., D'Errico, E., Tortelli, R., Distaso, E., Cortese, R., Tursi, M., . . . Simone, I. L. (2013). Cortical thinning and clinical heterogeneity in amyotrophic lateral sclerosis. *PLoS One, 8*(11), e80748. doi:10.1371/journal.pone.0080748

Miller, R. G., Jackson, C. E., Kasarskis, E. J., England, J. D., Forshew, D., Johnston, W., . . . Quality Standards Subcommittee of the American Academy of Neurology. (2009). Practice parameter update: The care of the patient with amyotrophic lateral sclerosis:

Multidisciplinary care, symptom management, and cognitive/behavioral impairment (an evidence-based review): Report of the Quality Standards Subcommittee of the American Academy of Neurology. *Neurology, 73*(15), 1227–1233. doi:10.1212/WNL.0b013e3181bc01a4

Miller, R. G., Mitchell, J. D. & Moore, D. H. (2012). Riluzole for amyotrophic lateral sclerosis (ALS)/motor neuron disease (MND). *Cochrane Database of Systematic Reviews, 3*, CD001447.

Neumann, M., Sampathu, D. M., Kwong, L. K., Truax, A. C., Micsenyi, M. C., Chou, T. T., . . . Lee, V. M. (2006). Ubiquitinated TDP-43 in frontotemporal lobar degeneration and amyotrophic lateral sclerosis. *Science, 314*(5796), 130–133. doi:10.1126/science.1134108

Niven, E., Newton, J., Foley, J., Colville, S., Swingler, R., Chandran, S., . . . Abrahams, S. (2015). Validation of the Edinburgh Cognitive and Behavioural Amyotrophic Lateral Sclerosis Screen (ECAS): A cognitive tool for motor disorders. *Amyotrophic Lateral Sclerosis and Frontotemporal Degeneration, 16*(3–4), 172–179. doi:10.3109/21678421.2015.1030430

Olney, R. K., Murphy, J., Forshew, D., Garwood, E., Miller, B. L., Langmore, S., . . . Lomen-Hoerth, C. (2005). The effects of executive and behavioral dysfunction on the course of ALS. *Neurology, 65*(11), 1774–1777. doi:10.1212/01.wnl.0000188759.87240.8b

Pagani, M., Chio, A., Valentini, M. C., Oberg, J., Nobili, F., Calvo, A., . . . Cistaro, A. (2014). Functional pattern of brain FDG-PET in amyotrophic lateral sclerosis. *Neurology, 83*(12), 1067–1074. doi:10.1212/WNL.0000000000000792

Peretti-Viton, P., Azulay, J. P., Trefouret, S., Brunel, H., Daniel, C., Viton, J. M., . . . Salamon, G. (1999). MRI of the intracranial corticospinal tracts in amyotrophic and primary lateral sclerosis. *Neuroradiology, 41*(10), 744–749.

Pettit, L. D., Bastin, M. E., Smith, C., Bak, T. H., Gillingwater, T. H. & Abrahams, S. (2013). Executive deficits, not processing speed relates to abnormalities in distinct prefrontal tracts in amyotrophic lateral sclerosis. *Brain, 136*(Pt 11), 3290–3304. doi:10.1093/brain/awt243

Phukan, J., Elamin, M., Bede, P., Jordan, N., Gallagher, L., Byrne, S., . . . Hardiman, O. (2012). The syndrome of cognitive impairment in amyotrophic lateral sclerosis: A population-based study. *Journal of Neurology Neurosurgery & Psychiatry, 83*(1), 102–108. doi:10.1136/jnnp-2011-300188

Pierrot-Deseilligny, E. & Burke, D. (eds). (2005). *The Circuitry of the Human Spinal Cord: Its Role in Motor Control and Movement Disorders* (vol. 1). Cambridge: Cambridge University Press.

Raaphorst, J., Beeldman, E., De Visser, M., De Haan, R. J. & Schmand, B. (2012). A systematic review of behavioural changes in motor neuron disease. *Amyotrophic Lateral Sclerosis, 13*(6), 493–501. doi:10.3109/17482968.2012.656652

Raaphorst, J., de Visser, M., Linssen, W. H., de Haan, R. J. & Schmand, B. (2010). The cognitive profile of amyotrophic lateral sclerosis: A meta-analysis. *Amyotrophic Lateral Sclerosis, 11*(1–2), 27–37. doi:10.3109/17482960802645008

Radakovic, R., Stephenson, L., Newton, J., Crockford, C., Swingler, R., Chandran, S. & Abrahams, S. (2017). Multidimensional apathy and executive dysfunction in amyotrophic lateral sclerosis. *Cortex, 94*, 142–151. doi:10.1016/j.cortex.2017.06.023

Renton, A. E., Chio, A. & Traynor, B. J. (2014). State of play in amyotrophic lateral sclerosis genetics. *Nature Neuroscience, 17*(1), 17–23. doi:10.1038/nn.3584

Renton, A. E., Majounie, E., Waite, A., Simon-Sanchez, J., Rollinson, S., Gibbs, J. R., . . . Traynor, B. J. (2011). A hexanucleotide repeat expansion in C9ORF72 is the cause of chromosome 9p21-linked ALS-FTD. *Neuron, 72*(2), 257–268. doi:10.1016/j.neuron.2011.09.010

Robberecht, W. & Philips, T. (2013). The changing scene of amyotrophic lateral sclerosis. *Nature Reviews Neuroscience, 14*(4), 248–264. doi:10.1038/nrn3430

Rocha, A. J. & Maia Junior, A. C. (2012). Is magnetic resonance imaging a plausible biomarker for upper motor neuron degeneration in amyotrophic lateral sclerosis/primary lateral sclerosis or merely a useful paraclinical tool to exclude mimic syndromes? A critical review of imaging applicability in clinical routine. *Arquivos de Neuro-Psiquiatria, 70*(7), 532–539.

Rosen, D. R. (1993). Mutations in Cu/Zn superoxide dismutase gene are associated with familial amyotrophic lateral sclerosis. *Nature, 364*(6435), 362. doi:10.1038/364362c0

Sabatelli, M., Conte, A. & Zollino, M. (2013). Clinical and genetic heterogeneity of amyotrophic lateral sclerosis. *Clinical Genetics, 83*(5), 408–416. doi:10.1111/cge.12117

Sancho, J., Servera, E., Banuls, P. & Marin, J. (2010). Prolonging survival in amyotrophic lateral sclerosis: Efficacy of noninvasive ventilation and uncuffed tracheostomy tubes. *American Journal of Physical Medicine & Rehabilitation, 89*(5), 407–411.

Schoenfeld, M. A., Tempelmann, C., Gaul, C., Kuhnel, G. R., Duzel, E., Hopf, J. M., . . . Vielhaber, S. (2005). Functional motor compensation in amyotrophic lateral sclerosis. *Journal of Neurology, 252*(8), 944–952. doi:10.1007/s00415-005-0787-y

Shiozawa, Z., Shindo, K., Ohta, E., Ohushi, K., Nagamatsu, M. & Nagasaka, T. (2000). A concise overview of recent breakthroughs in imaging of ALS. *Amyotrophic Lateral Sclerosis and Other Motor Neuron Disorders, 1 Suppl 2*, S3–6.

Simon, N. G., Huynh, W., Vucic, S., Talbot, K. & Kiernan, M. C. (2015). Motor neuron disease: Current management and future prospects. *Internal Medicine Journal, 45*(10), 1005–1013. doi:10.1111/imj.12874

Simon, N. G., Lomen-Hoerth, C. & Kiernan, M. C. (2014). Patterns of clinical and electrodiagnostic abnormalities in early amyotrophic lateral sclerosis. *Muscle and Nerve, 50*(6), 894–899. doi:10.1002/mus.24244

Simon, N. G., Turner, M. R., Vucic, S., Al-Chalabi, A., Shefner, J., Lomen-Hoerth, C. & Kiernan, M. C. (2014). Quantifying disease progression in amyotrophic lateral sclerosis. *Annals of Neurology, 76*(5), 643–657. doi:10.1002/ana.24273

Spataro, R., Ficano, L., Piccoli, F. & La Bella, V. (2011). Percutaneous endoscopic gastrostomy in amyotrophic lateral sclerosis. *Journal of the Neurological Sciences, 304*, 44–48.

Statland, J. M., Barohn, R. J., Dimachkie, M. M., Floeter, M. K. & Mitsumoto, H. (2015). Primary lateral sclerosis. *Neurologic Clinics, 33*(4), 749–760. doi:10.1016/j.ncl.2015.07.007

Strong, M. J., Abrahams, S., Goldstein, L. H., Woolley, S., McLaughlin, P., Snowden, J., . . . Turner, M. R. (2017). Amyotrophic lateral sclerosis – frontotemporal spectrum disorder (ALS-FTSD): Revised diagnostic criteria. *Amyotrophic Lateral Sclerosis and Frontotemporal Degeneration, 18*(3–4), 153–174. doi:10.1080/21678421.2016.1267768

Swash, M. (2012). Why are upper motor neuron signs difficult to elicit in amyotrophic lateral sclerosis? *Journal of Neurology, Neurosurgery & Psychiatry, 83*(6), 659–662. doi:10.1136/jnnp-2012-302315

Swinnen, B. & Robberecht, W. (2014). The phenotypic variability of amyotrophic lateral sclerosis. *Nature Reviews Neurology, 10*(11), 661–670. doi:10.1038/nrneurol.2014.184

Talbot, K. (2014). Should all patients with ALS have genetic testing? *Journal of Neurology, Neurosurgery & Psychiatry, 85*(5), 475. doi:10.1136/jnnp-2013-305727

Talbott, E. O., Malek, A. M. & Lacomis, D. (2016). The epidemiology of amyotrophic lateral sclerosis. *Handbook of Clinical Neurology, 138*, 225–238. doi:10.1016/B978-0-12-802973-2.00013-6

Taylor, J. P., Brown, R. H., Jr. & Cleveland, D. W. (2016). Decoding ALS: From genes to mechanism. *Nature, 539*(7628), 197–206. doi:10.1038/nature20413

Taylor, L. J., Brown, R. G., Tsermentseli, S., Al-Chalabi, A., Shaw, C. E., Ellis, C. M., . . . Goldstein, L. H. (2013). Is language impairment more common than executive dysfunction in amyotrophic lateral sclerosis? *Journal of Neurology Neurosurgery & Psychiatry*, *84*(5), 494–498. doi:10.1136/jnnp-2012-303526

Thorns, J., Jansma, H., Peschel, T., Grosskreutz, J., Mohammadi, B., Dengler, R. & Munte, T. F. (2013). Extent of cortical involvement in amyotrophic lateral sclerosis: An analysis based on cortical thickness. *BMC Neurology*, *13*, 148. doi:10.1186/1471-2377-13-148

Tremolizzo, L., Pellegrini, A., Susani, E., Lunetta, C., Woolley, S. C., Ferrarese, C. & Appollonio, I. (2016). Behavioural but not cognitive impairment is a determinant of caregiver burden in amyotrophic lateral sclerosis. *European Neurology*, *75*(3–4), 191–194. doi:10.1159/000445110

Turner, M. R., Hardiman, O., Benatar, M., Brooks, B. R., Chio, A., de Carvalho, M., . . . Kiernan, M. C. (2013). Controversies and priorities in amyotrophic lateral sclerosis. *Lancet Neurology*, *12*(3), 310–322. doi:10.1016/S1474-4422(13)70036-X

Turner, M. R., Kiernan, M. C., Leigh, P. N. & Talbot, K. (2009). Biomarkers in amyotrophic lateral sclerosis. *Lancet Neurology*, *8*(1), 94–109. doi:10.1016/S1474-4422(08)70293-X

Turner, M. R. & Talbot, K. (2012). Motor neurone disease is a clinical diagnosis. *Practical Neurology*, *12*(6), 396–397. doi:10.1136/practneurol-2012-000374

Van Blitterswijk, M., van Es, M. A., Hennekam, E. A., Dooijes, D., van Rheenen, W., Medic, J., . . . van den Berg, L. H. (2012). Evidence for an oligogenic basis of amyotrophic lateral sclerosis. *Human Molecular Genetics*, *21*(17), 3776–3784. doi:10.1093/hmg/dds199

Van den Berg, J. P., Klamijn, S., Lindeman, E., Veldink, J. H., de Visser, M., Van der Graaff, M. M., . . . Van den Berg, L. H. (2005). Multidisciplinary ALS care improves quality of life in patients with ALS. *Neurology*, *65*(8), 1264–1267.

Van Es, M. A., Hardiman, O., Chio, A., Al-Chalabi, A., Pasterkamp, R. J., Veldink, J. H. & van den Berg, L. H. (2017). Amyotrophic lateral sclerosis. *Lancet*, *390*(10107), 2084–2098. doi:10.1016/S0140-6736(17)31287-4

Van Laere, K., Vanhee, A., Verschueren, J., De Coster, L., Driesen, A., Dupont, P., . . . Van Damme, P. (2014). Value of 18fluorodeoxyglucose-positron-emission tomography in amyotrophic lateral sclerosis: A prospective study. *JAMA Neurology*, *71*(5), 553–561. doi:10.1001/jamaneurol.2014.62

Verstraete, E., Veldink, J. H., Hendrikse, J., Schelhaas, H. J., van den Heuvel, M. P. & van den Berg, L. H. (2012). Structural MRI reveals cortical thinning in amyotrophic lateral sclerosis. *Journal of Neurology Neurosurgery & Psychiatry*, *83*(4), 383–388. doi:10.1136/jnnp-2011-300909

Vucic, S. & Kiernan, M. C. (2006). Novel threshold tracking techniques suggest that cortical hyperexcitability is an early feature of motor neuron disease. *Brain*, *129*(Pt 9), 2436–2446. doi:10.1093/brain/awl172

Vucic, S. & Kiernan, M. C. (2013). Utility of transcranial magnetic stimulation in delineating amyotrophic lateral sclerosis pathophysiology. *Handbook of Clinical Neurology*, *116*, 561–575. doi:10.1016/B978-0-444-53497-2.00045-0

Vucic, S., Nicholson, G. A. & Kiernan, M. C. (2008). Cortical hyperexcitability may precede the onset of familial amyotrophic lateral sclerosis. *Brain*, *131*(Pt 6), 1540–1550. doi:10.1093/brain/awn071

Vucic, S., Ziemann, U., Eisen, A., Hallett, M. & Kiernan, M. C. (2013). Transcranial magnetic stimulation and amyotrophic lateral sclerosis: Pathophysiological insights. *Journal of Neurology Neurosurgery & Psychiatry*, *84*(10), 1161–1170. doi:10.1136/jnnp-2012-304019

Walhout, R., Verstraete, E., van den Heuvel, M. P., Veldink, J. H. & van den Berg, L. H. (2018). Patterns of symptom development in patients with motor neuron disease.

Amyotrophic Lateral Sclerosis and Frontotemporal Degeneration, 19(1–2), 21–28. doi:10.1080/ 21678421.2017.1386688

Walhout, R., Westeneng, H. J., Verstraete, E., Hendrikse, J., Veldink, J. H., van den Heuvel, M. P. & van den Berg, L. H. (2015). Cortical thickness in ALS: Towards a marker for upper motor neuron involvement. *Journal of Neurology, Neurosurgery & Psychiatry, 86*(3), 288–294. doi:10.1136/jnnp-2013-306839

Watermeyer, T. J., Brown, R. G., Sidle, K. C., Oliver, D. J., Allen, C., Karlsson, J., . . . Goldstein, L. H. (2015). Impact of disease, cognitive and behavioural factors on caregiver outcome in amyotrophic lateral sclerosis. *Amyotrophic Lateral Sclerosis and Frontotemporal Degeneration, 16*(5–6), 316–323. doi:10.3109/21678421.2015.1051990

Westeneng, H. J., Debray, T. P. A., Visser, A. E., van Eijk, R. P. A., Rooney, J. P. K., Calvo, A., . . . van den Berg, L. H. (2018). Prognosis for patients with amyotrophic lateral sclerosis: Development and validation of a personalised prediction model. *Lancet Neurology, 17*(5), 423–433. doi:10.1016/S1474-4422(18)30089-9

Wohlfart, G. (1958). Collateral regeneration in partially denervated muscles. *Neurology, 8*(3), 175–180.

Woolley, S. C., York, M. K., Moore, D. H., Strutt, A. M., Murphy, J., Schulz, P. E. & Katz, J. S. (2010). Detecting frontotemporal dysfunction in ALS: Utility of the ALS Cognitive Behavioral Screen (ALS-CBS). *Amyotrophic Lateral Sclerosis, 11*(3), 303–311. doi:10.3109/17482961003727954

Zhu, W., Fu, X., Cui, F., Yang, F., Ren, Y., Zhang, X., . . . Huang, X. (2015). ALFF Value in right parahippocampal gyrus acts as a potential marker monitoring amyotrophic lateral sclerosis progression: A neuropsychological, voxel-based morphometry, and resting-state functional MRI study. *Journal of Molecular Neuroscience, 57*(1), 106–113. doi:10.1007/s12031-015-0583-9

Zou, Z. Y., Zhou, Z. R., Che, C. H., Liu, C. Y., He, R. L. & Huang, H. P. (2017). Genetic epidemiology of amyotrophic lateral sclerosis: A systematic review and meta-analysis. *Journal of Neurology Neurosurgery & Psychiatry, 88*(7), 540–549. doi:10.1136/ jnnp-2016-315018

10

NEW CLINICAL NEUROSCIENCE TECHNOLOGIES FOR TREATING NEURODEGENERATIVE DISORDERS

Wei-Peng Teo, Alicia M. Goodwill and Peter G. Enticott

Introduction

The use of electricity and electromagnetism to probe neural activity and function has been described in fair detail even in ancient literature almost 2000 years ago (AD 43–48) (Ceccarelli, 1962). The earliest record for the use of electricity to treat ailments of the brain was by Scribonius Largus, Roman physician to the Emperor Claudius, who reported that placing a torpedo fish (a species of electric ray) over the heads of patients with headaches induced a transient period of stupor and analgesic effect. In a similar fashion, Muslim physician Ibn Sidah (AD 1007–1066) further suggested that placing a live electric catfish on the frontal bone of the skull may help to treat epilepsy (Kellaway, 1946). However, it was the work of Italian physician Luigi Galvani (de Micheli, 1991), who inadvertently discovered the phenomenon of 'animal electricity', and physicist Alessandro Volta (Pancaldi, 2003) that founded the field of electro-neurophysiology. Galvani's nephew, Giovanni Aldini in 1804, was one of the first to report the successful treatment of patients suffering from melancholia by applying direct electrical current over the head. Aldini further assessed the effects of direct electric currents applied to himself and reported an unpleasant sensation followed by insomnia for several days.

In the last two decades, advances in our understanding of electro-neurophysiology have led to the development and refinement of both invasive and non-invasive forms of brain stimulation to treat psychiatric and neurodegenerative diseases. In the field of non-invasive brain stimulation, transcranial magnetic stimulation, or TMS, has become a standard tool to probe cognitive functioning. Based on Faraday's law of electromagnetism, TMS is capable of stimulating cortical neurons so as to activate or inhibit specific regions of the brain (Ziemann, 2010). When applied repetitively with the appropriate pulse frequency, duration and intensity, repetitive TMS (rTMS) can exert a neuro-modulatory effect by which neural function and behaviour may be altered during (online) and after (offline) the stimulation period (Hallett, 2007; Thickbroom, 2007). Similar to TMS, another form of non-invasive brain stimulation, known as transcranial direct-current stimulation (tDCS), has in recent years received great attention (Nitsche et al., 2008; Tanaka & Watanabe, 2009). tDCS works by placing two electrodes (a positive anode and negative cathode in saline-soaked sponges) over the scalp of targeted brain regions. This method allows weak direct current (typically 0.5–2mA) to pass through the scalp from the cathode to anode non-invasively and safely to stimulate cortical regions of the brain. This effect of tDCS results in polarity-specific changes to brain activity (anodal/positive tDCS increases brain excitability; cathodal/negative tDCS, inhibits brain excitability) (Nitsche & Paulus, 2000; Priori, Berardelli, Rona, Accornero & Manfredi, 1998) that may have a follow-on effect on motor and/or cognitive performance.

While non-invasive brain stimulation techniques are capable of modulating cortical brain regions, their effects on subcortical structures are limited. In this sense, invasive techniques such as deep brain stimulation (DBS) may be used to target known neurological pathologies that stem from subcortical deficits, such as Parkinson's disease (PD). This procedure, while highly invasive in nature, produces almost immediate relief from PD-related motor symptoms such as resting tremors, muscle rigidity and gait disturbances. More recently, improvements in DBS therapy with the development of multi-directional electrical implant probes have a greater ability to deliver targeted, individualised DBS therapy to optimise treatment outcomes for people with PD.

While recent advances in non-invasive and invasive brain stimulation techniques have once again sparked renewed interest for its use to treat neurological and psychiatric disorders, its clinical efficacy and application are still unclear. In this chapter, we will highlight the current evidence for the efficacy of rTMS, tDCS and DBS as a treatment for neurodegenerative diseases. Further we will discuss some of the limitations with each method that may be used for future research and clinical considerations.

Transcranial magnetic stimulation in clinical neuroscience

Transcranial magnetic stimulation has emerged as a popular technique for treating physical, cognitive and behavioural symptomology in neurodegenerative disease. TMS is currently approved for treatment-resistant major depressive disorder (MDD) in many geographical locations including Australia, New Zealand, Japan, India, United States, Canada and Europe. Due to the non-invasive nature of this technique, scientists are continuing to uncover its therapeutic potential for relieving a range of symptoms in various neurodegenerative conditions, such as PD and Alzheimer's disease (AD).

The principles of TMS are derived from Faraday's law of induction, whereby a magnetic pulse is penetrated through the scalp perpendicular to a coil, eliciting a series of electrical currents. Traditional coils are circular or figure-of-eight in design, enabling widespread and more focal stimulation of brain regions respectively (Rossini et al., 2015). Newer H1 coils have also been developed, which can penetrate deeper neuronal regions (Tendler, Barnea Ygael, Roth & Zangen, 2016). TMS can be delivered through single-pulse, paired-pulse or repetitive rhythmic stimuli. Single- and paired-pulse methods provide transient stimulation and are generally utilised for assessment of the corticospinal pathway. In contrast, rTMS modulates underlying neuronal activity that outlasts the stimulation period (Rossini et al., 2015), providing an environment for the induction of brain plasticity.

The desired outcomes from rTMS can be manipulated primarily through the stimulation frequency. Higher rTMS frequencies ($\geq$ 5Hz) and intermittent theta-burst stimulation (iTBS) facilitate cortical excitability, whereas lower rTMS frequencies ($\leq$ 1Hz) and continuous theta-burst stimulation (cTBS) suppress cortical excitability (Rossini et al., 2015). Animal models have also suggested a neuroprotective role of rTMS (Lu et al., 2017). Collectively, the ability to manipulate these parameters holds promise for individualising treatment and specifically targeting symptoms that result from altered cortical neurotransmission and neurodegeneration.

Repetitive TMS is safe, non-invasive and may come with less adverse effects than many available pharmacological treatments. The most commonly reported side-effects include mild headaches following stimulation and a tingling sensation on the scalp. There is also a small (0.1%) risk of experiencing a seizure, however, this risk is low in people without history of epilepsy and can be mitigated through appropriate screening and adherence to the current safety guidelines for frequency and intensity of stimulation (Rossini et al., 2015).

The first insights into the benefits of rTMS in people with PD began over 20-years ago (Pascual-Leone et al., 1994). Since then numerous reports have highlighted its potential as a non-invasive adjunct to conventional physical and pharmacological therapy. The cardinal motor signs of PD can be examined via the United Parkinson's Disease Rating Scale subscale III (UPDRS III) and have been the most studied outcomes following rTMS. Pooled data from over 636 patients has showed improved UPDRS III scores (Goodwill et al., 2017; Xie et al., 2015) and gait (Goodwill et al., 2017) following both high- and low-frequency rTMS over the primary motor, supplementary motor and premotor cortical brain regions. The most recent large-scale clinical trial demonstrated the efficacy of high-frequency rTMS over bilateral motor cortices to improve bradykinesia and rigidity, but gait and tremor remained unchanged (Brys et al., 2016). This finding is perhaps expected considering the differing pathophysiology underpinning hypo- and hyperkinetic symptoms observed in PD. In this context, facilitated cortical excitability through the application of high-frequency rTMS may compensate for reduced output from the basal ganglia to motor cortical areas that plan and initiate voluntary movement.

Low-frequency rTMS has the potential to target hyperkinetic symptoms of PD and reduce neurodegeneration (Dong et al., 2015). Several studies have shown low-frequency rTMS to be effective in relieving levodopa-induced dyskinesias

(Filipovic, Rothwell, van de Warrenburg & Bhatia, 2009; Sayin et al., 2014; Wagle-Shukla et al., 2007) and improving hand dexterity (e.g. buttoning up clothes) (Ikeguchi et al., 2003), however changes on the UPDRS scale have been variable (Filipovic, Rothwell & Bhatia, 2010; Shimamoto et al., 2001).

Despite majority of the research regarding rTMS and PD focusing on motor symptoms, cognitive and mood disturbances, which are observed in up to 50% of people with PD (Cosgrove, Alty & Jamieson, 2015; Reijnders, Ehrt, Weber, Aarsland & Leentjens, 2008), may also benefit from this type of brain stimulation. Pooled data from 312 patients showed high-frequency rTMS improved depression on two clinical scales, to a similar magnitude as that observed from antidepressant selective serotonin re-uptake inhibitors (Xie et al., 2015). Following that report, two large randomised controlled trials have also demonstrated high-frequency rTMS over the motor cortex and dorsolateral prefrontal cortex effectively reduced depressive symptoms in people with PD (Makkos et al., 2016; Shin, Youn, Chung & Sohn, 2016). There is currently insufficient evidence in support of rTMS on cognition in PD (Goodwill et al., 2017). Of the few published studies, most have reported no marginal improvements in neuropsychological performance (Benninger et al., 2012; Sedlackova, Rektorova, Srovnalova & Rektor, 2009) or mild cognitive impairment (Buard et al., 2018) following high-frequency rTMS over the motor and/or dorsolateral prefrontal cortex.

In addition to cognitive dysfunction associated with PD, rTMS has been identified as an efficacious therapy for people with mild cognitive impairment and AD. While its intended use is not to provide a cure, rTMS can modulate cortical networks in specific areas of cognitive processing and has been beneficial in improving cognitive functioning in patients with mild-moderate AD (Cheng et al., 2018). rTMS may also exert neuroprotective properties which aim to slow the progression of cognitive decline in people with AD, through upregulating brain-derived neurotrophic factor (BDNF) within the hippocampus (Yulug et al., 2017).

In a number of randomised controlled trials in AD, high-frequency rTMS applied over the dorsolateral prefrontal cortex improved naming ability (Cotelli, Manenti, Cappa, Zanetti & Miniussi, 2008), global cognition (Alcalá-Lozano et al., 2018; Zhao et al., 2017), episodic memory and verbal learning (Zhao et al., 2017) and activities of daily living (Ahmed, Darwish, Khedr, El Serogy & Ali, 2012). Preliminary evidence has also shown that these improvements in cognitive functioning can be retained up to a month post-treatment (Alcalá-Lozano et al., 2018). Longitudinal research is required to determine whether rTMS can be used to prevent cognitive decline and conversion from mild cognitive impairment to AD.

Repetitive TMS can also be applied as an adjunct to other therapeutic techniques, such as cognitive training (Bentwich et al., 2011; Nguyen et al., 2017; Rabey & Dobronevsky, 2016). Improvements on the Alzheimer's Disease Assessment Scale following high-frequency rTMS and cognitive training were also comparable to the magnitude of improvement seen from cholinesterase inhibitors (Bentwich et al., 2011). In some patients, improvements in cognition following high-frequency rTMS have lasted from up to nine to 12 months following stimulation (Nguyen et al., 2017; Rabey & Dobronevsky, 2016), however retention may be unique to strong rTMS responders (Nguyen et al., 2017). Of note is the absence of control groups in these previous studies, which makes it difficult to distinguish whether the benefits are due to rTMS, cognitive training, the concurrent application of these techniques, or placebo effects. This promising evidence should be confirmed in larger randomised controlled trials.

Repetitive TMS has also been shown to improve other neuropsychological symptoms in AD. rTMS applied concurrent with antipsychotic medications resulted in improved cognition, behavioural and psychological symptoms (Wu et al., 2015). Moreover, in patients with mild cognitive impairment, high-frequency rTMS improved apathy symptoms, which is a predictor of conversion to AD (Padala et al., 2018). This preliminary evidence highlights the potential for rTMS to be utilised as a preventative technique in the early stages of mild cognitive impairment, which could delay or prevent the conversion to full-blown AD.

There is preliminary evidence regarding the benefits of rTMS to improve symptoms in multiple sclerosis (MS). MS is characterised by demyelination of nerve fibres and impaired neurotransmission; accordingly, most of the research has utilised high-frequency rTMS to target motor symptoms. In early small-scale studies, high-frequency rTMS over the motor cortex reduced spasticity (Centonze, Koch et al., 2007) and urinary dysfunction (Centonze, Petta et al., 2007), while improving hand dexterity (Koch et al., 2008) and working memory (Hulst et al., 2017). There are also reports of deep rTMS and iTBS reducing fatigue (Gaede et al., 2018) and spasticity, respectively (Mori et al., 2010). rTMS has also been prescribed as an adjunct to exercise therapy in this population, with reports of concurrent iTBS and exercise therapy yielding greater improvements in spasticity symptoms, physical function and quality of life than either modality alone (Mori et al., 2011).

There is insufficient available data to draw conclusions about the efficacy of rTMS in other neurodegenerative conditions such as motor neuron disease (MND) and Huntington's disease. Two case-reports have documented improvements in Huntington's disease-related chorea symptoms (Berardelli & Suppa, 2013) and anxiety, memory and physical pain (Davis, Phillips, Tendler & Oberdeck, 2016). Two small studies in people with ALS have reported modest-to-insignificant slowing of decline on the Amyotrophic Lateral Sclerosis Deterioration Scale following cTBS (Di Lazzaro et al., 2006, 2009), while high-frequency rTMS improved maximal strength and quality of life. Considering the lack of treatment or cure for these conditions, ongoing investigation into the benefits of rTMS to manage symptoms in these populations is warranted.

rTMS is a promising therapeutic tool that can be utilised alongside traditional physical and pharmological therapies to manage physical, behavioural and cognitive symptoms in neurodegenerative conditions such as PD and AD. Given the inherently large variability in outcomes following rTMS, individually prescribed protocols are needed to maximise the efficacy and clinically utility of this technique.

Transcranial electrical stimulation: old application, new uses

The main mechanism of tDCS acts by inducing a subthreshold shift in resting membrane potential towards depolarisation or hyperpolarisation of neurons. As a result, this shift in resting membrane threshold increases or decreases the likelihood of an incoming action potential to result in post-synaptic firing. For instance, when delivered to the primary motor cortex (M1) of healthy participants, anodal tDCS increases the excitability of the underlying cortical neurons of the M1, as measured by an increase in TMS-induced motor-evoked potential (MEP) amplitude, whereas cathodal tDCS elicits an opposite effect (Nitsche & Paulus, 2000). Moreover, the application of tDCS over several minutes may induce changes in excitability that can outlast the period of stimulation (Nitsche & Paulus, 2001). While in most of these seminal studies the M1 was the target, similar effects were found when tDCS was applied over the visual (Antal, Kincses, Nitsche, Bartfai & Paulus, 2004; Chaieb, Antal & Paulus, 2008) and somatosensory (Dieckhofer et al., 2006; Matsunaga, Nitsche, Tsuji & Rothwell, 2004) cortices.

Due to its highly portable nature and ability to induce sustained changes in cortical excitability, tDCS offers the potential to be used as an adjuvant therapy in a clinical setting. In clinical populations, most tDCS studies to date have focused predominantly on the use of anodal or cathodal tDCS to improve motor or cognitive outcomes in chronic conditions such as stroke (Marquez, van Vliet, McElduff, Lagopoulos & Parsons, 2015), PD (Elsner, Kugler, Pohl & Mehrholz, 2016; Goodwill et al., 2017) and AD (Hsu, Ku, Zanto & Gazzaley, 2015). Other clinical conditions, such as chronic pain (Vaseghi, Zoghi & Jaberzadeh, 2014), dystonia (Franca et al., 2018) and epilepsy (Regner et al., 2018), have also been investigated. Based on collective evidence from meta-analyses of tDCS literature, the application of tDCS in neurodegenerative disorders such as PD and AD showed a modest but significant improvement in motor and cognitive outcomes. However, these improvements were highly dependent on several factors that are not limited to stimulation type (anodal vs cathodal), stimulation intensity (0.5–2 mA), site of stimulation, disease severity and duration, functional status at baseline and the nature of motor or cognitive test that was used. It should be noted that the two biggest limitations in tDCS research to date are the lack of consistency and standardisation of stimulation parameters (i.e. electrode size and placement and stimulation intensity) and the relatively small sample sizes (between 20–40 participants) used in randomised controlled trials, which often limit the interpretation and generalisability of the results.

A major advantage of tDCS over any other non-invasive brain stimulation techniques is its portability and capacity to be delivered in conjunction with other forms of therapy. This represents an attractive option to clinicians and patients as it is both cost- and time-effective. The rationale of combining tDCS with conventional therapy (most often physical or cognitive therapy) is two-fold: (1) using tDCS as a primer by increasing the brain's propensity to activate and (2) reinforcing accurate patterns of movement or cognitive activation through practice. Indeed, there is evidence to support the combined use of tDCS and cognitive/motor training as being superior to either tDCS or cognitive/motor training alone in a range of populations that include healthy subjects (Elmasry, Loo & Martin, 2015), people with PD (Lawrence, Gasson, Bucks, Troeung & Loftus, 2017) and AD (Hsu et al., 2015). Furthermore, studies in people with stroke suggest that combined tDCS with motor skills training may facilitate long-term retention of arm function than skills training alone (Goodwill, Teo, Morgan, Daly & Kidgell, 2016; Lefebvre et al., 2012).

While the vast majority of non-invasive transcranial electrical stimulation literature has so far focused primarily on tDCS, other variants of neuromodulatory electrical brain stimulation techniques such as transcranial alternating-current stimulation (tACS) and transcranial random-noise stimulation (tRNS) warrant discussion. Compared to tDCS, paradigms such as tACS and tRNS are considered to be true neuromodulation techniques as they are capable of eliciting functional changes in neuron activation. In particular, these hybrid forms of non-invasive transcranial electrical stimulation techniques have been designed to incorporate a 'temporal' application, much like rTMS, to induce a frequency-specific neuromodulatory effect that may be used to enhance or suppress neural oscillatory waves.

As the name implies, tACS produces a flow of electrical particles that alternates equally between the positive and negative charge (Paulus, 2011). This means that the net direct current component is zero and therefore, unlike tDCS, the aftereffects of tACS are not likely to be a result of polarity-specific neuromodulation. Instead the primary neuromodulatory effect of tACS appears to act by inducing frequency-specific neural entrainment of cortical oscillatory activity (see Teo, Hendy, Goodwill & Loftus, 2017 for brief review). In preliminary clinical studies, tACS has been used to attenuate resting tremors by up to 50% in people with PD by disrupting the timing of cortical oscillations responsible for resting tremors (i.e. cortical tremor frequency) (Brittain, Probert-Smith, Aziz & Brown, 2013). This was done by identifying and delivering tACS that would drift in and out of phase alignment with the cortical tremor frequency. A variation of tACS, known as tRNS, adopts the same alternating current principle (Terney, Chaieb, Moliadze, Antal & Paulus, 2008). However, instead of using a constant stimulation frequency and intensity throughout the duration of stimulation, tRNS uses a random stimulation frequency (between 0.1–640 Hz) and intensity (−500 to +500 mA) approach throughout the period of stimulation. This form of stimulation is thought to cause repetitive opening of sodium channels (Paulus, 2011) or cause an increase in sensitivity of neuronal networks to neuromodulation (Francis, Gluckman & Schiff, 2003). As with tACS, tRNS has only recently been applied to clinical populations to provide relief from pain in patients with multiple sclerosis (Palm et al., 2016), schizophrenia (Haesebaert, Mondino, Saoud, Poulet & Brunelin, 2014) and tinnitus (Joos, De Ridder & Vanneste, 2015).

Advances in deep brain stimulation in clinical neuroscience

The major neurotechnological advance in the treatment of PD over recent decades has been DBS. A highly invasive neurosurgical procedure requiring significant preparation, DBS for PD involves neurosurgical implantation of electrodes in one of two brain sites: the subthalamic nucleus (STN) or the globus pallidus interna (GPi) (Ramirez-Zamora & Ostrem, 2018). These electrodes are connected to a battery powered titanium device, the neurostimulator, that is implanted subcutaneously (typically below the clavicle) and connected via implanted leads. Although there are dopaminergic effects, the mechanisms of action for DBS are many and diffuse (Herrington, Cheng & Eskandar, 2016).

DBS is now a very well-established treatment, with tens of thousands of patients around the world having successfully undergone the surgery. DBS is intended to target cardinal motor symptoms of PD, and there have been several large-scale clinical trials reporting improvements in tremor, rigidity, bradykinesia, and quality of life equivalently for both target regions (Follett, 2010). While both sites appear to have similar effects on motor function, there are a number of differences in the broader effects exerted (Ramirez-Zamora & Ostrem, 2018). For instance, STN stimulation can produce a more rapid clinical effect, a reduced need for medication, and improvements in non-motor areas (e.g. depression, which affects up to 50% of people with PD; Gökbayrak, Piryatinsky, Gavett & Ahmed, 2014), while GPi may be better for bradykinesia and gait (Ramirez-Zamora & Ostrem, 2018). The decision as to where to implant the electrodes is often not entirely clear, and particular groups may favour stimulation of one site over another (ibid.).

While DBS is performed with respect to motor symptoms of PD, there have been reports of other beneficial effects, including non-motor domains. For instance, depression, which affects around 50% of those diagnosed with PD, has been reported as reduced in PD following DBS, although results are inconsistent. STN stimulation has also been linked to improved sleep quality (Eugster, Bargiotas, Bassetti & Michael Schuepbach, 2016).

Perhaps unsurprisingly given the invasive nature of this approach, there have been a number of adverse events associated with DBS. Intraoperatively, there is a small risk of a number of complications, including stroke, infection, or seizure. STN stimulation has been linked to increased gait freezing (Cossu & Pau, 2017; although see Schlenstedt et al., 2017), disruption of speech (e.g. articulation) (Aldridge, Theodoros, Angwin & Vogel, 2016), and impulsiveness (Callesen, Scheel-Krüger, Kringelbach & Møller, 2013). There have also been reports of increased suicide attempts after DBS, particularly for STN DBS (Voon et al., 2008). Cognitive decline has been inconsistently reported, more so for STN (Combs et al., 2015), although a recent meta-analysis suggests no difference between stimulation sites on most neuropsychological measures (Elgebaly, Elfil, Attia, Magdy & Negida, 2018). It is important to note that while DBS for PD has been associated with consistent benefits in the motor domain, there is much that we do not know about the full range of side-effects, and how to best predict these at an individual level.

The success of DBS for PD has led to the exploration of DBS for particularly intractable cases of some neuropsychiatric disorders. For instance, DBS has been performed for major depressive disorder (MDD), with electrodes implanted within one of several cortico-limbic pathway regions including nucleus accumbens, the ventral capsule/ventral striatum, the subcallosal cingulate, and the medial forebrain bundle (Fitzgerald & Segrave, 2015). A very recent meta-analysis found general support for the efficacy of sham-controlled DBS trials in MDD, but serious adverse events were common (Kisely, Li, Warren & Siskind, 2018).

DBS has also been performed for obsessive-compulsive disorder, Tourette's syndrome, and anorexia nervosa, with all showing some degree of promise (Graat, Figee & Denys, 2017). Needless to say, a highly invasive treatment such as DBS will only be considered where (a) there is a serious decrement in quality of life and/or risk of suicide and (b) conventional treatments, including psychotherapy, pharmacology, repetitive transcranial magnetic stimulation (rTMS), and electro-convulsive therapy (ECT), have proven ineffective or intolerable.

Concluding remarks

Advancements in brain stimulation technologies provide an exciting opportunity to reinstate motor and cognitive functions in people with neurodegenerative disease. Invasive techniques like DBS are typically reserved for cases that have been resistant to traditional physical and pharmacological treatment, while non-invasive methods (rTMS and TMS) can be prescribed as an adjunct therapy in the early to moderate stages of disease. Challenges still remain for the clinical utility of non-invasive brain stimulation, including homogenisation of research protocols and establishment of optimal stimulation parameters for targeting various symptoms. Importance should also be placed on longitudinal follow-ups to establish whether changes observed from experimental protocols generate lasting clinical improvements in people with neurodegenerative disease.

Abbreviations and glossary

AD   Alzheimer's disease.

ALS   Amyotrophic lateral sclerosis.

BDNF   Brain-derived neurotrophic factor. Protein implicated in learning, memory, and associated neuroplastic processes.

cTBS   Continuous theta burst stimulation. Form of high frequency, low intensity electromagnetic brain stimulation that typically produces an inhibitory neuroplastic response.

DBS   Deep brain stimulation. Invasive therapeutic brain stimulation technique that involves neurosurgical implanting of stimulating microelectrodes.

EMG   Electroencephalogram. Provides an index of corticospinal excitability.

GPi   Globus pallidus interna. Part of the striatum/basal ganglia that may be a target of DBS for Parkinson's disease.

iTBS   Intermittent theta burst stimulation. Form of high frequency, low intensity electromagnetic brain stimulation that typically produces an excitatory neuroplastic response.

MDD   Major depressive disorder.

MEP   Motor-evoked potential. Response to single TMS pulse to motor cortex as measured via electroencephalogram.

PD   Parkinson's disease.

rTMS   Repetitive transcranial magnetic stimulation. Repeated delivery of non-invasive brain stimulation technique that involves the delivery of strong magnetic pulses to the scalp, which induces current in the cortex, and can produce lasting modulation of brain activity.

STN   Subthalamic nucleus. Part of the basal ganglia (ventral to thalamus) that may be a target of DBS for Parkinson's disease.

tACS   Transcranial alternating current stimulation. Non-invasive brain stimulation technique that modulates cortical activity by using oscillatory electrical stimulation in different frequency bands via scalp electrodes.

tDCS   Transcranial direct current stimulation. Non-invasive brain stimulation technique that modulates cortical activity by delivering weak electrical current to the brain via scalp electrodes.

TMS   Transcranial magnetic stimulation. Non-invasive brain stimulation technique that involves the delivery of strong magnetic pulses to the scalp, which induces current in the cortex and activates neurons and interneurons.

tRNS   Transcranial random noise stimulation. Non-invasive brain stimulation technique that modulates cortical activity by delivering variable intensity and polarity electrical current to the brain via scalp electrodes.

UPDRS   United Parkinson's Disease Rating Scale.

References

Ahmed, M. A., Darwish, E. S., Khedr, E. M., El Serogy, Y. M. & Ali, A. M. (2012). Effects of low versus high frequencies of repetitive transcranial magnetic stimulation on cognitive function and cortical excitability in Alzheimer's dementia. *Journal of Neurology, 259*(1), 83–92. doi:10.1007/s00415-011-6128-4

Alcalá-Lozano, R., Morelos-Santana, E., Cortés-Sotres, J. F., Garza-Villarreal, E. A., Sosa-Ortiz, A. L. & González-Olvera, J. J. (2018). Similar clinical improvement and maintenance after rTMS at 5 Hz using a simple vs. complex protocol in Alzheimer's disease. *Brain Stimulation, 11*(3), 625–627. doi:10.1016/j.brs.2017.12.011

Aldini, G. (1804). *Essai théorique et expérimental sur le galvanisme, avec une série d'expériences faites devant des commissaires de l'Institut national de France, et en divers amphithéâtres anatomiques de Londres.* Paris: Fournier Fils.

Aldridge, D., Theodoros, D., Angwin, A. & Vogel, A. P. (2016). Speech outcomes in Parkinson's disease after subthalamic nucleus deep brain stimulation: A systematic review. *Parkinsonism and Related Disorders, 33*, 3–11. doi:10.1016/j.parkreldis.2016.09.022

Antal, A., Kincses, T. Z., Nitsche, M. A., Bartfai, O. & Paulus, W. (2004). Excitability changes induced in the human primary visual cortex by transcranial direct current stimulation: Direct electrophysiological evidence. *Investigative Ophthalmology & Visual Science, 45*(2), 702–707.

Benninger, D. H., Iseki, K., Kranick, S., Luckenbaugh, D. A., Houdayer, E. & Hallett, M. (2012). Controlled study of 50-Hz repetitive transcranial magnetic stimulation for the treatment of Parkinson disease. *Neurorehabilitation and Neural Repair, 26*(9), 1096–1105. doi:10.1177/1545968312445636

Bentwich, J., Dobronevsky, E., Aichenbaum, S., Shorer, R., Peretz, R., Khaigrekht, M., . . . Rabey, J. M. (2011). Beneficial effect of repetitive transcranial magnetic stimulation combined with cognitive training for the treatment of Alzheimer's disease: A proof of concept study. *Journal of Neural Transmission (Vienna, Austria: 1996), 118*(3), 463–471. doi:10.1007/s00702-010-0578-1

Berardelli, A. & Suppa, A. (2013). Noninvasive brain stimulation in Huntington's disease. *Handbook of Clinical Neurology, 116*, 555–560. doi:10.1016/b978-0-444-53497-2.00044-9

Brittain, J. S., Probert-Smith, P., Aziz, T. Z. & Brown, P. (2013). Tremor suppression by rhythmic transcranial current stimulation. *Current Biology, 23*(5), 436–440. doi:10.1016/j. cub.2013.01.068

Brys, M., Fox, M. D., Agarwal, S., Biagioni, M., Dacpano, G., Kumar, P., . . . Pascual-Leone, A. (2016). Multifocal repetitive TMS for motor and mood symptoms of Parkinson disease: A randomized trial. *Neurology, 87*(18), 1907–1915. doi:10.1212/wnl.0000000000003279

Buard, I., Sciacca, D. M., Martin, C. S., Rogers, S., Sillau, S. H., Greher, M. R., . . . Kluger, B. M. (2018). Transcranial magnetic stimulation does not improve mild cognitive impairment in Parkinson's disease. *Movement Disorders, 33*(3), 489–491. doi:10.1002/mds.27246

Callesen, M. B., Scheel-Krüger, J., Kringelbach, M. L. & Møller, A. (2013). A systematic review of impulse control disorders in Parkinson's disease. *Journal of Parkinson's Disease, 3*(2), 105–138. doi:10.3233/JPD-120165

Ceccarelli, U. (1962). [The 1st pharmacopoeia: The 'De compositionibus medicamentorum' of Scribonio Largo]. *Minerva Med, 53*, 2398–2402.

Centonze, D., Koch, G., Versace, V., Mori, F., Rossi, S., Brusa, L., . . . Bernardi, G. (2007). Repetitive transcranial magnetic stimulation of the motor cortex ameliorates spasticity in multiple sclerosis. *Neurology, 68*(13), 1045–1050. doi:10.1212/01. wnl.0000257818.16952.62

Centonze, D., Petta, F., Versace, V., Rossi, S., Torelli, F., Prosperetti, C., . . . Finazzi-Agro, E. (2007). Effects of motor cortex rTMS on lower urinary tract dysfunction in multiple sclerosis. *Multiple Sclerosis, 13*(2), 269–271. doi:10.1177/1352458506070729

Chaieb, L., Antal, A. & Paulus, W. (2008). Gender-specific modulation of short-term neuroplasticity in the visual cortex induced by transcranial direct current stimulation. *Vision Neuroscience, 25*(1), 77–81. doi:10.1017/S0952523808080097

Cheng, C. P. W., Wong, C. S. M., Lee, K. K., Chan, A. P. K., Yeung, J. W. F. & Chan, W. C. (2018). Effects of repetitive transcranial magnetic stimulation on improvement of cognition in elderly patients with cognitive impairment: A systematic review and meta-analysis. *International Journal of Geriatric Psychiatry, 33*(1), e1–e13. doi:10.1002/gps.4726

Combs, H. L., Folley, B. S., Berry, D. T. R., Segerstrom, S. C., Han, D. Y., Anderson-Mooney, A. J., . . . van Horne, C. (2015). Cognition and depression following deep brain stimulation of the subthalamic nucleus and globus pallidus pars internus in Parkinson's disease: A meta-analysis. *Neuropsychology Review, 25*(4), 439–454. doi:10.1007/s11065-015-9302-0

Cosgrove, J., Alty, J. E. & Jamieson, S. (2015). Cognitive impairment in Parkinson's disease. *Postgraduate Medical Journal, 91*(1074), 212–220. doi:10.1136/postgradmedj-2015-133247

Cossu, G. & Pau, M. (2017). Subthalamic nucleus stimulation and gait in Parkinson's disease: A not always fruitful relationship. *Gait and Posture, 52,* 205–210. doi:10.1016/j.gaitpost.2016.11.039

Cotelli, M., Manenti, R., Cappa, S. F., Zanetti, O. & Miniussi, C. (2008). Transcranial magnetic stimulation improves naming in Alzheimer disease patients at different stages of cognitive decline. *European Journal of Neurology, 15*(12), 1286–1292. doi:10.1111/j.1468-1331.2008.02202.x

Davis, M., Phillips, A., Tendler, A. & Oberdeck, A. (2016). Deep rTMS for neuro-psychiatric symptoms of Huntington's disease: Case report. *Brain Stimulation, 9*(6), 960–961. doi:10.1016/j.brs.2016.09.002

De Micheli, A. (1991). [From Galvani's De viribus electricitatis . . . to modern electrovec-torcardiography]. *Arch Inst Cardiol Mex, 61*(1), 7–13.

Di Lazzaro, V., Dileone, M., Pilato, F., Profice, P., Ranieri, F., Musumeci, G., . . . Tonali, P. A. (2006). Repetitive transcranial magnetic stimulation for ALS: A preliminary controlled study. *Neuroscience Letters, 408*(2), 135–140. doi:10.1016/j.neulet.2006.08.069

Di Lazzaro, V., Pilato, F., Profice, P., Ranieri, F., Musumeci, G., Florio, L., . . . Dileone, M. (2009). Motor cortex stimulation for ALS: A double blind placebo-controlled study. *Neuroscience Letters, 464*(1), 18–21. doi:10.1016/j.neulet.2009.08.020

Dieckhofer, A., Waberski, T. D., Nitsche, M., Paulus, W., Buchner, H. & Gobbele, R. (2006). Transcranial direct current stimulation applied over the somatosensory cortex: Differential effect on low and high frequency SEPs. *Clinical Neurophysiology, 117*(10), 2221–2227. doi:10.1016/j.clinph.2006.07.136

Dong, Q., Wang, Y., Gu, P., Shao, R., Zhao, L., Liu, X., . . . Wang, M. (2015). The neuropro-tective mechanism of low-frequency rTMS on nigral dopaminergic neurons of Parkinson's disease model mice. *Parkinsons Disorders, 2015,* 564095. doi:10.1155/2015/564095

Elgebaly, A., Elfil, M., Attia, A., Magdy, M. & Negida, A. (2018). Neuropsychological performance changes following subthalamic versus pallidal deep brain stimulation in Parkinson's disease: A systematic review and metaanalysis. *CNS Spectrums, 23*(1), 10–23. doi:10.1017/S1092852917000062

Elmasry, J., Loo, C. & Martin, D. (2015). A systematic review of transcranial electrical stim-ulation combined with cognitive training. *Restorative Neurology and Neuroscience, 33*(3), 263–278. doi:10.3233/RNN-140473

Elsner, B., Kugler, J., Pohl, M. & Mehrholz, J. (2016). Transcranial direct current stimula-tion (tDCS) for idiopathic Parkinson's disease. *Cochrane Database of Systematic Reviews, 7,* CD010916. doi:10.1002/14651858.CD010916.pub2

Eugster, L., Bargiotas, P., Bassetti, C. L. & Michael Schuepbach, W. M. (2016). Deep brain stimulation and sleep-wake functions in Parkinson's disease: A systematic review. *Parkinsonism and Related Disorders, 32,* 12–19. doi:10.1016/j.parkreldis.2016.08.006

Filipovic, S. R., Rothwell, J. C. & Bhatia, K. (2010). Low-frequency repetitive transcranial magnetic stimulation and off-phase motor symptoms in Parkinson's disease. *Journal of Neurological Sciences, 291*(1–2), 1–4. doi:10.1016/j.jns.2010.01.017

Filipovic, S. R., Rothwell, J. C., van de Warrenburg, B. P. & Bhatia, K. (2009). Repetitive transcranial magnetic stimulation for levodopa-induced dyskinesias in Parkinson's dis-ease. *Movement Disorders, 24*(2), 246–253. doi:10.1002/mds.22348

Fitzgerald, P. B. & Segrave, R. A. (2015). Deep brain stimulation in mental health: Review of evidence for clinical efficacy. *Australian and New Zealand Journal of Psychiatry, 49*(11), 979–993. doi:10.1177/0004867415598011

Franca, C., de Andrade, D. C., Teixeira, M. J., Galhardoni, R., Silva, V., Barbosa, E. R. & Cury, R. G. (2018). Effects of cerebellar neuromodulation in movement disorders: A systematic review. *Brain Stimulation, 11*(2), 249–260. doi:10.1016/j.brs.2017.11.015

Francis, J. T., Gluckman, B. J. & Schiff, S. J. (2003). Sensitivity of neurons to weak electric fields. *Journal of Neuroscience, 23*(19), 7255–7261.

Gaede, G., Tiede, M., Lorenz, I., Brandt, A. U., Pfueller, C., Dörr, J., . . . Paul, F. (2018). Safety and preliminary efficacy of deep transcranial magnetic stimulation in MS-related fatigue. *Neurology Neuroimmunology and Neuroinflammation, 5*(1). doi:10.1212/nxi.00000 00000000423

Gökbayrak, N. S., Piryatinsky, I., Gavett, R. A. & Ahmed, O. J. (2014). Mixed effects of deep brain stimulation on depressive symptomatology in Parkinson's disease: A review of randomized clinical trials. *Frontiers in Neurology,* 5 August. doi:10.3389/fneur.2014.00154

Goodwill, A. M., Lum, J. A. G., Hendy, A. M., Muthalib, M., Johnson, L., Albein-Urios, N. & Teo, W. P. (2017). Using non-invasive transcranial stimulation to improve motor and cognitive function in Parkinson's disease: A systematic review and meta-analysis. *Scientific Reports, 7*(1), 14840. doi:10.1038/s41598-017-13260-z

Goodwill, A. M., Teo, W. P., Morgan, P., Daly, R. M. & Kidgell, D. J. (2016). Bihemispheric-tDCS and upper limb rehabilitation improves retention of motor function in chronic stroke: A pilot study. *Frontiers in Human Neuroscience, 10*, 258. doi:10. 3389/fnhum.2016.00258

Graat, I., Figee, M. & Denys, D. (2017). The application of deep brain stimulation in the treatment of psychiatric disorders. *International Review of Psychiatry, 29*(2), 178–190. doi: 10.1080/09540261.2017.1282439

Haesebaert, F., Mondino, M., Saoud, M., Poulet, E. & Brunelin, J. (2014). Efficacy and safety of fronto-temporal transcranial random noise stimulation (tRNS) in drug-free patients with schizophrenia: A case study. *Schizophrenia Research, 159*(1), 251–252. doi:10.1016/j.schres.2014.07.043

Hallett, M. (2007). Transcranial magnetic stimulation: A primer. *Neuron, 55*(2), 187–199.

Herrington, T. M., Cheng, J. J. & Eskandar, E. N. (2016). Mechanisms of deep brain stimulation. *Journal of Neurophysiology, 115*(1), 19–38. doi:10.1152/jn.00281.2015

Hsu, W. Y., Ku, Y., Zanto, T. P. & Gazzaley, A. (2015). Effects of noninvasive brain stimulation on cognitive function in healthy aging and Alzheimer's disease: A systematic review and meta-analysis. *Neurobiology of Aging, 36*(8), 2348–2359. doi:10.1016/j. neurobiolaging.2015.04.016

Hulst, H. E., Goldschmidt, T., Nitsche, M. A., de Wit, S. J., van den Heuvel, O. A., Barkhof, F., . . . Geurts, J. J. G. (2017). rTMS affects working memory performance, brain activation and functional connectivity in patients with multiple sclerosis. *Journal of Neurology Neurosurgery and Psychiatry, 88*(5), 386–394. doi:10.1136/jnnp-2016-314224

Ikeguchi, M., Touge, T., Nishiyama, Y., Takeuchi, H., Kuriyama, S. & Ohkawa, M. (2003). Effects of successive repetitive transcranial magnetic stimulation on motor performances and brain perfusion in idiopathic Parkinson's disease. *Journal of the Neurological Sciences, 209*(1–2), 41–46.

Joos, K., De Ridder, D. & Vanneste, S. (2015). The differential effect of low- versus high-frequency random noise stimulation in the treatment of tinnitus. *Experimental Brain Research, 233*(5), 1433–1440. doi:10.1007/s00221-015-4217-9

Kellaway, P. (1946). The part played by electric fish in the early history of bioelectricity and electrotherapy. *Bulletin of the History of Medicine, 20*(2), 112–137.

Kisely, S., Li, A., Warren, N. & Siskind, D. (2018). A systematic review and meta-analysis of deep brain stimulation for depression. *Depression and Anxiety, 35*(5), 468–480. doi:10.1002/da.22746

Koch, G., Rossi, S., Prosperetti, C., Codeca, C., Monteleone, F., Petrosini, L., . . . Centonze, D. (2008). Improvement of hand dexterity following motor cortex rTMS in multiple sclerosis patients with cerebellar impairment. *Multiple Sclerosis, 14*(7), 995–998. doi:10.1177/1352458508088710

Lawrence, B. J., Gasson, N., Bucks, R. S., Troeung, L. & Loftus, A. M. (2017). Cognitive training and noninvasive brain stimulation for cognition in Parkinson's disease: A meta-analysis. *Neurorehabilitation and Neural Repair, 31*(7), 597–608. doi:10.1177/1545968317712468

Lefebvre, S., Laloux, P., Peeters, A., Desfontaines, P., Jamart, J. & Vandermeeren, Y. (2012). Dual-tDCS enhances online motor skill learning and long-term retention in chronic stroke patients. *Frontiers in Human Neuroscience, 6*, 343. doi:10.3389/fnhum.2012.00343

Lu, X., Bao, X., Li, J., Zhang, G., Guan, J., Gao, Y., . . . Wang, R. (2017). High-frequency repetitive transcranial magnetic stimulation for treating moderate traumatic brain injury in rats: A pilot study. *Experimental and Therapeutic Medicine, 13*(5), 2247–2254. doi:10.3892/etm.2017.4283

Makkos, A., Pál, E., Aschermann, Z., Janszky, J., Balázs, É., Takács, K., . . . Kovács, N. (2016). High-frequency repetitive transcranial magnetic stimulation can improve depression in Parkinson's disease: A randomized, double-blind, placebo-controlled study. *Neuropsychobiology, 73*(3), 169–177. doi:10.1159/000445296

Marquez, J., van Vliet, P., McElduff, P., Lagopoulos, J. & Parsons, M. (2015). Transcranial direct current stimulation (tDCS): Does it have merit in stroke rehabilitation? A systematic review. *International Journal of Stroke, 10*(3), 306–316. doi:10.1111/ijs.12169

Matsunaga, K., Nitsche, M. A., Tsuji, S. & Rothwell, J. C. (2004). Effect of transcranial DC sensorimotor cortex stimulation on somatosensory evoked potentials in humans. *Clinical Neurophysiology, 115*(2), 456–460.

Mori, F., Codeca, C., Kusayanagi, H., Monteleone, F., Boffa, L., Rimano, A., . . . Centonze, D. (2010). Effects of intermittent theta burst stimulation on spasticity in patients with multiple sclerosis. *European Journal of Neurology, 17*(2), 295–300. doi:10.1111/j.1468-1331.2009.02806.x

Mori, F., Ljoka, C., Magni, E., Codeca, C., Kusayanagi, H., Monteleone, F., . . . Centonze, D. (2011). Transcranial magnetic stimulation primes the effects of exercise therapy in multiple sclerosis. *Journal of Neurology, 258*(7), 1281–1287. doi:10.1007/s00415-011-5924-1

Nguyen, J.-P., Suarez, A., Kemoun, G., Meignier, M., Le Saout, E., Damier, P., . . . Lefaucheur, J.-P. (2017). Repetitive transcranial magnetic stimulation combined with cognitive training for the treatment of Alzheimer's disease. *Neurophysiologie Clinique = Clinical Neurophysiology, 47*(1), 47–53. doi:10.1016/j.neucli.2017.01.001

Nitsche, M. A., Cohen, L. G., Wassermann, E. M., Priori, A., Lang, N., Antal, A., . . . Pascual-Leone, A. (2008). Transcranial direct current stimulation: State of the art 2008. *Brain Stimulation, 1*(3), 206–223. doi:10.1016/j.brs.2008.06.004

Nitsche, M. A. & Paulus, W. (2000). Excitability changes induced in the human motor cortex by weak transcranial direct current stimulation. *Journal of Physiology, 527*(Pt 3), 633–639.

Nitsche, M. A. & Paulus, W. (2001). Sustained excitability elevations induced by transcranial DC motor cortex stimulation in humans. *Neurology, 57*(10), 1899–1901.

Padala, P. R., Padala, K. P., Lensing, S. Y., Jackson, A. N., Hunter, C. R., Parkes, C. M., . . . Sullivan, D. H. (2018). Repetitive transcranial magnetic stimulation for apathy in mild cognitive impairment: A double-blind, randomized, sham-controlled, cross-over pilot study. *Psychiatry Research, 261*, 312–318. doi:10.1016/j.psychres.2017.12.063

Palm, U., Chalah, M. A., Padberg, F., Al-Ani, T., Abdellaoui, M., Sorel, M., . . . Ayache, S. S. (2016). Effects of transcranial random noise stimulation (tRNS) on affect, pain and attention in multiple sclerosis. *Restorative Neurology and Neuroscience, 34*(2), 189–199. doi:10.3233/RNN-150557

Pancaldi, G. (2003). *Volta: Science and Culture in the Age of Enlightenment*. Princeton, NJ: Princeton University Press.

Pascual-Leone, A., Valls-Sole, J., Brasil-Neto, J. P., Cammarota, A., Grafman, J. & Hallett, M. (1994). Akinesia in Parkinson's disease. II. Effects of subthreshold repetitive transcranial motor cortex stimulation. *Neurology, 44*(5), 892–898.

Paulus, W. (2011). Transcranial electrical stimulation (tES - tDCS; tRNS, tACS) methods. *Neuropsychol Rehabil, 21*(5), 602–617. doi:10.1080/09602011.2011.557292

Priori, A., Berardelli, A., Rona, S., Accornero, N. & Manfredi, M. (1998). Polarization of the human motor cortex through the scalp. *Neuroreport, 9*(10), 2257–2260.

Rabey, J. M. & Dobronevsky, E. (2016). Repetitive transcranial magnetic stimulation (rTMS) combined with cognitive training is a safe and effective modality for the treatment of Alzheimer's disease: Clinical experience. *Journal of Neural Transmission (Vienna, Austria: 1996), 123*(12), 1449–1455.

Ramirez-Zamora, A. & Ostrem, J. L. (2018). Globus pallidus interna or subthalamic nucleus deep brain stimulation for Parkinson disease: A review. *JAMA Neurology, 75*(3), 367–372. doi:10.1001/jamaneurol.2017.4321

Regner, G. G., Pereira, P., Leffa, D. T., de Oliveira, C., Vercelino, R., Fregni, F. & Torres, I. L. S. (2018). Preclinical to clinical translation of studies of transcranial direct-current stimulation in the treatment of epilepsy: A systematic review. *Frontiers in Neuroscience, 12*, 189. doi:10.3389/fnins.2018.00189

Reijnders, J. S. A. M., Ehrt, U., Weber, W. E. J., Aarsland, D. & Leentjens, A. F. G. (2008). A systematic review of prevalence studies of depression in Parkinson's disease. *Movement Disorders, 23*(2), 183–189. doi:10.1002/mds.21803

Rossini, P. M., Burke, D., Chen, R., Cohen, L. G., Daskalakis, Z., Di Iorio, R., . . . Ziemann, U. (2015). Non-invasive electrical and magnetic stimulation of the brain, spinal cord, roots and peripheral nerves: Basic principles and procedures for routine clinical and research application. An updated report from an IFCN Committee. *Clinical Neurophysiology, 126*(6), 1071–1107. doi:10.1016/j.clinph.2015.02.001

Sayin, S., Cakmur, R., Yener, G. G., Yaka, E., Ugurel, B. & Uzunel, F. (2014). Low-frequency repetitive transcranial magnetic stimulation for dyskinesia and motor performance in Parkinson's disease. *Journal of Clinical Neuroscience, 21*(8), 1373–1376. doi:10.1016/j.jocn.2013.11.025

Schlenstedt, C., Shalash, A., Muthuraman, M., Falk, D., Witt, K. & Deuschl, G. (2017). Effect of high-frequency subthalamic neurostimulation on gait and freezing of gait in Parkinson's disease: A systematic review and meta-analysis. *European Journal of Neurology, 24*(1), 18–26. doi:10.1111/ene.13167

Sedlackova, S., Rektorova, I., Srovnalova, H. & Rektor, I. (2009). Effect of high frequency repetitive transcranial magnetic stimulation on reaction time, clinical features and cognitive functions in patients with Parkinson's disease. *Journal of Neural Transmission (Vienna), 116*(9), 1093–1101. doi:10.1007/s00702-009-0259-0

Shimamoto, H., Takasaki, K., Shigemori, M., Imaizumi, T., Ayabe, M. & Shoji, H. (2001). Therapeutic effect and mechanism of repetitive transcranial magnetic stimulation in Parkinson's disease. *Journal of Neurology, 248 Suppl 3*, III48–52.

Shin, H.-W., Youn, Y. C., Chung, S. J. & Sohn, Y. H. (2016). Effect of high-frequency repetitive transcranial magnetic stimulation on major depressive disorder in patients with Parkinson's disease. *Journal of Neurology, 263*(7), 1442–1448. doi:10.1007/s00415-016-8160-x

Tanaka, S. & Watanabe, K. (2009). [Transcranial direct current stimulation – a new tool for human cognitive neuroscience]. *Brain and Nerve, 61*(1), 53–64.

Tendler, A., Barnea Ygael, N., Roth, Y. & Zangen, A. (2016). Deep transcranial magnetic stimulation (dTMS) – beyond depression. *Expert Review of Medical Devices, 13*(10), 987–1000. doi:10.1080/17434440.2016.1233812

Teo, W. P., Hendy, A. M., Goodwill, A. M. & Loftus, A. M. (2017). Transcranial alternating current stimulation: A potential modulator for pathological oscillations in Parkinson's disease? *Frontiers in Neurology, 8*, 185. doi:10.3389/fneur.2017.00185

Terney, D., Chaieb, L., Moliadze, V., Antal, A. & Paulus, W. (2008). Increasing human brain excitability by transcranial high-frequency random noise stimulation. *Journal of Neuroscience, 28*(52), 14147–14155. doi:10.1523/JNEUROSCI.4248-08.2008

Thickbroom, G. W. (2007). Transcranial magnetic stimulation and synaptic plasticity: Experimental framework and human models. *Experimental Brain Research, 180*(4), 583–593. doi:10.1007/s00221-007-0991-3

Vaseghi, B., Zoghi, M. & Jaberzadeh, S. (2014). Does anodal transcranial direct current stimulation modulate sensory perception and pain? A meta-analysis study. *Clinical Neurophysiology, 125*(9), 1847–1858. doi:10.1016/j.clinph.2014.01.020

Voon, V., Krack, P., Lang, A. E., Lozano, A. M., Dujardin, K., Schüpbach, M., . . . Moro, E. (2008). A multicentre study on suicide outcomes following subthalamic stimulation for Parkinson's disease. *Brain, 131*(10), 2720–2728. doi:10.1093/brain/awn214

Wagle-Shukla, A., Angel, M. J., Zadikoff, C., Enjati, M., Gunraj, C., Lang, A. E. & Chen, R. (2007). Low-frequency repetitive transcranial magnetic stimulation for treatment of levodopa-induced dyskinesias. *Neurology, 68*(9), 704–705. doi:10.1212/01. wnl.0000256036.20927.a5

Wu, Y., Xu, W., Liu, X., Xu, Q., Tang, L. & Wu, S. (2015). Adjunctive treatment with high frequency repetitive transcranial magnetic stimulation for the behavioral and psychological symptoms of patients with Alzheimer's disease: A randomized, double-blind, sham-controlled study. *Shanghai Archives of Psychiatry, 27*(5), 280–288. doi:10.11919/j. issn.1002-0829.215107

Xie, C.-L., Chen, J., Wang, X.-D., Pan, J.-L., Zhou, Y., Lin, S.-Y., . . . Wang, W.-W. (2015). Repetitive transcranial magnetic stimulation (rTMS) for the treatment of depression in Parkinson disease: A meta-analysis of randomized controlled clinical trials. *Neurological Sciences: Official Journal of the Italian Neurological Society and of the Italian Society of Clinical Neurophysiology, 36*(10), 1751–1761. doi:10.1007/s10072-015-2345-4

Yulug, B., Hanoglu, L., Ksanmemmedov, E., Duz, O. A., Polat, B., Hanoglu, T., . . . Kilic, E. (2017). Beyond the therapeutic effect of rTMS in Alzheimer's disease: A possible neuroprotective role of hippocampal BDNF? A mini review. *Mini Reviews in Medicinal Chemistry*. doi:10.2174/1389557517666170927162537

Zhao, J., Li, Z., Cong, Y., Zhang, J., Tan, M., Zhang, H., . . . Shan, P. (2017). Repetitive transcranial magnetic stimulation improves cognitive function of Alzheimer's disease patients. *Oncotarget, 8*(20), 33,864–33,871. doi:10.18632/oncotarget.13060

Ziemann, U. (2010). TMS in cognitive neuroscience: Virtual lesion and beyond. *Cortex, 46*(1), 124–127. doi:10.1016/j.cortex.2009.02.020

11

CONCLUSIONS AND LAST THOUGHTS

John L. Bradshaw

Humankind has long been preoccupied with several great mysteries: the origin of matter and the universe, the origin of life, and our position within the *scala naturae*, the ordered, as was long believed, hierarchy of all living things, from the 'lowest' possible living creatures, to ourselves, at the 'summit'; in particular, white Anglo-Saxon or Aryan males. Evolutionary theory deposed such an ordered and directed striving to the summit, and via the genetic code, itself a later additional wonder, saw the emergence and continued existence of all living things as being in large part subject to random influences and selective pressures. Human consciousness is an even later mystery, the Hard Question. Our possible uniqueness in terms of thought, problem solving, insight, self-awareness, language, tool manufacture and use, and appreciation of the aesthetic, though a comparatively recent concept, is nowadays itself being doubted on all fronts. That said, while we clearly lie on several continua in such contexts with other species, particularly the primates and, interestingly, the birds, our capacity for language and tool manufacture and deployment (praxis), certainly puts us quantitatively ahead of the pack.

As far back as several millennia before the Common Era, ancient Egyptian medical papyri recognised that the human brain is the seat, if not of the soul, then certainly of thought, consciousness, movement and speech. Though much relevant evidence has been lost, writers in the Hippocratic tradition of classical Greece, around the fifth or sixth century BCE, recognised and extended such thinking, and at least intuitively seemed aware that a study of brain pathology or injury could inform us about the organisation and operation of the normal brain, and that such knowledge could, in turn, also inform us about proper management of injury and disease.

In the context of ageing and other degenerative processes, the truly modern era may be seen as beginning around the early to middle of the nineteenth century. Thus in 1817 one James Parkinson, born in 1755, a Londoner who had in 1784 been approved by the City of London Corporation as a surgeon, and nowadays the equivalent of a modern GP, wrote his ground-breaking 'Essay on the shaking Palsy', which eponymously bears his name. However, during his life, he was probably better known for his writings on fossils and the emerging fields of geology and palaeontology. Indeed, his book *Organic Remains of a Former World* made him world famous. Ironically, in view of his far more important contributions to modern neurology, his death in 1824 was consequent upon a stroke, which had brought about, before his death, symptoms of what we nowadays would term 'aphasia'.

Parkinson's essay is so insightful, so accurate and comprehensive that it bears comparison with a modern account, clinical or academic, of his disease, though it must be acknowledged that nearly 2,000 years ago Galen had described the shaking palsy, and even earlier similar mention is made in the Ayurvedic texts of ancient India.

Another medical practitioner, George Huntington, in 1872 wrote an equally clear and perceptive account of the disorder, which similarly bears his name. In particular, he was able accurately to describe three main peculiarities of the disease: its heritability (which of course is in contrast, generally, to Parkinson's disease), the fact that it usually manifests in adult life, and the tendency in its sufferers to insanity and suicide. Its exact genetic origin was not unravelled until a couple of decades ago, when a talented geneticist, herself born of a family where the disease was manifest, studied patients in an area (Lake Maracaibo, Venezuela) where due to unique historical and geomorphological factors the disorder was particularly prevalent.

While we should not ignore the many fundamental contributions to modern neurology by the French physician Charcot, who died in 1893, perhaps the third 'big name' in ageing and neurodegeneration has to be Alois Alzheimer, again one after whom the disorder is eponymously known. Born in 1864, he died aged only 51 in 1915. His was the first published (1906) case of 'presenile dementia', though it was not until 1910 that this modern appellation was given. His lecture in 1906 was very poorly attended, unlike the crowds who flocked to the immediately subsequent talk, upon masturbation in all its forms.

Aging *per se*, at least from the time of Classical Rome, has been a preoccupation of human kind. *Eheu fugaces, labuntur anni*, 'Alas, the fleeting years slip by', was the plangent regret of the Roman poet Horace. Writing roughly contemporaneously with Horace, the sophisticated lawyer, politician, orator and writer Cicero wrote, in impeccable Latin, a model for all young classical aspirants today, his dialogue on old age, *De Senectute*. He deals with the burdens of advancing years, how best to bear them, their compensations and consolations, often with surprisingly modern insights. A century or so later, the historian Tacitus notes with economical prose the '*curvata senio membra, fluxa senio mens*', 'the bow-legged stance, the failing intellect', of our senior years.

Nor need one necessarily live to a very advanced age to experience dementia, as Jonathan Swift in writing *Gulliver's Travels* knew all too well over 250 years ago:

When they (come) to fourscore years . . . they have no Remembrance of anything but what they learned and observed in their Youth and middle Age, and even that is very imperfect . . . In talking they forget the common Appellation of things, and the names of Persons, even of those who are their nearest Friends and Relations. For the same reason they can never amuse themselves with Reading, because their Memory will not serve to carry them from the Beginning of a Sentence to the End . . . neither are they able . . . to hold any Conversation (farther than a few general Words).

Swift himself suffered progressive memory loss in his later years, protracted bouts of walking, a progressive loss of speech, and an inability to recognised acquaintances, all clear signs of Alzheimer's.

Around the time of Freud, and almost certainly as a consequence of his thinking, the two disciplines which we now know as psychiatry and neurology parted company, developing each according to its emerging canons, often it being almost arbitrary whether a given condition was studied and/or managed by one or other proponent. Nowadays we see both disorders, Parkinson's and Huntington's, as archetypically movement disorders, even though traditionally Parkinson's has been managed by neurologists, and Huntington's by psychiatrists – even though there are emotional disturbances accompanying both disorders, if of very different types. Different vocabularies, moreover, have developed between the two disciplines, often for closely similar or even identical symptom patterns, for example, perhaps, catatonia and akinesia. It is only nowadays that this convergence is being recognised, with the advent of biological psychiatry and biological psychology, and their offspring neuropsychiatry and neuropsychology.

At the same time, there is the closely similar emerging discipline of cognitive and behavioural neuroscience, often attempting to bridge the two parent disciplines. Moreover, a plethora of otherwise unrelated disciplines has rushed with almost unseemly haste to prefix with 'neuro-', as with neuroforensics, neuroeconomics, neurolinguistics, neurophilosophy. . ., leading to a kind of commodification, with often unreasonable expectations. Psychology, the original offspring of physiology and philosophy, is nowadays generally the study of behaviour, *sensu lato*. Neuropsychology is seen as the domain of the underlying neural determinants.

Neuropsychology, as a discipline in its own right, has tended in turn to develop along two broad fronts, roughly the clinical and the experimental, though with the advent of sophisticated new imaging techniques, the above two branches are again beginning to converge, just like neurology and psychiatry before them. The very title of the journal *The Journal of Neurology, Neurosurgery and Psychiatry* anticipated such trends.

This book's earlier companion volume, *Developmental Disorders of the Brain*, emphasised the contribution of two great neural systems, the basal-ganglia/frontostriatal (movement initiation and sequencing, in large part), and the fronto-parieto-cerebellar (largely target acquisition and end-point accuracy, at least in the movement domain), along with corresponding cognitive analogues. Many if not most neurodevelopmental disorders seemed to be in part determined by developmental anomalies in one or other (occasionally both, particularly perhaps as in autism), systems. With largely age-related degenerative disorders, much more, even the whole brain, may be involved, and the prior distinction loses much of its heuristic relevance. We made no attempt in this book to include stroke, partly because strokes can occur at any age, and in almost any locus, and partly because of their heterogeneity, each stroke often being associated with a particular loss or alteration of function. Stroke merits, and has merited, treatment in its own right.

The neurodevelopmental disorders were often seen to be characterised by a spectral presentation, from 'normal' to frankly pathological, often with societal norms and expectations determining whether the proband was to be 'diagnosed' or deemed as abnormal. This may not be so true with, for example, Parkinson's and Huntington's diseases, where 'gold-standard' diagnoses are possible, unlike, however, Alzheimer's, though progress is indeed nowadays being made with blood assays. Indeed, with continuing cognitive decline and frank Alzheimer's, a continuous distribution of functionality along a spectrum between 'normality' and pathology is characteristic of the disorder. Another difference between neuro-degenerative and neurodevelopmental disorders is the considerable extent of the overlap between the disorders, a case in point being the group autism, schizophrenia, obsessive-compulsive disorder and bipolar disorder in the neurodevelopmental realm; there is very little such overlap in the case of the neurodegenerative disorders. Note, however, that in its later stages Huntington's may increasingly involve Parkinsonian rigidity. On the other hand, it is not always clear whether Friedreich's ataxia, or schizophrenia, should both be seen as predominantly neurodegenerative or neurodevelopmental.

What is however evident in both domains, the developmental and the degenerative, is the often extreme heterogeneity in presentation. The brain is, of course, after all said to be the single most complex system in the known universe, so heterogeneity is perhaps only to be expected, even maybe in single gene disorders like Huntington's, where environmental and epigenetic differences may have increasing impact over an extensive lifetime. That said, Alzheimer's, Parkinson's and multiple sclerosis are particularly heterogeneous in their presentations.

An important distinction, always perhaps to be borne in mind, lies between *trait* (risk of a disorder manifesting), *state* (the actual diagnosis of the disorder occurring), and *rate* (its progress and development, fast or slow). Progression can of course be either relentlessly continuous, or episodic with remissions and relapses or exacerbations. While Alzheimer's tends to be the former, multiple sclerosis, at least with a subset of patients, may be episodic, with a waxing and waning course.

The epidemiology of a disorder is a significant factor, whether it is more or less common, similarly or instead differently presenting, as between the sexes or over the age range. Parkinson's disease is a particularly relevant instance of both points, sex and age. Race, politically an undeservedly 'dirty' word nowadays, is not to be ignored either; different races do seem to be differentially subject to various degenerative conditions, whether in prevalence or in rate or mode of decline, and differences at simply an environmental level are not necessarily responsible. Age of onset is certainly an important factor in how Parkinson's continues to develop, and also in Friedreich's ataxia, though whether or not this is simply a consequence of heterogeneity in a disorder is a moot point.

Age is clearly an important risk factor; so too are the environmental aspects, such as smoking, exposure to pesticides, alcohol, drugs, traumatic brain injury (a single major instance, or cumulative exposure over a lifetime, as with footballers prone to 'heading' the ball). The presence of other disorders, such as diabetes, itself often a degenerative condition, is another risk factor. Then there is the question as to whether comorbid depression, itself viewed as a neurodevelopmental condition, can predispose one maybe after many years to dementia, or whether the former is just a consequence of the very early stages of declining cognitive function. Indeed, is age itself just another disease?

The relative contributions of environmental and genetic factors is a long-standing controversy. One's progress in life is clearly not totally determined by one's genes; biology need not entirely mean destiny, except maybe in single-gene disorders (Huntington's, fragile X, maybe some of the ataxias). With the recent emphasis on epigenetics, we see how environmental influences can be encoded, via methylation switches, into the non-protein-coding genome of later generations, via the abiding influence of stress, deprivation, starvation and other environmental influences. It is therefore clearly useless to continue to debate the relative importance of genes versus environment, nature versus nurture, just as the distinction between brain and mind is largely chimerical, however philosophers might wish to argue the point. What *is*, however, important to note is that age-related disorders may largely, though not entirely, escape the constraints of selective processes, since reproduction typically takes place *before* the clinical manifestations develop. However, some disorders (e.g. Parkinson's) may have long lead times, maybe 20 years, before overt clinical signs may manifest. Conversely, other disorders, such as Huntington's, maybe via disinhibition, can sometimes be associated with high reproductive success, in terms of perpetuating the responsible genes.

The important contribution of the chapter by Mees et al. is the increasingly evident emphasis and importance of epigenetic factors in influencing the progress, detrimentally or beneficially, in altering the otherwise inevitable unfolding and progress of a neurodegenerative disorder. Exercise, cognitive or physical, not too much and not too little, in accordance with the classical inverted-U shape characterising behavioural consequences of arousal and stress, can be extraordinarily beneficial in modulating, slowing, pathological processes. The true genius lies in identifying the mediating chemicals, at various levels, in a search for a treating substance whereby to minimise the need for, or even to replace, the actual exercise protocol, by the provision of a finely calibrated mediating neurochemical substitute. Again, genes must not be seen as inexorable determinants of one's fate, determining our susceptibility or resistance to degenerative disease. Originally conceived within the context of Huntington's, the concept and approach is clearly applicable to many if not most degenerative disorders; it costs little, and largely obviates the need for new or the infringement of existing patents.

A possible commonality between the various neurodegenerative conditions, related to the common, in both senses of the word, is the occurrence of inflammatory processes, oxidative stress, possibly involving iron metabolism, cell-membrane and DNA changes, and immunological anomalies. A fascinating extension of this argument is the possible involvement of prion-like particles, self-replicating 'patches' of misfolded proteins, self-perpetuating cascade-fashion throughout the CNS. Originally conceptualised in the context of certain rare forms of dementia (kuru, bovine spongiform encephalopathy, Creutzfeldt–Jakob disease), the mechanism may even operate in Alzheimer's and Parkinson's diseases, among possibly many others.

Clearly, diagnosis should aim to go beyond 'mere' symptom evaluation; this is the importance of determining possible *biomarkers* as gold-standards. Thus, compensatory mechanisms can cloud observation, or description, or evaluation of symptoms. Such confounding compensation may involve adoption of new cognitive strategies by the patient, or 'enrolment' of fresh or additional neural circuits, either of which can mask symptomatology. Conversely, loss of function may 'merely' involve diminution of activation. Subsequent apparent recovery of function may thus involve the newly emergent emphasis upon brain plasticity: other areas taking over, spare capacity, regrowth, co-opting alternative pathways or mechanisms.

At the end of the day, the clinician must operate within the hopefully expanding limits upon the patient's activities of daily living. The neuropsychologist will need to address, quantify, and possibly rectify deficits in perceptual, cognitive, attentional (holding, shifting, dividing), motor, linguistic and emotional features – all involving extensive team work and job specialisation. Motor features, of course, involve upper-limb dexterity and praxis, lower-limb gait, articulatory and phonological performance, and oculomotor mechanisms. Mechanisms which are affected may be localised to specific regions, where imaging and electrophysiology may come into play, or more diffusely represented within whole circuits or systems, where diffusion tensor imaging (DTI) or correlational procedures of simultaneous pathway activation, may need deployment.

The idea that cognitive (or indeed any other) mechanisms involved in a particular task, situation or function may be mediated by the temporary functional linkage of discrete circuits, any one or more of which may also play contributory roles in other such tasks, situations or functions, is an increasingly appealing one. Thus for task A, synchronised, coordinated activity may involve circuits 1, 3, 4, 9, 11 and 14; for task B, circuits 1, 2, 5, 9, 10 and 16 may be called into play, and for task C, it may be circuits or regions 2, 4, 9, and 11. Such an arrangement may of course also help explain why performing two very similar tasks simultaneously or closely sequentially, is often harder, and may involve more mutual interference, than when performing two quite different tasks. Is this why we find tongue twisters so confusing? Functional near-infrared spectroscopy (fNIRS) with correlational analysis may be required to address this issue.

Two other such glimpses into the future involve, on the one hand, possibly greater use of virtual reality, whereby a far wider and better control of subjective experience may be possible, both for purposes of pure research and for clinical therapeutics. Likewise, algorithms borrowed from currently developing applications of machine learning may greatly facilitate resolution of questions in pure research, in assessment, diagnosis and clinical management, whether via online presentation of appropriate stimulus material, or in the detection or identification of critical symptomatology. Nor should we forget the potentially fruitful possibilities, in the future, of deployment of electrostimulation, optogenetics and gene editing techniques, both for clinical management and research.

Clinicians should at all times, however, bear in mind that behind every exciting new finding or syndrome, lies someone's, or some family's, personal tragedy.

INDEX